AF578219

Lifestyle Modification for the Prevention and Treatment of Hypertension

Lifestyle Modification for the Prevention and Treatment of Hypertension

edited by

Paul K. Whelton
Tulane University Health Sciences Center
Tulane University School of Public Health and Tropical Medicine, and
Tulane University School of Medicine
New Orleans, Louisiana, U.S.A.

Jiang He
Gail T. Louis
Tulane University School of Public Health and Tropical Medicine
New Orleans, Louisiana, U.S.A.

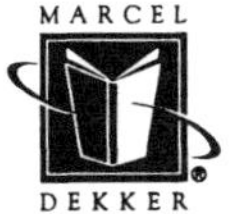

MARCEL DEKKER, INC. NEW YORK • BASEL

Library of Congress Cataloging-in-Publication Data
A catalog record for this book is available from the Library of Congress.

ISBN: 0-8247-4118-8

This book is printed on acid-free paper.

Headquarters
Marcel Dekker, Inc.
270 Madison Avenue, New York, NY 10016
tel: 212-696-9000; fax: 212-685-4540

Eastern Hemisphere Distribution
Marcel Dekker AG
Hutgasse 4, Postfach 812, CH-4001 Basel, Switzerland
tel: 41-61-260-6300; fax: 41-61-260-6333

World Wide Web
http://www.dekker.com

The publisher offers discounts on this book when ordered in bulk quantities. For more information, write to Special Sales/Professional Marketing at the headquarters address above.

Current printing (last digit):
10 9 8 7 6 5 4 3 2 1

PRINTED IN THE UNITED STATES OF AMERICA

Preface

Hypertension is an important public health challenge in the world because of its high prevalence and the concomitant increase in risk of cardiovascular–renal disease. In the United States and other economically developed countries, hypertension represents a major health and financial burden. For example, as many as 43 million Americans have hypertension, defined as having a systolic blood pressure ≥140 mmHg and/or diastolic blood pressure ≥90 mmHg and/or taking antihypertensive medications. According to the National Heart, Lung, and Blood Institute and the American Heart Association, in 2003 the estimated direct health expenditures (physician or other health care provider visits, hospital/nursing home stays, and antihypertensive medications) for care of patients with hypertension in the United States were $37.2 billion and the associated indirect costs (lost productivity due to morbidity and mortality) were $13.1 billion. In many economically developing countries, hypertension has become a significant cause of mortality and disability. In the People's Republic of China the estimated number of hypertensive cases has increased from 30 million in the 1960s to 94 million in the 1990s. Similar trends have been shown in other developing regions.

Hypertension is the most important modifiable risk factor for coronary heart disease, stroke, congestive heart failure, end-stage renal disease, and peripheral vascular disease. Prospective studies have repeatedly identified an increasing risk of cardiovascular disease, stroke, and renal insufficiency with progressively higher levels of both systolic and diastolic blood pressure. These studies have demonstrated a positive, continuous, and independent association between blood pressure and the incidence of coronary heart disease, stroke, congestive heart failure, and end-stage renal disease. They have shown no evidence of a J-shaped relationship or a threshold below which increasing levels of blood pressure are not associated with a corresponding increase in the risk of stroke, coronary heart disease, and renal disease. Randomized controlled trials have demonstrated that antihypertensive drug therapy reduces the risk of cardiovascular disease and stroke among patients with hypertension. However, antihypertensive medications are also associated with increased health care costs and adverse effects. Furthermore, treatment of hypertension cannot entirely eliminate the risk of cardiovascular–renal disease associated with elevated blood pressure. *Lifestyle Modification for the Prevention and Treatment of Hypertension* therefore provides an attractive complementary approach to dealing with the societal burden of hypertension.

Substantial achievements have been made in the identification of effective lifestyle modification approaches for the prevention and treatment of hypertension over the past 20 years. However, the totality of clinical and epidemiological evidence supporting these approaches, as well as the feasibility and cost-effectiveness of each approach, has not been previously synthesized and made widely available to health care providers in office and community settings. This book attempts to fill these gaps by providing a compendium of the scientific evidence on the efficacy of lifestyle modification, while focusing on the interventional techniques and skills necessary to help clinicians implement the interventions that have been proven to be efficacious in treatment trials. Chapters by leading authorities in clinical hypertension and public health provide valuable insights and the strategies necessary to translate the theory of lifestyle modification intervention into practice. This book is written primarily for health care providers, including general internists, family physicians, geriatricians, nurse practitioners, and physician assistants, as well as medical subspecialists, such as cardiologists and nephrologists. It will also be invaluable to dietitians, psychologists, and epidemiologists, as well as students, practitioners, and researchers in preventive medicine and public health.

Jiang He
Paul K. Whelton
Gail T. Louis

Contents

Contributors

Lawrence J. Appel, M.D., M.P.H. Department of Medicine, Johns Hopkins University School of Medicine, Baltimore, Maryland, U.S.A.

William B. Applegate, M.D., M.P.H. Department of Internal Medicine, Wake Forest University School of Medicine, Winston-Salem, North Carolina, U.S.A.

Lawrence J. Beilin, M.B., B.S., M.D. Department of Medicine, The University of Western Australia and the West Australian Heart Research Institute, Perth, Australia

Gerald S. Berenson, M.D. Department of Epidemiology, Tulane University School of Public Health and Tropical Medicine, New Orleans, Louisiana, U.S.A.

Francesco P. Cappuccio, M.D., M.Sc. Department of General Practice and Primary Care, St. George's Hospital Medical School, London, England

William C. Cushman, M.D. Department of Preventive Medicine, University of Tennessee Health Science Center, Memphis, Tennessee, U.S.A.

Jeffrey A. Cutler, M.D., M.P.H. Division of Epidemiology and Clinical Applications, National Heart, Lung, and Blood Institute, Bethesda, Maryland, U.S.A.

Paul Elliott, Ph.D. Department of Epidemiology and Public Health, Imperial College of Science, Technology, and Medicine, London, England

Edward D. Frohlich, M.D. Alton Ochsner Medical Foundation, New Orleans, Louisiana, U.S.A.

Jiang He, M.D., Ph.D. Department of Epidemiology and Medicine, Tulane University School of Public Health and Tropical Medicine, New Orleans, Louisiana, U.S.A.

Nayyar Iqbal, M.D. Department of Medicine, University of Pennsylvania School of Medicine, Philadelphia, Pennsylvania, U.S.A.

Kazuko Ishikawa-Takata, Ph.D. Division of Health Promotion and Exercise, National Institute of Health and Nutrition, Shinjyuku, Tokyo, Japan

Daniel W. Jones, M.D. Division of Hypertension, University of Mississippi Medical Center, Jackson, Mississippi, U.S.A.

Norman M. Kaplan, M.D. Department of Internal Medicine, The University of Texas Southwestern Medical School, Dallas, Texas, U.S.A.

Patricia M. Kearney, M.D., M.P.H. Department of Epidemiology, Tulane University School of Public Health and Tropical Medicine, New Orleans, Louisiana, U.S.A.

Shiriki Kumanyika, Ph.D. Department of Biostatistics and Epidemiology, University of Pennsylvania School of Medicine, Philadelphia, Pennsylvania, U.S.A.

Claude Lenfant, M.D. National Heart, Lung, and Blood Institute, Bethesda, Maryland, U.S.A.

Trevor A. Mori, Ph.D., C.P.Chem. Department of Medicine, The University of Western Australia and the West Australian Heart Research Institute, Perth, Australia

Paul Muntner, Ph.D. Department of Epidemiology and Medicine, Tulane University School of Public Health and Tropical Medicine, New Orleans, Louisiana, U.S.A.

Eva Obarzanek, Ph.D., M.P.H., R.D. Division of Epidemiology and Clinical Applications, National Heart, Lung, and Blood Institute, Bethesda, Maryland, U.S.A.

Toshiki Ohta, M.D. Division of Health Promotion, National Institute of Health and Nutrition, Shinjyuku, Tokyo, Japan

Thomas G. Pickering, M.D., D.Phil. Department of Medicine, Mount Sinai Medical Center, New York, New York, U.S.A.

Ian B. Puddey, M.B., B.S., M.D. Department of Medicine, The University of Western Australia and the West Australian Heart Research Institute, Perth, Australia

Mohammad Rafey, M.D. Department of Medicine, Mount Sinai Medical Center, New York, New York, U.S.A.

Edward J. Roccella, Ph.D., M.P.H. National Heart, Lung, and Blood Institute, Bethesda, Maryland, U.S.A.

Sathanur R. Srinivasan, Ph.D. Department of Epidemiology, Tulane University School of Public Health and Tropical Medicine, New Orleans, Louisiana, U.S.A.

Jeremiah Stamler, M.D. Emeritus, Department of Preventive Medicine, Northwestern University Medical School, Chicago, Illinois, U.S.A.

Elaine Urbina, M.D. Department of Pediatrics, Tulane University School of Medicine, New Orleans, Louisiana, U.S.A.

Paul K. Whelton, M.D., M.Sc. Department of Epidemiology and Medicine, Tulane University School of Public Health and Tropical Medicine, New Orleans, Louisiana, U.S.A.

Jeff D. Williamson, M.D., M.H.S. Department of Medicine, Wake Forest University School of Medicine, Winston-Salem, North Carolina, U.S.A.

Marion R. Wofford, M.D. Division of Hypertension, University of Mississippi Medical Center, Jackson, Mississippi, U.S.A.

1

Hypertension as an Important Public Health Challenge

Jiang He, Patricia M. Kearney, and Paul K. Whelton
Tulane University School of Public Health and Tropical Medicine,
New Orleans, Louisiana, U.S.A.

INTRODUCTION

Hypertension is an important public health challenge worldwide because of its high prevalence and the concomitant increase in risk of cardiovascular and renal disease [1,2]. According to data from the Third National Health and Nutrition Examination Survey (NHANES III), which was conducted from 1988 to 1992, as many as 42.3 million adult residents of the United States have hypertension, defined as having a systolic blood pressure ≥140 mmHg and/or a diastolic blood pressure ≥90 mmHg and/or taking antihypertensive medications. In addition, there are 7.7 million U.S. residents who have been told at least twice by a health professional that they have hypertension. Overall, there are about 50 million adult hypertensives in the United States [3]. Hypertension is also a major health burden in other economically developed and developing countries [4–6]. For example, based on data from a recent study, there are approximately 130 million hypertensives aged 35 to 74 years in China [6]. Hypertension is not only the most common, but also the most important modifiable risk factor for coronary heart disease, stroke, congestive heart failure, chronic renal failure, and peripheral vascular disease [7–16]. Observational epidemiologic studies have demonstrated that elevated blood pressure is related to an increased risk of cardiovascular and renal disease [9–12]. Randomized controlled trials have also shown that antihypertensive drug treatment reduces the morbidity and mortality of cardiovascular and renal disease among patients with hypertension [13–16]. Hypertension and blood pressure-related cardiovascular disease represent a huge financial burden for society. The overall estimated cost of hypertension in the United States in 2002 probably exceeds $47.2 billion, including direct health expenditure for the treatment of hypertension ($34.4 billion) and indirect costs from lost productivity due to morbidity and mortality ($12.8 billion) [17]. In summary, both health statistics and economic analyses indicate that hypertension is a serious public health problem in the world.

BLOOD PRESSURE AND AGE

Blood Pressure in Western Populations

In most societies mean blood pressure rises with increasing age [2,18]. As a consequence there is a concomitant increase in the incidence and prevalence of hypertension with age. The age-related increase in blood pressure, however, varies considerably, depending on the individual's stage of life, gender, race/ethnicity, initial level of blood pressure, and exposure to environmental factors.

Childhood and Adolescence

Information on the pattern of blood pressure in children and adolescents is provided by the *Report of the Second Task Force on Blood Pressure Control in Children* [19]. This report is based on data from blood pressure measurements on over 70,000 children who participated in nine cross-sectional surveys conducted in the United States and the United Kingdom. At birth average systolic and diastolic pressures were 70 mmHg and 50 mmHg, respectively. Shortly thereafter, there is a rise in systolic blood pressure, so that by the end of the first year of life it approximates 94 mmHg. Diastolic blood pressure rises by only 2 mmHg over the same time period. For the next 2 to 3 years, systolic and diastolic blood pressures remain stable. Thereafter, there is a tendency for blood pressure to rise with increasing age throughout the remainder of childhood and adolescence. The slope for age-related change in blood pressure is much steeper for systolic (1 to 2 mmHg/year) than for diastolic (0.5 to 1 mmHg/year) blood pressure.

The task force database provided information on an approximately equal number of boys and girls. There is little evidence of a difference in pattern of average blood pressure between the sexes until adolescence. During the teenage years, average blood pressure is consistently higher for boys than for girls. This is particularly true for systolic blood pressure. By age 18, boys have average systolic and diastolic blood pressures that are almost 10 mmHg and 5 mmHg higher than the corresponding values for girls. There was no evidence for a systematic difference in average blood pressure among white, black, and Mexican-American children in the task force database. Data from the Bogalusa Heart Study and the Child and Adolescent Trial for Cardiovascular Health, however, indicate that mean blood pressure level is higher in black compared to white children and lower in Mexican-American compared to black and white children [20,21].

Adults and the Elderly

There is a general tendency for both systolic and diastolic blood pressure to rise during adulthood [2,18]. The age-related rate of rise is consistently higher for systolic than for diastolic blood pressure. Systolic blood pressure tends to rise until the eighth or ninth decade, whereas diastolic blood pressure tends to remain constant or decline after the fifth decade. As a consequence, pulse pressure increases progressively with aging. This is particularly true during the latter part of life.

The pattern of blood pressure change with age is modified to a certain extent by gender and race. In young adults systolic and diastolic blood pressures tend to be higher in men than in women. The age-related rise in blood pressure with age is steeper for women than for men, however. As a result, by the seventh decade women tend to have levels of systolic blood pressure that equal or exceed those seen in men. Selective survivorship may explain part of this gender-related difference in blood pressure, as men with high blood pressure earlier on may be less likely to survive and contribute to average blood pressure later in life. Longitudinal analysis of the Framingham cohort and other data sets suggests, however, that selective survivorship only explains a portion of these age-related trends [22].

Race also influences age-related change in blood pressure. This has been well documented in NHANES III (Fig. 1). In both men and women, non-Hispanic blacks had the highest and non-Hispanic whites had the lowest average systolic blood pressure until the end of the fifth decade. In the sixth and later decades, among men, Mexican Americans tended to have the highest average systolic blood pressure, although the differences among the three race/ethnicity groups were small. In women, non-Hispanic blacks continued to have the highest and non-Hispanic whites continued to have the lowest average systolic blood pressure during the sixth decade. By the seventh decade, however, the three race/ethnicity groups had similar average systolic blood pressure levels. Throughout adult life, men had a slightly higher

Men
160
150
140
130
120
110
100
90
80
70
60
mmHg
Systolic blood pressure
Diastolic blood pressure
Non-Hispanic white
Non-Hispanic black
Mexican American
18-29
30-39
40-49
50-59
60-69
70-79
80+
Age (years)

(a)

Women
160
150
140
130
120
110
100
90
80
70
60
mmHg
Systolic blood pressure
Diastolic blood pressure
Non-Hispanic white
Non-Hispanic black
Mexican American
18-29
30-39
40-49
50-59
60-69
70-79
80+
Age (years)

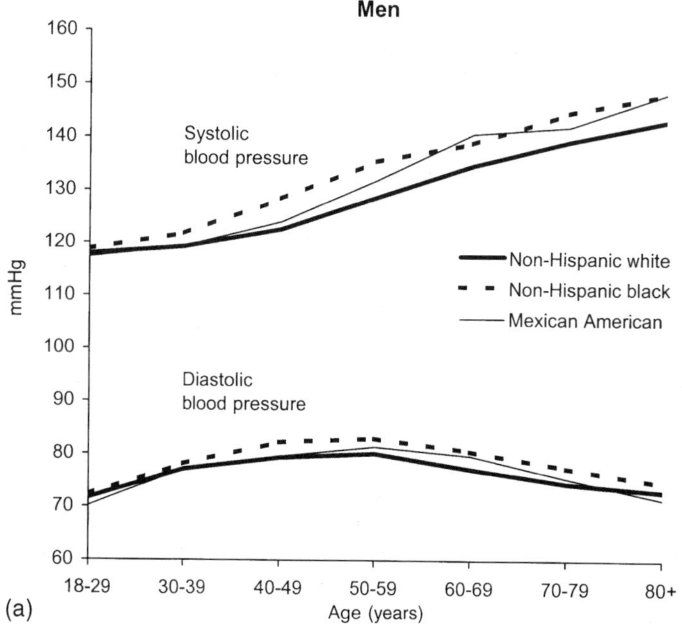

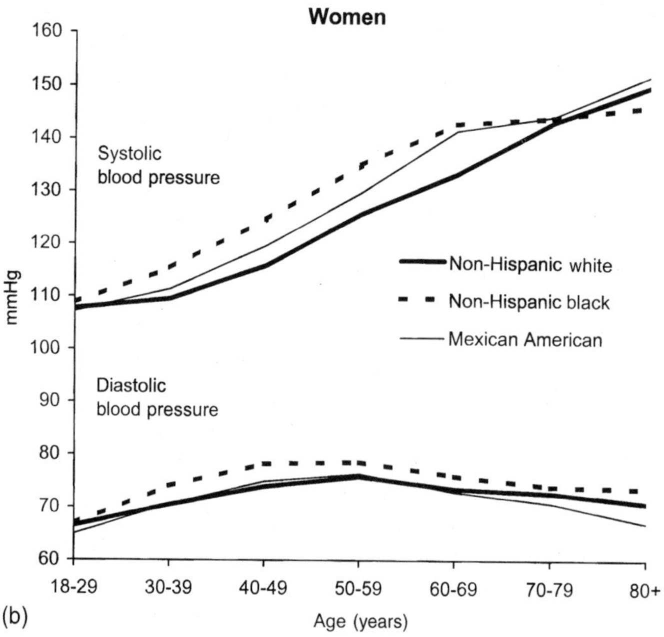

(b)

average level of diastolic blood pressure than women did. Non-Hispanic black women had a higher average diastolic blood pressure than non-Hispanic white or Mexican-American women. The same was true in men until the end of the fifth decade. Thereafter, diastolic blood pressures were similar in the three race/ethnicity groups.

Blood Pressure in Isolated Populations

The rise in blood pressure with age that has been observed in many populations around the world is not universal. Some isolated populations have not been found to have the same age-related increase in blood pressure [23–25]; instead their blood pressure remains relatively constant throughout life and hypertension is almost absent. When individuals from these environments migrate to less isolated areas they are found to develop the age-related rise in blood pressure and hypertension that is so common in economically developed countries [23–25]. Such a rapid change in the pattern of a biological trait suggests that environmental factors play a key role in determining age-related changes in blood pressure.

CLASSIFICATION OF HYPERTENSION

The *Sixth Report of the Joint National Committee on Prevention Detection, Evaluation, and Treatment of High Blood Pressure* (JNC VI) was published in 1997 and recommended a classification of blood pressure that was adopted by the World Health Organization–International Society of Hypertension (Table 1) [26,27]. These criteria are for individuals who are not on antihypertensive medication and who are not acutely ill. The classification is based on the average of two or more blood pressure readings after an initial screening visit. When systolic blood pressure and diastolic blood pressure fall into different categories, the higher category should be selected to classify the individual's blood pressure.

According to JNC VI criteria, optimal blood pressure is defined as a systolic blood pressure less than 120 mmHg and a diastolic blood pressure less than 80 mmHg. Those with a systolic blood pressure between 130 mmHg and 139 mmHg or diastolic blood pressure between 85 and 89 mmHg are designated as having a high normal blood pressure. Hypertension is charac-

FIGURE 1 Mean systolic and diastolic blood pressure by age and race\ethnicity for men (a) and women (b) 18 years of age and older in the United States. *Source*: The National Health and Nutrition Examination III, 1988–92.

TABLE 1 Classification of Blood Pressure for Adults Age 18 and Older

Category	Systolic blood pressure (mmHg)		Diastolic blood pressure (mmHg)
Optimal[a]	<120	and	<80
Normal	<130	and	<85
High-normal	130–139	or	85–89
Hypertension[b]			
Stage 1	140–159	or	90–99
Stage 2	160–179	or	100–109
Stage 3	≥180	or	≥110

Not taking antihypertensive drugs and not acutely ill. When systolic and diastolic pressures fall into different categories, the higher category should be selected to classify the individual's blood pressure status. Isolated systolic hypertension is defined as systolic blood pressure of 140 mmHg or greater and diastolic blood pressure below 90 mmHg and staged appropriately.

[a] Optimal blood pressure with respect to cardiovascular disease risk is below 120/80 mmHg. Unusually low readings should be evaluated for clinical significance, however.

[b] Based on the average of two or more readings taken at each of two or more visits after an initial screening.

Source: Ref. 26.

terized by a confirmed elevation of systolic (≥140 mmHg) or diastolic (≥90 mmHg) blood pressure. Hypertension is further characterized into three stages according to the patient's level of systolic and diastolic blood pressure. Stage 1 is the mildest (systolic 140 to 159 mmHg and diastolic < 100 mmHg or diastolic 90 to 99 mmHg and systolic < 160 mmHg) and most common form of hypertension. It accounts for 80% of hypertension. Stage 2 hypertension includes those with systolic blood pressure 160 to 179 mmHg and diastolic blood pressure 100 to 109 mmHg. Stage 3 hypertension is defined as systolic blood pressure ≥180 mmHg or diastolic blood pressure ≥110 mmHg. Isolated systolic hypertension is defined as systolic blood pressure of 140 mmHg or greater and diastolic blood pressure below 90 mmHg and staged appropriately.

DISTRIBUTION OF HYPERTENSION IN POPULATIONS

The distribution of hypertension in general populations is influenced by a number of factors. The incidence and prevalence of hypertension varies by age, gender, and racial composition of the population under study. The

TABLE 2 Percentage of Prevalence of Hypertension in the United States (1989–1994)

	All races[a]			White			Black		
Age (years)	Total	Men	Women	Total	Men	Women	Total	Men	Women
18–24	2.6	4.6	0.7	2.5	4.6	0.5	2.6	4.1	1.4
25–34	5.4	8.4	2.4	4.9	8.1	1.6	8.2	10.6	6.2
35–44	13.0	16.0	10.2	11.3	14.3	8.5	25.9	29.5	22.9
45–54	27.6	30.0	25.2	25.8	29.1	22.6	46.9	44.3	48.8
55–64	43.7	44.2	43.2	42.1	43.0	41.4	60.0	58.0	63.0
65–74	59.6	55.8	62.7	58.6	54.9	61.7	71.0	65.2	75.6
≥75	70.3	60.5	76.2	69.7	59.0	76.1	75.5	71.3	77.9
Total	23.4	23.5	23.3	23.2	23.4	23.1	28.1	27.9	28.2

[a] Includes race and ethnic groups not shown separately due to small sample sizes.
Source: Ref. 3.

incidence and prevalence of hypertension are also affected by environmental exposures, such as intake of dietary sodium and potassium, body weight, alcohol consumption, and physical activity. We will only discuss age, gender, and race/ethnicity distribution of hypertension in this section.

Age

There is a large body of data available from western populations that demonstrates that mean blood pressure rises with increasing age, consequently the prevalence of hypertension increases with age. In NHANES III, the prevalence of hypertension increased with increasing age (Table 2). In the 18 to 24 age group the overall prevalence of hypertension was only 2.6%. The prevalence of hypertension increased to 5.4% in 25 to 34-year-olds and 13.0% in 35 to 44-year-olds. The prevalence rates continued to rise with 27.6% of 45 to 54-year-olds affected and 43.7% of 55 to 64-year olds. In 65 to 74-year olds the overall prevalence was 59.6%, and in over 75-year-olds it was 70.3%. Several longitudinal cohort studies have also documented that the incidence of hypertension increases with age [28–30].

Gender

Overall the prevalence and incidence of hypertension are slightly higher in men compared to women. In NHANES III, the age-adjusted prevalence of hypertension for all races was 23.5% in men and 23.3% in women. In whites the prevalence was 23.4% in men and 23.1% in women. In blacks the prevalence was slightly higher in women than in men, 28.2% and 27.9%, respectively. The relationship between gender and hypertension is modified by age. In young adults, the prevalence and incidence rates of hypertension are higher in men than in women. By their 60s, however, women tend to have levels of blood pressure that equal or exceed those seen in men, consequently the prevalence of hypertension is higher in women than in men late in life.

Race/Ethnicity

In NHANES III the prevalence of hypertension in different racial groups was compared. It was found that in the 18 to 49 age group, non-Hispanic blacks had a prevalence of hypertension of 15% in men and 8% in women and non-Hispanic whites had a prevalence of hypertension of 11% in men and 4% in women. Mexican Americans had the highest prevalence of hypertension in men of 20%, while in women it was only 3% [31]. In the 50 to 69-year age group, the prevalence was 45% in men and 43% in women among non-Hispanic blacks, 35% in men and 29% in women among non-Hispanic whites, and 37% in both men and women among Mexican Americans, respectively. Overall the prevalence of hypertension is highest in male and female African Americans. The prevalence of hypertension is higher in white men than in Mexican-American men, while the prevalence is higher in Mexican-American women than white women.

Several longitudinal cohort studies have also shown that African Americans have a higher incidence of hypertension than whites [28,30, 32,33]. In the Atherosclerosis Risk in Communities Study, the 6-year incidence of hypertension was 13.9% and 12.6% in white men and women, and 24.9% and 30.3% in African-American men and women aged 45 to 49 years [31]. The corresponding incidence of hypertension among participants aged 50 to 64 years was 18.0% and 17.0% in white men and women, and 28.3% and 29.9% in African-American men and women, respectively. Other longitudinal cohort studies indicated that the incidence of hypertension in African Americans was an average of two times higher than in whites [28,32,33].

LIFETIME RISK OF HYPERTENSION

Although the prevalence of hypertension is a useful indicator of burden of disease in the community, it does not tell us about the risk for developing hypertension in individuals. The individual risk for developing hypertension is best described by incidence or lifetime cumulative incidence statistics. Limited information is available about the incidence of hypertension

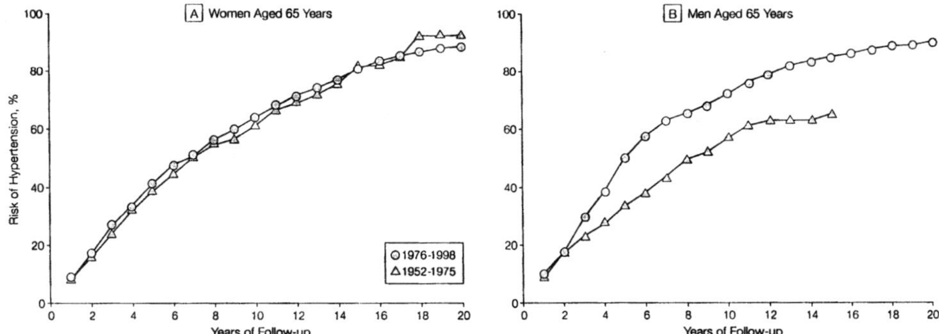

FIGURE 2 Residual lifetime risk of hypertension in women and men aged 65 years. Cumulative incidence of hypertension in 65-year-old women and men. Data for 65-year-old men in the 1952–1975 period is truncated at 15 years since there were few participants in this age category who were followed beyond this time interval. *Source*: Ref. 34.

because it requires follow-up of a large population for a prolonged period of time [28–30,32,33].

The lifetime risk for developing hypertension was estimated among 1298 study participants who were aged 55 to 65 years and free of hypertension at baseline during the 1976-to-1998 period [34]. For 55-year-old participants, the cumulative risk for developing hypertension was calculated through age 80 years, while for 65-year-old participants, the risk for developing hypertension was calculated through age 85 years. These follow-up time intervals (25 years for 55-year-olds and 20 years for 65-year-olds) correspond to the current mean residual life expectancies for white individuals at these two ages in the United States. The lifetime risks for developing hypertension were 90% in both 55-year-old and 65-year-old participants (Fig. 2). The lifetime probability of receiving antihypertensive medication was 60% [34].

GLOBAL BURDEN OF HYPERTENSION

The prevalence of hypertension varies widely worldwide. National studies have been reported from a variety of countries in different world regions (Table 3). The definition of hypertension, blood pressure measurement methodology, and the standard population for age adjustment differs among studies, however, making direct comparisons difficult. Using JNC VI criteria, the overall prevalence of hypertension worldwide in the adult population is approximately 25% [35].

TABLE 3 Percentage of Prevalence of Hypertension Among Economically Developed and Developing Countries

Country	Study year	Sample size	Age	Hypertension definition	Prevalence of hypertension		
					Men	Women	Total
Canada	1986–1992	23,129	18–74	≥140/90 or meds	26.0	18.0	22.0
England	1998	11,529	≥16	≥140/90 or meds	41.5	33.3	37.0
USA	1988–1994	17,752	≥18	≥140/90 or meds	23.5	23.3	23.4
China	1991	949,370	≥15	≥140/90 or meds	14.4	12.8	13.6
Egypt	1991	6,733	25–95	≥140/90 or meds	25.7	26.9	26.3
Mexico	1992–1993	14,657	20–69	≥140/90 or meds	37.5	28.1	—
South Africa	1998	13,802	15–65	≥140/90 or meds	22.9	24.6	23.9

Economically Developed Countries

According to data from NHANES III, which was conducted from 1988 to 1992, as many as 42.3 million adult residents of the United States have hypertension, defined as having a systolic blood pressure ≥140 mmHg and/or a diastolic blood pressure ≥90 mmHg and/or taking antihypertensive medications. In addition, there are 7.7 million U.S. residents who have been told at least twice by a health professional that they have hypertension. Overall, there are about 50 million adult hypertensives in the United States [3]. A similar prevalence of hypertension was reported in the Canadian Heart Health Survey, a cross-sectional population-based survey that collected data in each of the 10 Canadian provinces between 1986 and 1992 [36]. The study reported an overall prevalence of hypertension of 26% in men and 18% in women, which represents 4.1 million Canadian adults.

Many studies have estimated the prevalence of hypertension in Europe, although there are relatively few national studies. The reported prevalence tends to be higher than equivalent studies in the United States. The Health Survey for England 1998 is a cross-sectional household-based nationwide survey of English adults aged 16 years or older [37]. According to the study, 41.5% of men and 33.3% of women had a systolic and/or diastolic blood pressure ≥140/90 mmHg and/or were receiving antihypertensive therapy.

The prevalence of hypertension in Australia's general population was estimated as part of the National Heart Foundation's Risk Factor Prevalence Study, which was conducted from 1980 to 1989 [38]. The survey was administered to a randomly selected sample as a multicenter cross-sectional survey in 1980, 1983, and 1989. The Australian Institute of Health and Welfare analyzed the data from the National Risk Factor Prevalence Study to obtain estimates of the prevalence of hypertension, defined as systolic blood pressure ≥140 mmHg and/or diastolic blood pressure ≥90 mmHg and/or receiving treatment for high blood pressure. The prevalence of hypertension in Australian adults aged 25 to 64 was 31.9% in men and 20.7% in women, according to this study [39].

Economically Developing Countries

Several large national hypertension surveys have been conducted in China during the past several decades [40,41]. The 1991 Chinese National Hypertension Survey included a representative sample of the general Chinese population of 950,000 individuals aged 15 years or older. Three blood pressure measurements were obtained at a single visit, and hypertension was defined as a mean systolic blood pressure ≥140 mmHg and/or diastolic blood pressure ≥90 mmHg and/or taking antihypertensive medications. The overall prevalence of hypertension was 13.6% in the Chinese population

(14.4% in men and 12.8% in women). Hypertension was less prevalent in the rural than the urban areas, with prevalence rates of 11.4% and 10.9% for men and women in rural China and 17.7% and 15.0% in urban China, respectively [40,41]. A recently completed national survey indicated that 27.2% of the Chinese adult population aged 35 to 74 years, representing 129,824,000 persons, had hypertension [6].

The Egyptian National Hypertension Project estimated the prevalence of hypertension in the Egyptian population [42]. The survey, which was initiated in 1991, was a national probability sample of adults aged 25 years or older conducted in six Egyptian governorates. Hypertension was defined according to JNC VI criteria. The estimated overall prevalence of hypertension was 26.3%. Hypertension was slightly more common in women than in men (26.9% versus 25.7%, respectively) [40].

Studies from Latin America have generally found a high prevalence of hypertension. In the 1992-to-1993 Mexican national survey of chronic diseases, a multistage sampling method was used to select a national representative sample of the urban population [43]. The blood pressure of 14,657 individuals (6053 men and 8604 women) aged 20 to 69 years was measured using standard methods, and hypertension was defined by the JNC VI criteria. The crude prevalence of hypertension was 28.1% in women and 37.5% in men. When the results were standardized using the Mexican 1990 census data, the prevalence was 27.2% in women and 37.1% in men (representing over 12 million hypertensive patients) [43].

The prevalence of hypertension in South Africa was estimated in the Demographic and Health Survey in 1998 [44]. This study was conducted on 13,802 randomly selected South Africans 15 years and older who were visited in their homes. When using a cutoff point of 140/90 mmHg and/or antihypertension treatment, the prevalence of hypertension was 22.9% in men and 24.6% in women. When the data were age-standardized to the South African population census of 1996 the estimated prevalence of hypertension was—21% for both men and women.

SECULAR TRENDS IN THE PREVALENCE OF HYPERTENSION

Repeated independent cross-sectional surveys in the same populations over time provide information about secular trends in blood pressure and hypertension. Attention must be paid, however, to the comparability of the methods on sampling and blood pressure measurement as well as the definition of hypertension between surveys. Few national data are available to examine the secular trend of hypertension in the general population.

Generally speaking, the prevalence of hypertension has declined in most western populations but increased in economically developing regions.

The U.S. National Health and Nutritional Examination Surveys may provide the best data to examine the secular trends of hypertension, although there was variation in sample size within each subgroup of the population, in the protocol for blood pressure measurement, and in the potential for measurement error [45]. Overall, hypertension prevalence in the United States has declined progressively since 1971, and the distributions of systolic and diastolic blood pressures have shifted downward during the approximately 30-year period between 1960 to 1962 and 1988 to 1991 [45]. The decline in the prevalence of hypertension has been consistent across age, gender, and racial groups (Fig. 3). For example, the age-adjusted prevalence of hypertension, defined as blood pressure $\geq$140/90 mmHg and/or current use of antihypertensive medication, peaked at 36.3% in the period from 1971 to 1974 and declined to 20.4% in the period from 1988 to 1991. Between 1976 to 1980 and 1988 to 1991, the prevalence of hypertension among black men age 50 to 59 years remained relatively stable at 54.7% and 53.3%, respectively. The prevalence for black men aged 60 to 74 increased from 67.0% to 71.2%. In every other age-specific and ethnic group, hypertension prevalence between 1976 to 1980 and 1988 to 1991 declined markedly. The proportionate

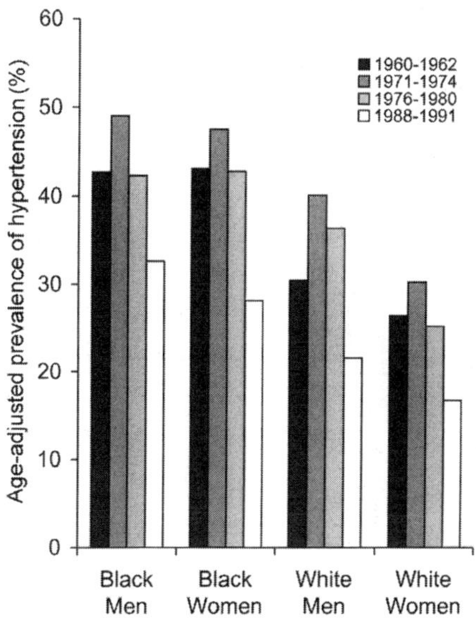

FIGURE 3 Age-adjusted prevalence of hypertension in black men, black women, white men, and white women (1960–1990). *Source*: Ref. 45.

decrease was greatest among the 18 to 29-year group and least among the 60 to 74-year group.

Age-adjusted mean systolic blood pressures decreased from 131 mmHg in 1971 to 1974 to 119 mmHg in the period from 1988 to 1991 in the U.S. general population [45]. Mean diastolic pressure decreased from 83 mmHg to 73 mmHg over the same time period. For black men and women, the decline in age-specific systolic blood pressure tended to be steepest between 1971 to 1974 and 1976 to 1980; the decline in white men and women was greatest between 1976 to 1980 and 1988 to 1991 for most age groups. Age-adjusted diastolic pressures decreased in all subgroups between 1971 to 1974 and 1988

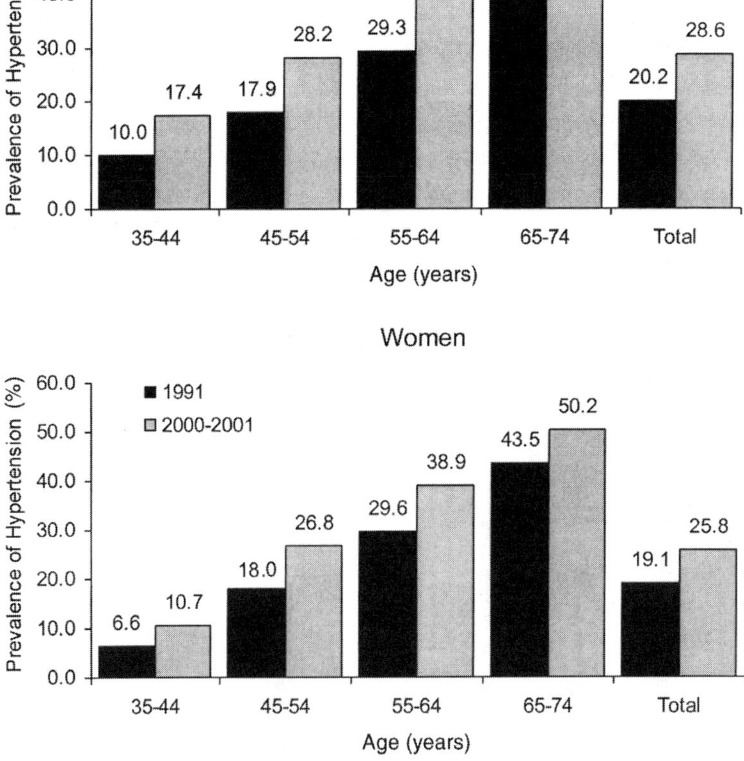

FIGURE 4 Prevalence of hypertension among Chinese aged 34–74 years in the 1991 Chinese National Hypertension Survey and 2000–2001 InterASIA Study.

to 1991. Age-specific diastolic blood pressure also declined markedly and progressively between 1971 to 1974 and 1988 to 1991 for every group.

Several national surveys of hypertension have been conducted in China over the past few decades and these surveys indicate that the prevalence of hypertension has progressively increased in China [41,46]. These surveys, however, have used different methods for selecting study participants and blood pressure measurement. The blood pressure cut points for the definition of hypertension have also varied, therefore caution should be observed in comparison of findings from these surveys. With this in mind, the most recently completed InterASIA study and the 1991 Chinese National Hypertension Survey may provide the most valid comparison regarding blood pressure measurement methods and definition of hypertension [41,46]. These data indicate that the prevalence of hypertension may have increased from 20.2% to 28.6% (a 42% increase) in men and from 19.1% to 25.8% (a 35% increase) in women, aged 35 to 74 years, respectively, during the past decade (Fig. 4). More troublesome, the trend of increase in prevalence was much greater in younger age groups compared to older age groups. For example, the percentage increase was 74% in men and 62% in women aged 35 to 44 years and 18% in men and 15% in women aged 65 to 74 years.

TREATMENT AND CONTROL OF HYPERTENSION IN THE COMMUNITY

Treatment and control of hypertension in the community requires that elevated blood pressure be recognized and that individuals with hypertension receive adequate treatment. The degree of awareness, treatment, and control of hypertension varies considerably between countries (Table 4). In addition, hypertension control rates are varied by age, gender, race/ethnicity, socioeconomic status, education, and quality of health care within countries [47].

Economically Developed Countries

In the United States there has been a trend toward greater awareness, treatment, and control of hypertension in the community (Fig. 5). During the 12-year interval between NHANES II and III, the proportion of hypertensive patients who are aware of their condition has increased from 51–73%. Increases in awareness were greater for whites than blacks during this time period. Awareness was higher for women than men among both blacks and whites. For example, 67% of black and white men with hypertension were aware of their diagnosis, while 79% and 82% of black and white women were aware at the NHANES III.

TABLE 4 Percentages of Awareness, Treatment, and Control of Hypertension Among Countries by World Region

Country	Study year	Age	Hypertension control definition		Hypertensives			Treated hypertensives
					Aware	Treated	Controlled	Controlled
Canada	1986–1992	18–74	≤140/90 or meds	Total	58.0	39.0	16.0	41.0
England	1998	16–75	≤140/90 or meds	Total	46.2	31.8	9.3	29.4
United States	1988–1991	18–80+	≤140/90 or meds	Total	69.0	53.0	24.0	45.0
China	1991	15–75	≤140/90 or meds	Total	26.3	12.1	2.8	23.1
Egypt	1991	25–95	≤140/90 or meds	Total	37.5	23.9	8.0	33.5
Mexico	1992–1993	20–69	≤140/90 or meds	Total	28.2	10.7	2.3	21.8
South Africa	1998	15–65	≤140/90 or meds	Total	41.0	30.0	14.8	49.3

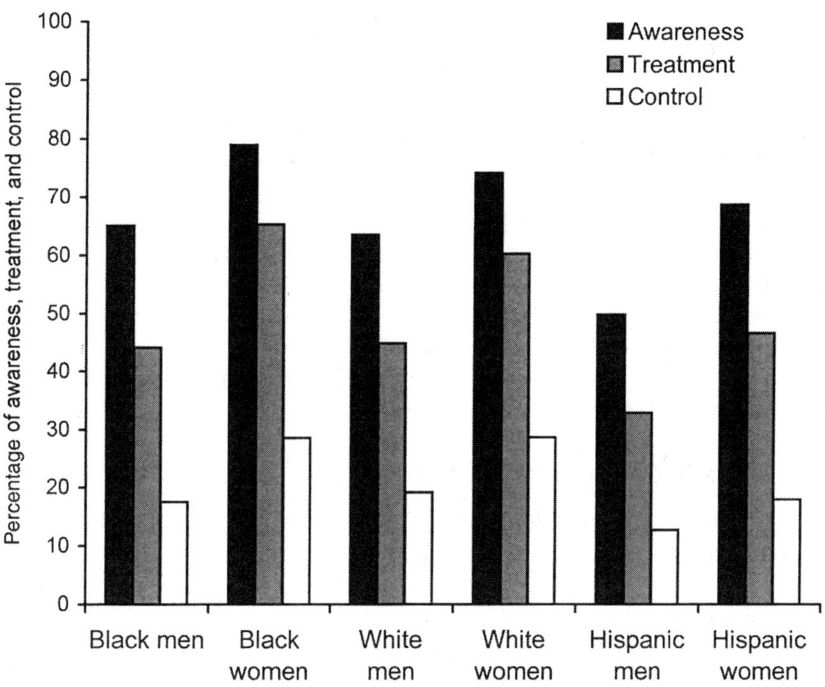

FIGURE 5 The percentages of awareness, treatment, and control of hypertension in U.S. populations (1988–1992). *Source:* Ref. 45.

The increase in awareness of hypertension between 1976 to 1980 and 1988 to 1991 has been accompanied by an increase in the proportion of hypertensives receiving treatment with antihypertensive medications. Overall the percentage of hypertensives receiving treatment increased from 31% in 1976 to 1980 to 55% in 1988 to 1991 in the U.S. population. The large difference in awareness of hypertension between men and women in NHANES III is mirrored by a 19% difference in treatment rates. Less than half of male hypertensives receive treatment (46%), while almost two-thirds of women were on treatment for their high blood pressure (65%). For both genders, the percentage of treatment increased by over 20% between 1976 to 1980 and 1988 to 1991; from 21–46% in men, and from 43–65% in women. The percentages of treatment were virtually identical during NHANES III for black and white men at 46% and 47%, respectively, and both black and white women at 65%.

The proportion of controlled hypertension increased nearly threefold at the 140/90 mmHg cut point during the 12 years between NHANES II and III.

The control rate of hypertension, however, remains low at 29%. The control rate is higher in women at 38% than in men at 22%. A greater percentage of whites achieves control than blacks—31% and 26%, respectively. The control rate among treated hypertensives is also higher in women than in men and in blacks than in whites. The overall percentage of treated hypertensives with controlled blood pressure increased from 32% in 1976 to 1980 to 55% in 1988 to 1991 in the U.S. general population.

The high rates of awareness of hypertension that have been achieved in the United States have not yet been achieved in other developed countries. The most recent European national study was conducted in England in 1998 [37]. While the rates of awareness, treatment and control had improved since the previous health survey for England (from 26–32% for treatment and from 6–9% for control), the rates remain low.

Economically Developing Countries

The percentages of hypertension awareness, treatment, and control are low in economically developing countries and regions. In China, the percentage of awareness, treatment, and control of hypertension is over twice as high in urban than in rural areas [40,41]. Based on data from the 1991 Chinese National Hypertension Survey, only 13.9% of hypertensive patients are aware of their diagnosis, 5.4% are receiving treatment, and 1.2% are achieving control of their hypertension in rural China. The awareness, treatment, and control rates were 35.6%, 17.1%, and 4.1%, respectively, in urban China. The recent InterASIA study findings indicate that among Chinese hypertensive patients, 44.7% were aware of their high blood pressure, 28.2% were taking antihypertensive medication, and 8.1% achieved blood pressure control [42].

Results from the Egyptian National Hypertension Project (NHP) showed that slightly more than one-third of all Egyptians who could be classified as hypertensive were aware that they had high blood pressure [43]. Women (46.3%) were more aware of their diagnosis than men (28.0%), and those in the 55 to 64 age group (43.5%) were more aware than their counterparts in either the youngest (20.7%) or oldest (34.3%) age group. The estimated percentage of hypertensive individuals receiving pharmacological treatment in Egypt was 23.9%. The estimated percentage of hypertensive individuals whose blood pressures were under control was 8.0%. The control rates were higher in women than men (10.9% and 4.8%, respectively).

CONCLUSION

Hypertension is a common public health problem throughout the world. It often goes undiagnosed, and even when it is identified and treated, few hypertensives achieve adequate control of their blood pressure. The improvements in the awareness, treatment, and control of blood pressure in the United States provide hope that similar strides may be made elsewhere. Given the high prevalence of hypertension in the community and the difficulties in achieving and maintaining the goals of therapy, however, lifestyle modification remains an attractive therapeutic option. The rising prevalence of hypertension in the developing world, that has accompanied the adoption of a more western-type lifestyle illustrates the importance of lifestyle approaches in the prevention and treatment of hypertension.

ACKNOWLEDGMENTS

The authors would like to acknowledge Ms. Megan Whelton and Ms. Kristi Reynolds for their contributions to this project. This work was supported in part by grant RO1HL60300 from the National Heart, Lung and Blood Institute of the National Institutes of Health, in Bethesda, Maryland.

REFERENCES

1. He J, Whelton PK. Epidemiology and prevention of hypertension. Med Clin Am 1997;81:1077–1097.
2. Whelton PK. Epidemiology of hypertension. Lancet 1994;344:101–106.
3. Wolz M, Cutler J, Roccella EJ, Rohde F, Thom T, Burt V. Statement from the National High Blood Pressure Education Program: prevalence of hypertension. AJH 2000;13:103–104.
4. Fuentes R, Ilmaniemi N, Laurikainen E, Tuomilehto J, Nissinen A. Hypertension in developing economies: a review of population-based studies carried out from 1980 to 1998. J Hypertens 2000;18:521–529.
5. Singh RB, Suh IL, Singh VP, Chaithiraphan S, Laothavorn P, Sy RG, Babilonia NA, Rahman AR, Sheikh S, Tomlinson B, Sarraf-Zadigan N. Hypertension and stroke in Asia: prevalence, control and strategies in developing countries for prevention. J Human Hypertens 2000;14:749–763.
6. Gu D, Reynolds K, Wu X, Chen J, Duan X, Muntner P, Huang G, Reynolds RF, Su S, Whelton PK, He J. Prevalence, awareness, treatment, and control of hypertension in China. Hypertension 2002;40:920–927.
7. Kannel WB. Blood pressure as a cardiovascular risk factor: prevention and treatment. JAMA 1996;275:1571–1576.
8. He J, Whelton PK. Systolic blood pressure and risk of cardiovascular and renal disease: an overview of evidence from observational epidemiologic studies and randomized controlled trials. Am Heart J 1999;138:S211–S219.
9. MacMahon S, Peto R, Cutler J, Collins R, Sorlie P, Neaton J, Abbott R, Godwin J, Dyer A, Stamler J. Blood pressure, stroke, and coronary heart disease. Part 1. Prolonged differences in blood pressure: prospective observational studies corrected for the regression dilution bias. Lancet 1990;335:765–774.

10. Stamler J, Stamler R, Neaton JD. Blood pressure, systolic and diastolic, and cardiovascular risks. US population data. Arch Int Med 1993;153:598–615.
11. Klag MJ, Whelton PK, Randall BL, Neaton JD, Brancati FL, Ford CE, Shulman NB, Stamler J. Blood pressure and end-stage renal disease in men. N J Med 1996;334:13–18.
12. He J, Ogden LG, Bazzano LA, Vupputuri S, Loria C, Whelton PK. Risk factors for congestive heart failure in U.S. general population: NHANES I Epidemiologic Follow-Up Study. Arch Int Med 2001;161:996–1002.
13. Whelton PK, He J. Blood pressure reduction. In: Hennekens CH, Buring JE, Manson JE, Ridker PM, eds. Clinical Trials in Cardiovascular Disease. A Companion to Braunwald's Heart Disease. Philadelphia: Saunders, 1999.
14. Collins R, Peto R, MacMahon S, Hebert P, Fiebach NH, Eberlein KA, Godwin J, Qizibash N, Taylor JO, Hennekens CH. Blood pressure, stroke, and coronary heart disease. II. short-term reductions in blood pressure: overview of randomized drug trials in their epidemiological contest. Lancet 1990; 335:827–838.
15. Hebert P, Moser M, Mayer J, Glynn RJ, and Hennekens CH. Recent evidence on drug therapy of mild to moderate hypertension and decreased risk of coronary heart disease. Arch Int Med 1993;153:578–581.
16. He J, Whelton PK. Selection of initial antihypertensive drug therapy. Lancet 2000;356:1942–1943.
17. American Heart Association. 2002 Heart and Stroke Statistical Update. Dallas, TX: American Heart Association, 2002.
18. Whelton PK, He J, Klag MJ. Blood pressure in westernized populations. In: Swales JD, ed. Textbook of Hypertension. Oxford: Blackwell Scientific, 1994: 11–21.
19. Task Force on Blood Pressure Control in Children. Report of the Second Task Force on Blood Pressure Control in Children—1987. Pediatrics 1987;79: 1–25.
20. Berenson GS, Wattigney WA, Webber LS. Epidemiology of hypertension from childhood to young adulthood in black, white, and Hispanic population samples. Pub Health Rep. 1996;111(suppl. 2):3–6.
21. Kelder SH, Osganian SK, Feldman HA, Webber LS, Parcel GS, Leupker RV, Wu MC, Nader PR. Tracking of physical and physiological risk variables among ethnic subgroups from third to eighth grade: the Child and Adolescent Trial for Cardiovascular Health cohort study. Preventive Med 2002; 34:324–333.
22. Kannel WB, Gordon T. Evaluation of cardiovascular risk in the elderly: the Framingham Study. Bull NY Acad Med 1978;54:573–591.
23. Poulter NR, Sever PS. Low blood pressure populations and impact of rural-urban migration. In: Swales JD, ed. Textbook of Hypertension. Oxford: Blackwell Scientific, 1994:22–36.
24. He J, Tell GS, Tang YC, Mo PS, He GQ. Effect of migration on blood pressure: the Yi People Study. Epidemiology 1991;2:88–97.

25. He J, Klag MJ, Whelton PK, Chen JY, Mo JP, Qian MC, Mo PS, He GQ. Migration, blood pressure pattern and hypertension: the Yi Migrant Study. Am J Epidem 1991;134:1085–1101.
26. Sixth Report of the Joint National Committee on the Detection, Evaluation, and Treatment of High Blood Pressure (JNC VI). Arch Int Med 1997;157: 2413–2446.
27. Guidelines Subcommittee. 1999 World Health Organization–International Society of Hypertension guidelines for the management of hypertension. J Hypertens 1999;17:151–183.
28. Cornoni-Huntley J, LaCroix AZ, Havlik RJ. Race and sex differentials in the impact of hypertension in the United States: the National Health and Nutrition Examination Survey I Epidemiologic Follow-up Study. Arch Intern Med. 1989;149:780–788.
29. Vasan RS, Larson MG, Leip EP, Kannel WB, Levy D. Assessment of frequency of progression to hypertension in non-hypertensive participants in the Framingham Heart Study: a cohort study. Lancet 2001;358:1682–1686.
30. Fuchs FD, Chambless LE, Whelton PK, Nieto FJ, Heiss G. Alcohol consumption and the incidence of hypertension: the Atherosclerosis Risk in Communities Study. Hypertension. 2001;37:1242–1250.
31. Burt VL, Whelton PK, Roccella EJ, Brown C, Cutler JA, Higgins M, Horan MJ, Labarthe D. Prevalence of hypertension in the US adult population: results from the third National Health and Nutrition Examination Survey, 1988–1991. Hypertension 1995;25:305–313.
32. Apostolides AY, Cutter G, Daugherty SA, Detels R, Kraus J, Wassertheil-Smoller S, Ware J. Three-year incidence of hypertension in thirteen US communities. Prevent Med 1982;11:487–499.
33. Manolio TA, Burke GL, Savage PJ, Sidney S, Gardin JM, Oberman A. Exercise blood pressure response and 5-year risk of elevated blood pressure in a cohort of young adults: the CARDIA Study. Am J Hypertens 1994;7:234–241.
34. Vasan RS, Beiser A, Seshadri S, Larson MG, Kannel WB, D'Agostino RB, Levy D. Residual lifetime risk for developing hypertension in middle-aged women and men: the Framingham Heart Study. JAMA, 2002;287:1003–1010.
35. Mulrow PJ. Hypertension: a worldwide epidemic. In Izzo JL, Black HR, eds. Hypertension Primer. 2nd Ed. Dalls: American Heart Association, 1999;271–273.
36. Joffres MR, Ghadirian P, Fodor JG, Petrasovits A, Chockalingam A, Hamet P. Awareness, treatment, and control of hypertension in Canada. Am J Hypertens. 1997;10:1097–1102.
37. Primatesta P, Brookes M, Poulter NR. Improved hypertension management and control: results from the health survey for England 1998. Hypertension 2001;38:827–832.
38. Bennett SA, Magnus P. Trends in cardiovascular risk factors in Australia. Results from the National Heart Foundation's Risk Factor Prevalence Study, 1980–1989. Med J Aust. 1994;161:519–527.

39. http://www.aihw.gov.au/pls/cvd/cvd_risk.show_form.
40. Tao S, Wu X, Duan X, Fang W, Hao J, Fan D, Wang W, and Li Y. Hypertension prevalence and status of awareness, treatment and control in China. Chinese Med J 1995;108:483–489.
41. Wu X, Duan X, Gu D, Hao J, Tao S, Fan D. Prevalence of hypertension and its trends in Chinese populations. Internat J Cardiol 1995;52:39–44.
42. Ibrahim MM, Rizk H, Appel LJ, Aroussy W, Helmy S, Sharaf Y, Ashour Z, Kandil H, Roccella E, Whelton PK, Hypertension prevalence, awareness, treatment, and control in Egypt. Results from the Egyptian National Hypertension Project (NHP). NHP Investigative Team. Hypertension 1995; 26:886–890.
43. Arroyo P, Fernandez V, Loria A, Kuri-Morales P, Orozco-Rivadeneyra S, Olaiz G, Tapia-Conyer R. Hypertension in urban Mexico: the 1992–93 national survey of chronic diseases. J Human Hypertens 1999;13:671–675.
44. Steyn K, Gaziano TA, Bradshaw D, Laubscher R, Fourie J. South African Demographic and Health Coordinating Team. Hypertension in South African adults: results from the Demographic and Health Survey, 1998. J Hypertens 2001;19:1717–1725.
45. Burt VL, Cutler JA, Higgins M, Horan MJ, Labarthe D, Whelton PK, Brown C, Roccella EJ. Trends in the prevalence, awareness, treatment, and control of hypertension in the adult US population. Data from the health examination surveys, 1960 to 1991. Hypertension 1995;26:60–69.
46. He J, Whelton PK, Wu X, Burt VL, Tao S, Roccella EJ, Klag MJ. Comparison of secular trends in prevalence of hypertension in the People's Republic of China and the United States of America. Am J Hypertens. 1996;9:74A.
47. He J, Muntner P, Chen J, Roccella EJ, Streiffer RH, Whelton PK. Factors associated with hypertension control in the general population of the United States. Arch Int Med 2002;162:1051–1058.

2

Blood Pressure and Risk of Vascular Disease

Jiang He, Patricia M. Kearney, and Paul Muntner
Tulane University School of Public Health and Tropical Medicine, New Orleans, Louisiana, U.S.A.

INTRODUCTION

Hypertension is the most important modifiable risk factor for cardiovascular, cerebrovascular, and renal disease. Most evidence regarding the effects of blood pressure on the risk of cardiovascular-renal disease derives from two principal sources: prospective observational studies of the incidence of or mortality from coronary heart disease, stroke, congestive heart failure, and end-stage renal disease, and randomized controlled trials of antihypertensive therapy. The positive relationship between systolic and diastolic blood pressure and the risk of cardiovascular-renal disease has been documented by numerous prospective cohort studies. This relationship is strong, continuous, graded, consistent, independent, predictive, and etiologically significant for those with and without a previous history of coronary heart disease [1,2]. Furthermore, randomized controlled trials have demonstrated that antihypertensive drug therapy reduces the risk of cardiovascular and renal disease [3,4].

OBSERVATIONAL STUDIES

Results from several prospective cohort studies indicate that elevated blood pressure level is associated with an increased risk of coronary heart disease, stroke, congestive heart failure, and chronic kidney failure [5–7]. This increased risk is continuous throughout a wide range of blood pressures, even at a "normal" level, and independent from other established cardiovascular risk factors. Furthermore, these studies suggest that the association of systolic blood pressure with cardiovascular and renal disease is stronger than that of diastolic blood pressure.

Coronary Heart Disease and Stroke

Coronary heart disease and stroke are the leading causes of death and long-term disability in the United States and other countries [8]. A number of prospective cohort studies have examined the relationship between blood pressure and the risk of coronary heart disease and stroke, and the findings from these studies have been combined in several pooling projects [5–7]. MacMahon and colleagues conducted a pooled analysis of nine prospective observational studies with 418,343 participants aged 25 to 84 years [6]. None of the study participants had clinical evidence of coronary heart disease or stroke at baseline, and they were followed for an average of 10 years. The combined results demonstrated a positive, continuous, and independent association between diastolic blood pressure and the incidence of coronary heart disease and stroke (Fig. 1). The risk of coronary heart disease and stroke was approximately 5 times and 10 times higher in those at the highest end of the blood pressure range compared to those at the lowest. There was no evidence of a J-shaped relationship or a "threshold" below which lower levels of blood pressure were not associated with a lower risk of stroke and coronary heart disease. After correction for "regression dilution" bias, prolonged differences in usual diastolic blood pressure of 5, 7.5, and 10 mmHg were respectively associated with at least a 34%, 46%, and 56% lower incidence of stroke and at least a 21%, 29%, and 37% lower incidence of coronary heart disease [6].

The Prospective Studies Collaboration examined the association between diastolic blood pressure and subsequent risk of stroke by reviewing 45 prospective observational cohorts involving 450,000 individuals with 5 to 30 years of follow-up (mean 16 years, total 7.3 million person years of observation), during which 13,397 participants developed a stroke [7]. Blood pressure was measured in most studies with a standard mercury sphygmomanometer as either a single reading or the average of two consecutive readings at a single visit. When the highest and lowest of the six blood pressure categories were compared, the difference in usual

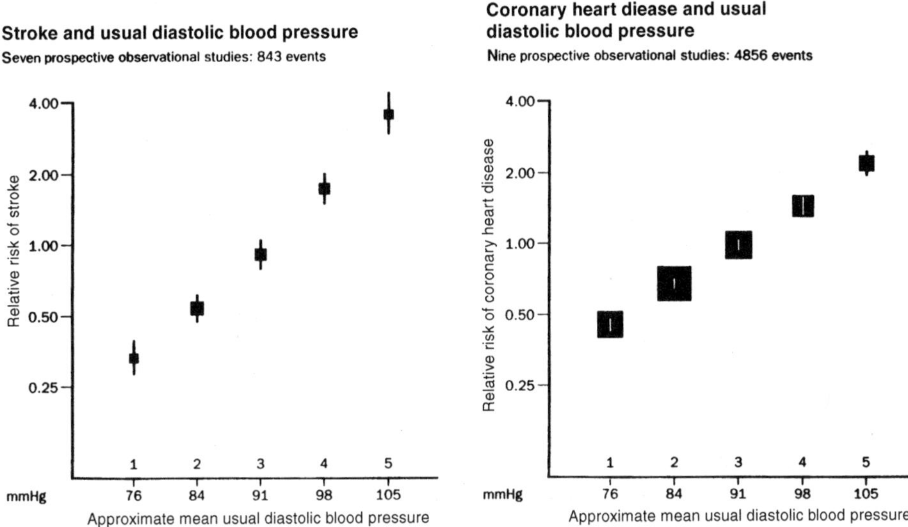

FIGURE 1 Relative risks of stroke and coronary heart disease estimated from combined results among seven prospective cohort studies. *Source*: Ref. 5.

diastolic blood pressure was 27 mmHg (102 vs. 75 mmHg), and there was a fivefold difference in stroke risk. This fivefold difference was seen in both those with and without a pre-existing history of coronary heart disease. For every 10 mmHg increase in usual diastolic blood pressure the risk of stroke increased by 80% after adjustment for total cholesterol, history of coronary heart disease, sex, age, and ethnicity. The positive relationship between diastolic blood pressure and the risk of stroke did not flatten out at blood pressure levels below 80 mmHg, indicating that there was no threshold below which the positive association between blood pressure and risk of stroke disappeared.

Stroke is a leading cause of death in eastern Asia. The incidence of both ischemic and hemorrhagic stroke is much higher than in Western Europe or North America, and a greater proportion of strokes is due to cerebral hemorrhage [7]. The relationship between blood pressure and stroke was examined in a pooled project of 18 cohorts from the People's Republic of China and Japan [7]. A total of 124,774 participants were included and were followed up for an average of 7 years. Within most individual cohorts there was evidence of a positive relationship between usual diastolic blood pressure and the relative risk of any type of stroke. Overall, individuals in the group with the highest baseline diastolic blood pressure had a risk of stroke about 13 times greater than those in the group with the lowest baseline diastolic blood pressure (Fig. 2). For a 5 mmHg higher usual diastolic blood pressure the risk of stroke was increased by 44% [8].

The role of systolic blood pressure in the development of coronary heart disease and stroke was demonstrated in several prospective cohort studies [9–11]. Data from 30 years of follow-up of the Framingham Heart Study cohort, comprising 5070 men and women who were aged 30 to 62 years and free of cardiovascular disease at their baseline examination, indicates that systolic blood pressure is a strong and consistent predictor of the development of coronary heart disease in both men and women within several age strata [9]. Individuals with a systolic blood pressure greater than 180 mmHg had a relative risk of coronary heart disease of more than 3 for men aged 35 to 64 years and 5 for women of the same age group compared to those with systolic blood pressure less than 120 mmHg. For stroke and transient ischemic attack, the contribution of systolic blood pressure to risk was even greater. Compared to those with systolic pressure less than 120 mmHg, the age-adjusted relative risk ranges from 3.25 for men aged > 65 years to 8.0 for men aged 35 to 64 years among those with pressures of 180 mmHg or greater. In the Italian RIFLE Pooling Project, Menotti and colleagues studied the association between systolic blood pressure and coronary death in 31,317 participants aged 30 to 69 years

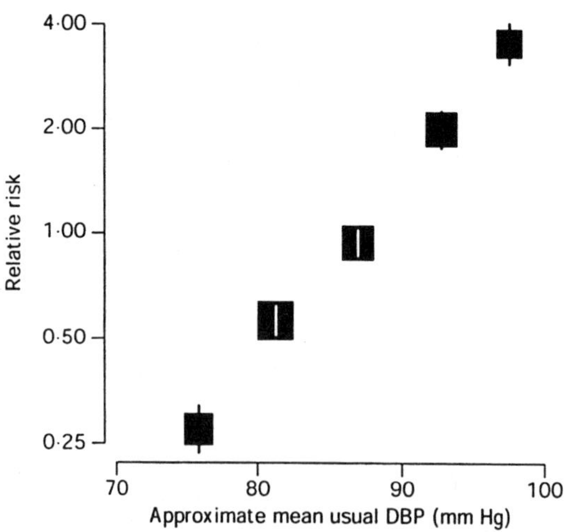

FIGURE 2 Overall relative risk of total stroke according to approximate usual diastolic blood pressure estimated from pooled results among 18 prospective cohort studies. *Source*: Ref. 7.

from 45 cohorts of men [10]. During an average follow-up of 6 years, 239 of the men died from coronary heart disease. In a multivariate Cox model, systolic blood pressure was positively and consistently associated with coronary heart disease deaths in each of the four age groups studied (30–39, 40–49, 50–59, and 60–69 years).

More recent studies have confirmed the importance of systolic blood pressure in determining the risk of cardiovascular events. The Cardiovascular Health Study examined the association between blood pressure level and the risk of myocardial infarction, stroke and total mortality among 5888 adults aged 65 years or older [11]. In the multivariate model for myocardial infarction, a one standard deviation higher systolic blood pressure, diastolic blood pressure and pulse pressure was associated with hazard ratios (95% confidence intervals) of 1.24 (1.15 to 1.35), 1.13 (1.04 to 1.22), and 1.21 (1.12 to 1.31), respectively. For stroke the hazard ratios (95% confidence intervals) were 1.34 (1.21 to 1.47), 1.29 (1.17 to 1.42), and 1.21 (1.10 to 1.34) with systolic, diastolic, and pulse pressure, respectively.

Although incidence and mortality of cardiovascular disease vary among populations in different parts of the world, the relationship between blood pressure and coronary heart disease seems similar. The Seven Countries Study examined the association between blood pressure and long-term mortality from coronary heart disease in 12,031 men (age range, 40 to 59 years) who were free of coronary heart disease at baseline [12]. The 25-year mortality rates from coronary heart disease in the United States and northern Europe were high (approximately 70 deaths per 10,000 person-years), while rates in Japan and Mediterranean southern Europe were low (approximately 20 deaths per 10,000 person years). The relative increase in 25-year mortality from coronary heart disease for a given increase in blood pressure was similar among the populations, however. For an increase of 10 mmHg in systolic blood pressure, the multivariate-adjusted relative risk of death from coronary heart disease ranged from 1.09 in inland southern Europe to 1.25 in Serbia and Japan [12]. The multivariate-adjusted relative risk for all the populations combined was 1.17 before adjustment for within-subject variability in blood pressure and 1.28 after adjustment. For an increase of 5 mmHg in diastolic blood pressure, the relative risk of death ranged from 1.06 in inland southern Europe to 1.19 in Mediterranean southern Europe, with a relative risk for the total population of 1.13 before adjustment for within-subject variation in blood pressure and 1.28 after adjustment. No significant differences were observed among the populations with respect to the relative risk of death from coronary heart disease over the 25-year period for these increments in blood pressure ($P > 0.1$ by the likelihood-ratio test for the interaction between the blood pressure variables and the ordinal population variable) [12].

End-Stage Renal Disease

The incidence of end-stage renal disease has been increasing during the past several decades in the United States, including the proportion that has been attributed to hypertension [13]. Prospective cohort studies have demonstrated that blood pressure is an important risk factor for the development of and progression to end-stage renal disease [14–16]. Klag and colleagues assessed the development of end-stage renal disease through 1990 in 332,544 men, 35 to 57 years of age, who were screened between 1973 and 1975 for entry into the Multiple Risk Factor Intervention Trial (MRFIT). During an average of 16 years of follow-up, 814 subjects either died of end-stage renal disease or were treated for that condition. A strong, graded relationship between both systolic and diastolic blood pressure and end-stage renal disease was identified, independent of age, race, income, use of medication for diabetes mellitus, history of myocardial infarction, serum cholesterol concentration, and cigarette smoking [14]. The risk of end-stage renal disease in men with hypertension as compared to men with optimal levels of blood pressure increased with each of the four successively more severe stages of hypertension. As compared with men with an optimal level of blood pressure, the relative risk (95% confidence interval) of end-stage renal disease for those with high normal, and stage 1, 2, 3, and 4 hypertension was 1.9 (1.4 to 2.7),

TABLE 1 Baseline Blood Pressure and the Incidence of End-Stage Renal Disease Due to Any Cause in 332,544 Men Screened for MRFIT

Blood pressure category	Age-adjusted rate per 100,000 person-years[a]	Adjusted relative risk (95% CI)[b]
Optimal (<120/80 mmHg)	5.3	1.0
Normal but not optimal (120–129/80-84 mmHg)	6.6	1.2 (0.8–1.7)
High Normal (130–139/85-89 mmHg)	11.1	1.9 (1.4–2.7)
Hypertension		
Stage 1 (140–160/90–100 mmHg)	21.0	3.1 (2.3–4.3)
Stage 2 (160–180/100–110 mmHg)	43.6	6.0 (4.3–8.4)
Stage 3 (180–200/110–120 mmHg)	96.1	11.2 (7.7–16.2)
Stage 4 (>200/120 mmHg)	187.1	22.1 (14.2–34.3)
Total	15.6	-

[a] Adjusted by the direct method for the age distribution of all men screened.

[b] Relative risks, with men with optimal blood pressure as the reference category, were estimated with use of a proportional-hazards regression model, with stratification according to clinic and adjustment for age, race, income, serum cholesterol concentration, number of cigarettes smoked per day, use of medication for diabetes mellitus, and previous myocardial infarction.

3.1 (2.3 to 4.3), 11.2 (7.7 to 16.2), and 22.1 (14.2 to 34.3), respectively (Table 1). These relations remained after excluding end-stage renal disease cases that occurred soon after screening and after taking into account the baseline serum creatinine concentration and urinary protein excretion. These data indicate that elevated blood pressure levels are a strong independent risk factor for end-stage renal disease and that interventions to prevent the disease need to emphasize the prevention and control of both high-normal and high blood pressure [14].

Perry and colleagues have also studied the predictive effect of blood pressure on end-stage renal disease in 5730 black and 6182 nonblack male veterans who had hypertension at their baseline examination [15]. Over an average follow-up of 15 years, 245 of the veterans developed end-stage renal disease. In a multiple Cox proportional hazards model, men with a baseline systolic blood pressure between 165 and 180 mmHg had a 2.8-fold higher risk of end-stage renal disease and men with a baseline systolic blood pressure greater than 180 mmHg had a 7.6-fold higher risk of end-stage renal disease compared to their counterparts who had a baseline systolic blood pressure of less than 140 mmHg [15]. This study indicates that pretreatment blood pressure level is an important risk factor for progression of renal disease in patients with hypertension.

Congestive Heart Failure

In contrast to other forms of cardiovascular disease that have declined in the U.S. population over the past two decades, both the incidence and prevalence of heart failure are increasing [17,18]. The relationship between blood pressure and heart failure has been examined in several large prospective cohort studies [19–23]. In the original Framingham Heart Study and Framingham Offspring Study cohorts, a total of 5143 participants aged 40 to 89 years and free of congestive heart failure at baseline examination were used to study the relative and population-attributable risks of hypertension for the development of congestive heart failure [20]. During up to 20 years of follow-up (mean, 14 years), there were 392 new cases of heart failure; in 91% (357/392), hypertension antedated the development of heart failure. After adjustment for age and heart failure risk factors in proportional hazards regression models, the hazard for developing heart failure in hypertensive compared with normotensive subjects was approximately two fold in men and three fold in women. Multivariable analyses revealed that hypertension had a high population-attributable risk for congestive heart failure, accounting for 39% of cases in men and 59% in women [20]. Among hypertensive subjects, myocardial infarction, diabetes, left ventricular hypertrophy, and valvular heart disease were important predictors for increased risk for congestive heart failure in both sexes [20]. This study indicated that hypertension was the most common risk factor for heart failure, and it contributed a large proportion of heart failure cases in this population-based sample. Preventive strategies directed toward earlier and more aggressive blood pressure control are likely to offer the greatest promise for reducing the incidence of congestive heart failure and its associated mortality.

The independent contribution of blood pressure to the risk of heart failure was also assessed in the National Health and Nutrition Examination I Epidemiologic Follow-up Study (NHEFS) [23]. This prospective cohort study included 13,643 individuals without a history of congestive heart failure at baseline who were followed up for an average of 19 years. A total of 1382 cases of heart failure were documented over this time period. After adjustment for age, race, and time-dependent history of coronary heart disease, there was a positive and significant association between hypertension and increased risk of subsequently developing congestive heart failure in men and women, relative risk 1.50 (95% confidence interval 1.34 to 1.68). In a multivariate model that simultaneously included all the significant risk factors identified in the previous model, hypertension remained a significant predictor of increased risk of congestive heart failure in men and women, relative risk 1.40 (95% confidence interval 1.24 to 1.59). As the NHEFS population is a representative sample of the U.S. general population, the population-attributable risk of various risk factors could be calculated. Hypertension accounted for 10.1% of the population-attributable risk for congestive heart failure, which was much lower than that estimated from the Framingham Heart Study.

Systolic, Diastolic, and Pulse Pressure

Most early studies of the relationship between blood pressure and the risk of cardiovascular disease have concentrated on diastolic blood pressure [6,7]. The emphasis on diastolic blood pressure was strengthened by trials that demonstrated the benefit of lowering elevated diastolic blood pressure [3,24,25]. It is now increasingly recognized, however, that systolic blood pressure and pulse pressure are more important determinants of cardiovascular and renal disease risk than diastolic blood pressure [2,4,26–29]. In the Honolulu Heart Program, 7591 middle-aged Hawaiian-Japanese men who were free of coronary heart disease and stroke at their initial examination were followed up for 18 years [26]. Both systolic and diastolic blood pressure were significantly and positively associated with the risk of sudden coronary death. The relative risk of coronary death associated with corresponding levels of systolic blood pressure was greater than that for diastolic blood pressure, however. For example, compared to the lowest quartile of systolic and diastolic blood pressure, the age-adjusted relative risk for the upper quartile of systolic and diastolic blood pressure was 4.46 and 3.36, respectively [26]. Other prospective studies have also indicated that systolic blood pressure is as strong as or even stronger than diastolic blood pressure as a predictor of coronary heart disease, stroke, congestive heart failure, and end-stage renal disease [2,14,27–30].

Data from the MRFIT screenee cohort provide the most precise and valid comparison of the associations of systolic and diastolic blood pressure with the risk of coronary heart disease and stroke [2]. The MRFIT screenee cohort consists of 347,978 men, 35 to 57 years of age, who were screened between 1973 and 1975 for possible entry into the MRFIT and did not report a previous hospitalization for coronary heart disease or stroke. During 11.6 years of follow-up, 7150 deaths from coronary heart disease and 733 deaths from stroke were identified. Given the large sample size of the MRFIT screenee cohort, it was possible to evaluate the relationship of systolic and diastolic blood pressure to coronary heart disease and stroke while concurrently stratifying for the level of blood pressure. As indicated in Fig. 3, compared to men with a systolic/diastolic blood pressure of less than

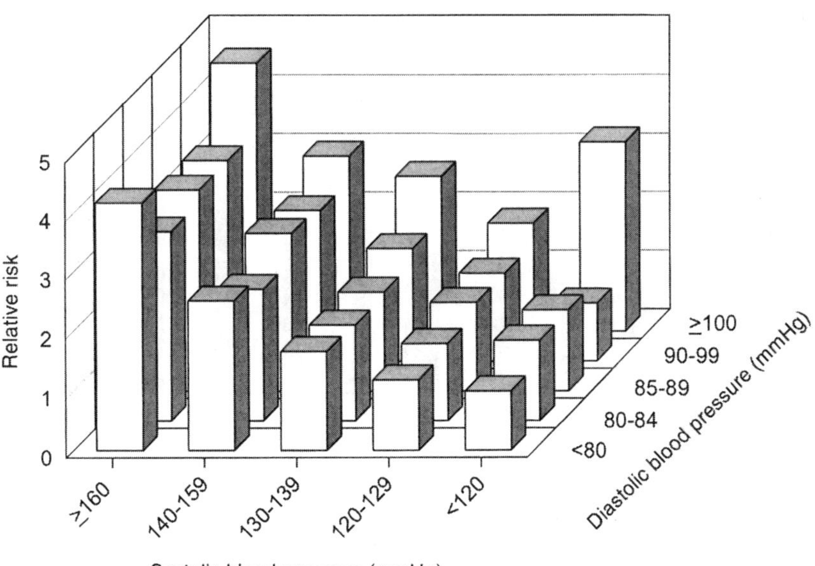

FIGURE 3 Adjusted relative risks of coronary heart disease death according to baseline systolic and diastolic blood pressure in men screened for the Multiple Risk Factor Intervention Trials. *Source*: Data from Ref. 2.

120/80 mmHg, all other strata were at a greater risk of subsequent coronary heart disease. Furthermore, a higher systolic blood pressure was related to a higher risk of coronary heart disease in a continuous and graded fashion at every level of diastolic blood pressure. Although the risk of coronary heart disease also increased with progressively higher levels of diastolic blood pressure at every level of systolic blood pressure, the magnitude of the increase in risk for diastolic blood pressure was not as steep or as consistent as that for systolic blood pressure. To compare systolic blood pressure with diastolic blood pressure in relation to the relative risks of coronary heart disease and stroke, blood pressure was divided into deciles in the MRFIT cohort [2]. In every decile, systolic blood pressure was more strongly related to the risk of coronary heart disease and stroke than was diastolic blood pressure (Figs. 4,5). For example, in a comparison of the highest decile vs. the lowest, the relative risk associated with systolic and diastolic blood pressure was 3.7 and 2.8, respectively, for coronary heart disease, and 8.2 and 4.4, respectively, for stroke [2].

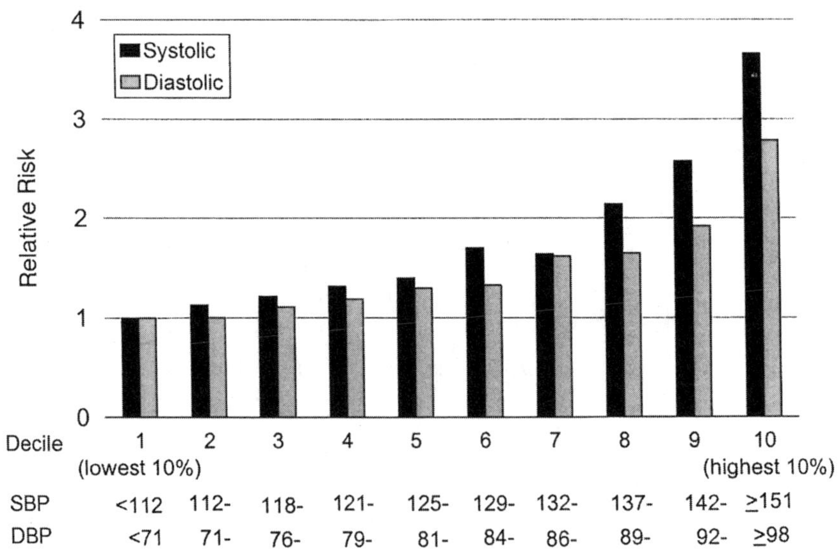

FIGURE 4 Adjusted relative risks of coronary heart disease death according to deciles of baseline systolic blood pressure (SBP) and diastolic blood pressure (DBP) in men screened for the Multiple Risk Factor Intervention Trials. *Source*: Data from Ref. 2.

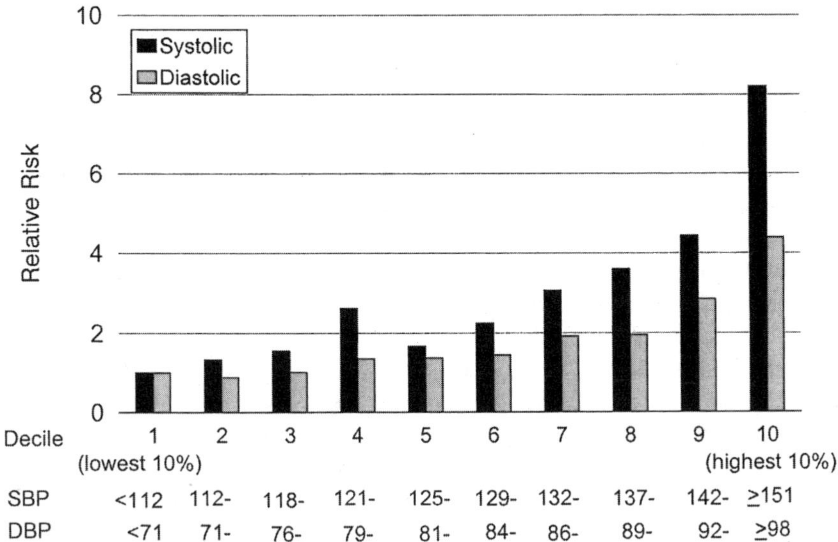

FIGURE 5 Adjusted relative risks of stroke death according to deciles of baseline systolic blood pressure (SBP) and diastolic blood pressure (DBP) in men screened for the Multiple Risk Factor Intervention Trials. *Source*: Data from Ref. 2.

To determine whether systolic or diastolic blood pressure is a stronger predictor of the risk of stroke, some investigators have included both variables simultaneously in regression models [31]. In the Copenhagen City Heart Study, 19,698 women and men aged 20 years or older were followed up for an average of 12 years. During the period of follow-up, a total of 631 strokes were identified [31]. Both systolic and diastolic blood pressure were positively and significantly associated with an increased risk of stroke, independent of age, sex, education, income, marital status, exercise, body mass index, smoking, alcohol consumption, diabetes, antihypertensive treatment, plasma cholesterol, and triglyceride [31]. When systolic and diastolic pressure were entered simultaneously into the Cox proportional hazards model, however, the effect of diastolic blood pressure diminished, while the pattern of the association between systolic pressure and stroke risk remained unchanged [31]. Again, this analysis suggests that systolic blood pressure is a stronger predictor of stroke than diastolic blood pressure.

The combined effects of various levels of systolic and diastolic blood pressure on the age-adjusted relative risk of end-stage renal disease using data from the MRFIT screenee cohort are shown in Fig. 6. The relative risks of end-stage renal disease associated with differences in diastolic blood pressure within each stratum of systolic blood pressure were far less marked than the steep risk gradient apparent for progressively higher levels of systolic blood pressure within each stratum of diastolic blood pressure. For example, among the men in whom the diagnosis of stage 1 hypertension was based on systolic blood pressure (140 to 159 mmHg), the relative risk for the four lower categories of diastolic blood pressure were similar. In contrast, for the men in whom the diagnosis of stage 1 hypertension was based on diastolic blood pressure (90 to 99mmHg), the relative risks of end-stage renal disease for increasing levels of systolic blood pressure rose sharply, from 1.8 to 27.1. Indeed, the increase in risk was present even across the three categories of systolic blood pressure within the normotensive range. A comparison of the relative risk of end-stage renal disease by quintile of systolic and diastolic blood pressure demonstrated that systolic blood pressure was a quantitatively more important predictor of subsequent end-stage renal disease than diastolic blood pressure. For example, compared to the corresponding lowest quintile,

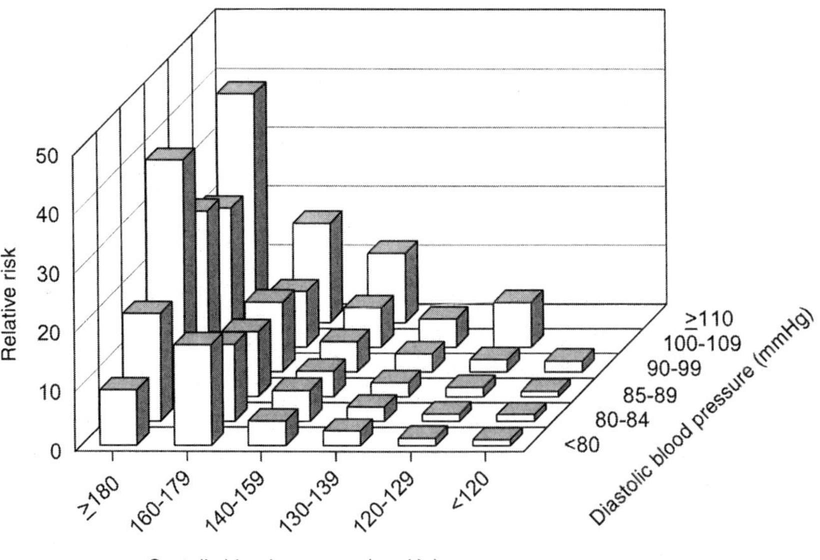

FIGURE 6 Age-adjusted relative risks of end-stage renal disease according to baseline levels of systolic and diastolic blood pressure in men screened for the Multiple Risk Factor Intervention Trial. *Source*: Data from Ref. 14.

the relative risks (95% confidence intervals) in the highest quintile were 5.0 (3.7 to 6.7) for systolic and 4.0 (3.0 to 5.2) for diastolic blood pressure, respectively [14]. Furthermore, in a Cox proportional hazards model in which systolic and diastolic blood pressure were considered together, a baseline systolic blood pressure that was higher by one standard deviation (15.8 mmHg) had more predictive power (relative risk, 1.6; 95% confidence interval, 1.5 to 1.7) than a one standard deviation (10.5 mmHg) increase in diastolic blood pressure (relative risk, 1.2; 95% confidence interval, 1.1 to 1.2). The MRFIT analysis provides strong evidence favoring the notion that systolic is a more important predictor of end-stage renal disease than diastolic blood pressure.

Several prospective cohort studies have reported recently that pulse pressure is an important independent risk factor for coronary heart disease, stroke, and heart failure, especially in older persons [32–35]. Glynn et al. examined which combinations of systolic, diastolic, pulse, and mean arterial pressure best predict total and cardiovascular mortality in 9431 older adults, aged 65 to 102 years, using data from the Established Populations for Epidemiologic Studies of the Elderly [32]. Over an average follow-up of 10.6 years among survivors, 4528 total deaths and 2304 cardiovascular deaths were documented. In the univariate and multivariate analyses, systolic and pulse pressure were much stronger predictors than diastolic or mean arterial pressure on cardiovascular and total mortality [32]. In the same study population, pulse pressure was an independent predictor of congestive heart failure, after controlling for age, sex, mean arterial pressure, history of coronary heart disease, diabetes mellitus, atrial fibrillation, valvular heart disease, and antihypertensive medication use [33]. For each 10-mmHg elevation in pulse pressure, there was a 14% increase in risk of congestive heart failure (95% confidence interval, 5–24%). Those in the highest tertile of pulse pressure (> 67 mmHg) had a 55% increased risk of congestive heart failure compared with those in the lowest (< 54 mmHg). This study indicated that pulse pressure was more predictive than systolic blood pressure alone and was independent of diastolic blood pressure [33]. In a meta-analysis that pooled individual patient data from the European Working Party on High Blood Pressure in the Elderly Trial (n = 840), the Systolic Hypertension in Europe Trial (n = 4695), and the Systolic Hypertension in China Trial (n = 2394), pulse pressure was a much stronger predictor than mean arterial pressure of cardiovascular disease outcomes [34]. Reanalysis of data from MRFIT, however, indicated that cardiovascular disease risk assessment was improved by considering both systolic and diastolic blood pressure, not just systolic, diastolic, or pulse pressure separately [35].

Overall observational studies have demonstrated that the association of systolic blood pressure with cardiovascular and renal disease is stronger than the corresponding relationship for diastolic blood pressure. This information is critical both in terms of developing guidelines for patient care and public health. The importance of systolic blood pressure in predicting hypertension-related risks of coronary heart disease, stroke, heart failure, and end-stage renal disease in the general population or hypertension patients was emphasized in the most recent report of the Joint National Committee on Prevention, Detection, Evaluation and Treatment of High Blood Pressure [1].

Relative, Absolute, and Population-Attributable Risk

It has been increasingly recognized that the individual risk for cardiovascular and renal disease in patients with hypertension or in the general population is determined not only by the level of blood pressure but also by the presence or absence of target organ damage or other risk factors, such as smoking, dyslipidemia, diabetes, obesity, and physical inactivity. Many prospective cohort studies have documented that these factors independently modify the risk of cardiovascular and renal disease associated with blood pressure [1,9,36–39]. Traditionally, blood pressure levels alone were used to make treatment decisions in patients with hypertension. This approach was based on the fact that the relative risk of cardiovascular and renal disease increased continuously and in a graded manner among hypertensive patients. The approach worked well for treatment decisions made in patients with moderate or more severe forms of hypertension (stages 2 to 3), but it is less well suited for treatment decisions in patients with milder elevations of blood pressure. The most recent report of the Joint National Committee on the Prevention, Detection, Evaluation, and Treatment of High Blood Pressure has emphasized the importance of absolute, as opposed to relative, risk in clinical decision making [1]. For the first time, the national guideline has recommended therapeutic decisions regarding blood pressure treatment should be based not only on an individual's average blood pressure level, but also on the presence or absence of target organ damage or other risk factors. Lifestyle modification has been recommended as the first-line treatment for hypertension patients at low risk for cardiovascular and renal disease.

The burden of blood pressure-related vascular disease in the community depends on the prevalence of hypertension as well as on its importance as a predictor of risk in the individual. Figures 7 and 8 show the relative risk and population-attributable risk of hypertension on coronary heart disease and stroke, respectively. These estimates were derived from a 16-year follow-up experience among 347,978 men who were screened for inclusion in MRFIT [2]. After adjustment for age, race, income, serum

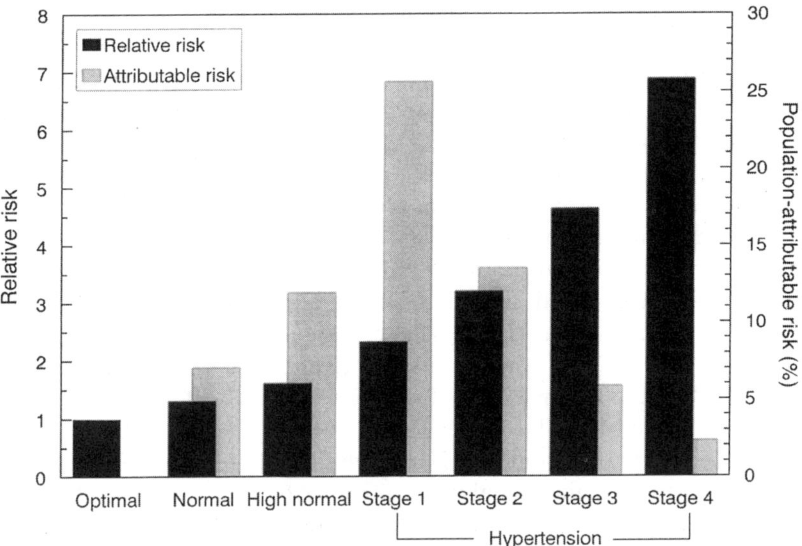

FIGURE 7 The relative risk and population-attributable risk of hypertension on coronary heart disease. *Source*: Data from Ref. 67.

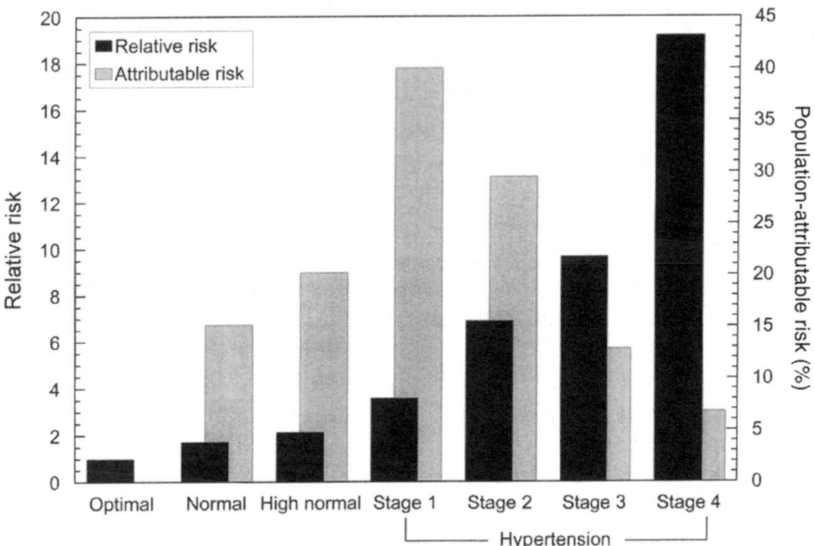

FIGURE 8 The relative risk and population-attributable risk of hypertension on stroke. *Source*: Data from Ref. 67.

cholesterol, cigarettes smoked, and use of medication for diabetes, the relative risks of coronary heart disease mortality were 2.3-, 3.2-, 4.6-, and 6.9-fold higher for those with hypertension of stage 1, 2, 3, or 4 at baseline compared to their counterparts with optimal blood pressure. The prevalence of stage 1 and stage 2 hypertension was more common than stage 3 and stage 4 hypertension in the general population, however. The population-attributable risks were therefore greater for stage 1 (25.6%) and stage 2 (13.5%) hypertension compared to stage 3 (5.8%) and stage 4 (2.3%) hypertension. Although stroke is a somewhat more blood pressure-dependant disease, the overall pattern for blood pressure-related population-attributable risk appears to be quite similar. For example, the relative risks of stroke were 3.6, 6.9, 9.7, and 19.2, and the population-attributable risks of stroke were 40.0%, 29.5%, 12.8%, and 6.8% for stage 1, 2, 3, and 4 hypertension, respectively, in the MRFIT cohort.

The recent paper from the Framingham Heart Study reported the association between high-normal blood pressure (systolic pressure of 130 to 139 and/or diastolic pressure of 85 to 89 mmHg) and risk of cardiovascular disease among 6859 persons who were initially free of hypertension and cardiovascular disease [40]. The 10-year cumulative incidence of cardiovascular disease in subjects 35 to 64 years of age who had high-normal blood pressure was 4% (95% confidence interval, 2–5%) for women and 8% (95% confidence interval, 6–10%) for men; in subjects 65 to 90 years of age, the incidence was 18% (95% confidence interval, 12–23%) for women and 25% (95% confidence interval, 17–34%) for men. As compared with optimal blood pressure, high-normal blood pressure was associated with a hazard ratio for cardiovascular disease of 2.5 (95% confidence interval, 1.6 to 4.1) in women and 1.6 (95% confidence interval, 1.1 to 2.2) in men after adjustment for important risk factors [40]. Because of a high proportion of persons in the United States with high-normal blood pressure [approximately 13% based on data from National Health and Nutrition Examination Survey (NHANES) III] [41], high-normal blood pressure will likely contribute substantially to cardiovascular disease risk in the community.

These data on the relative and absolute importance of blood pressure in determining the risk of blood pressure-related cardiovascular and renal disease have important implications for prevention of blood pressure-related disease. First, they provide a strong rationale for detection, treatment, and control of hypertension in the community. Second, they emphasize the importance of treating those with the least severe stage of hypertension because the majority of hypertension-related coronary heart disease and stroke occur within this range of blood pressure. Finally, the data indicate that treatment of hypertension represents only a partial response to the overall burden of blood pressure-related cardiovascular disease in the general population. Even individuals with so-called normal levels of blood pressure are at a increased risk of cardiovascular and renal disease [40]. Primary prevention strategies that target the entire population are required to lower the overall risk.

CLINICAL TRIALS

Over the past several decades, many antihypertensive drug treatment trials have been conducted to determine whether blood pressure reduction decreases the risk of cardiovascular disease [42,43]. Results from these trials have been pooled in several meta-analyses in order to obtain a more precise and accurate estimate of the effect of antihypertensive treatment on clinical outcomes [43–46].

Whelton and He pooled the results from 17 major randomized, controlled trials in which the effects of antihypertensive medication on cardiovascular disease were evaluated in 47,653 trial participants [47–66]. The number of participants enrolled in individual trials ranged from fewer than 100 to more than 17,000, with a median sample size of 840. An elevated diastolic blood pressure was the primary inclusion criterion in most studies, but in some trials participants were required to have both an elevated systolic and diastolic blood pressure at enrollment. The mean age was 56 years, with a range of 38 to 76 years. Men and women were represented in approximately equal numbers. In most trials, the participants were followed for 4 to 5 years. Treatment was double-blind in nine of the trials, single-blind in four trials, and open in the remaining four trials. Diuretics were used as first-step drug therapy in 12 of the 17 trials.

In most of the trials, the goal in the active treatment group was to achieve and maintain a diastolic blood pressure of 90 mmHg or less. Approximately one-quarter of the participants randomized to control therapy received antihypertensive drug therapy at some stage during their follow-up. The mean net reduction in diastolic blood pressure during follow-up for those assigned to active treatment compared to control ranged from 4 mmHg to 27 mmHg, with an overall average net reduction of 6.5 mmHg (weighted by sample size). The true overall net reduction in diastolic blood pressure may have been closer to about 5 to 6 mmHg, however, because blood pressure measurements were only obtained in those who continued to participate in the follow-up examinations. Information on systolic blood pressure during follow-up was available for nine of the 17 trials. In these studies, the overall weighted average net reduction in systolic blood pressure was 16 mmHg. For both systolic and diastolic blood pressure, the observed reduction in blood pressure was greater in trials in which the participants had a higher level of blood pressure at entry.

Coronary Heart Disease and Stroke

Overall, 934 coronary heart disease events occurred in the participants who were assigned to active treatment and 1104 in those who were allocated to control (Table 2). When results from the 17 trials were pooled, a highly significant reduction in the odds of total ($p<0.001$) and fatal ($p=0.006$) coronary heart disease was observed among the participants allocated to active treatment. The reduction in total coronary heart disease was 16% (95% confidence interval: 8–23%), as was the reduction in fatal coronary heart disease (95% confidence interval: 5–26%). As shown in Fig. 9, antihypertensive drug treatment was associated with a reduction in total coronary heart disease in 13 of the 17 trials. The reduction was statistically significant in only two of the trials, however. In the Hypertension Detection and Follow-up Program Cooperative Group trial, total coronary heart disease was reduced by 21% (95% confidence interval: 7–33%), and in the Systolic Hypertension in the Elderly Program trial, total coronary heart disease was reduced by 28% (95% confidence interval: 6–44%).

A total of 525 strokes occurred in participants who were allocated to active treatment and 768 occurred in those who were assigned to control (Table 2). Compared to control, those in active treatment experienced a 38% reduction in the odds of total stroke (95% confidence interval: 31–45%; $p<0.001$) and a 40% reduction in the odds of fatal stroke (95%

TABLE 2 Reduction in Risk for Coronary Heart Disease, Stroke, Cardiovascular Disease, and All-Cause Mortality: Results from 17 Randomized Trials with 23,847 Active Treatment and 23,806 Control Participants

	Number of events		Percentage risk reduction (95% CI)[a]	P value
	Active	Control		
Total coronary heart disease	934	1104	16 (8–23)	<0.001
Fatal coronary heart disease	470	560	16 (5–26)	0.006
Total stroke	525	835	38 (31–45)	<0.001
Fatal stroke	140	234	40 (26–51)	<0.001
Cardiovascular disease deaths	768	964	21 (13–28)	<0.001
All-cause deaths	1435	1634	13 (6–19)	<0.001

[a] Risk reduction = 1- odds ratio.

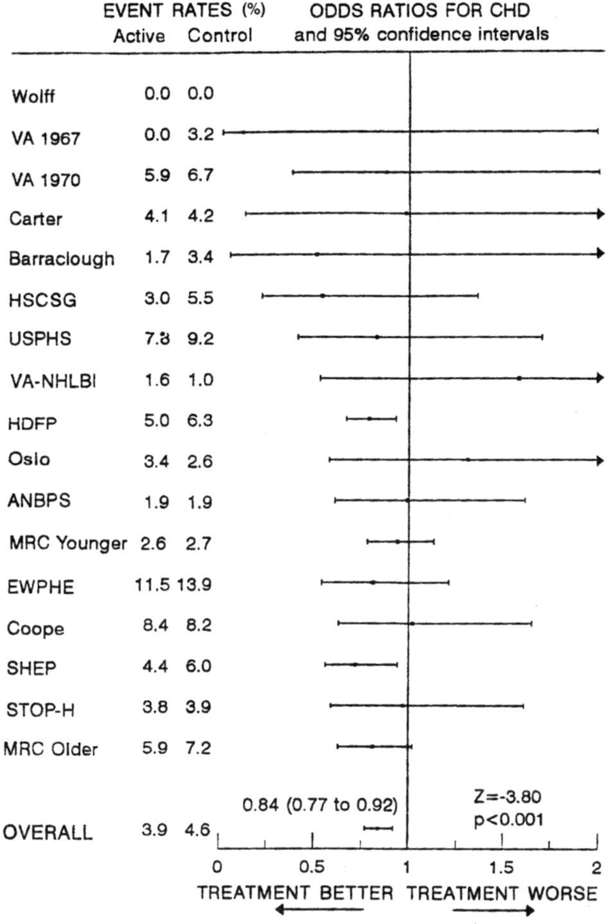

FIGURE 9 Odds ratios and 95% confidence intervals for total (fatal and nonfatal) coronary heart disease (CHD) related to antihypertensive drug treatment.

confidence interval: 26–51%; $p < 0.001$). In 14 of the 17 trials, the odds of total stroke were reduced for those assigned to active treatment compared to control, and in nine of the trials the reduction was statistically significant (Fig. 10).

While the relative reduction in coronary heart disease events was less than half that noted for stroke, the absolute reductions in outcomes were more similar. This is due to the greater frequency of coronary heart disease

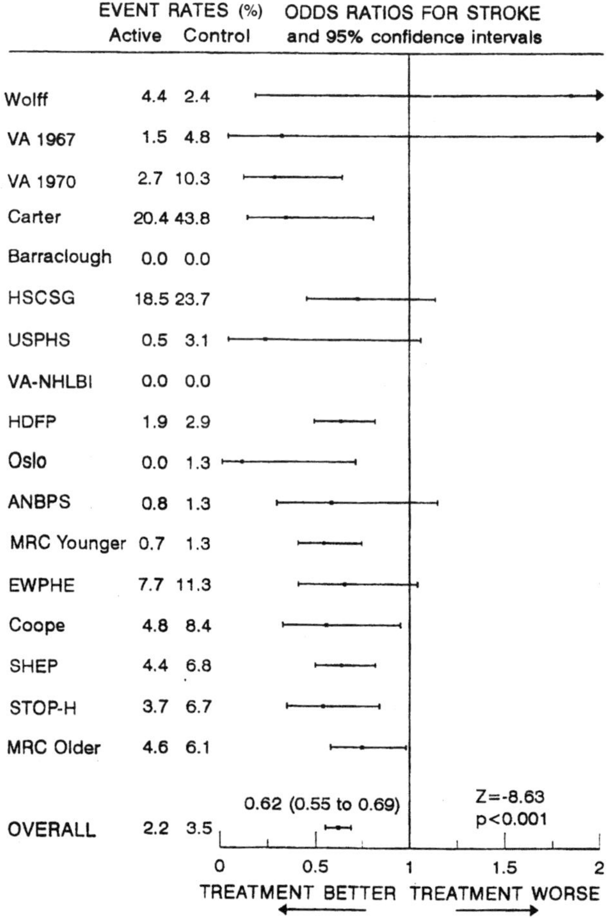

FIGURE 10 Odds ratios and 95% confidence intervals for total (fatal and nonfatal) stroke related to antihypertensive drug treatment.

among study participants. The absolute reductions in total and fatal coronary heart disease were 7 and 4 per 1000 persons, whereas the corresponding absolute reductions in total and fatal stroke were 13 and 4 per 1000 persons.

Cardiovascular Disease and Total Mortality

Overall, 768 deaths from cardiovascular disease occurred in the participants who were allocated to active treatment, and 964 deaths occurred in their counterparts who were allocated to control (Table 2). The overall reduction in cardiovascular disease mortality for active treatment compared to control was 21% (95% confidence interval: 12–28%; $p < 0.001$). In six of the 17 trials, the reduction in cardiovascular disease mortality was statistically significant (Fig. 11). Noncardiovascular disease mortality was evenly distributed between the treatment and control groups (667 vs. 670). All-cause mortality was reduced by 13% (95% confidence interval: 6–19%, $p < 0.001$) in those allocated to active compared to control treatment (Table 2; Fig. 12).

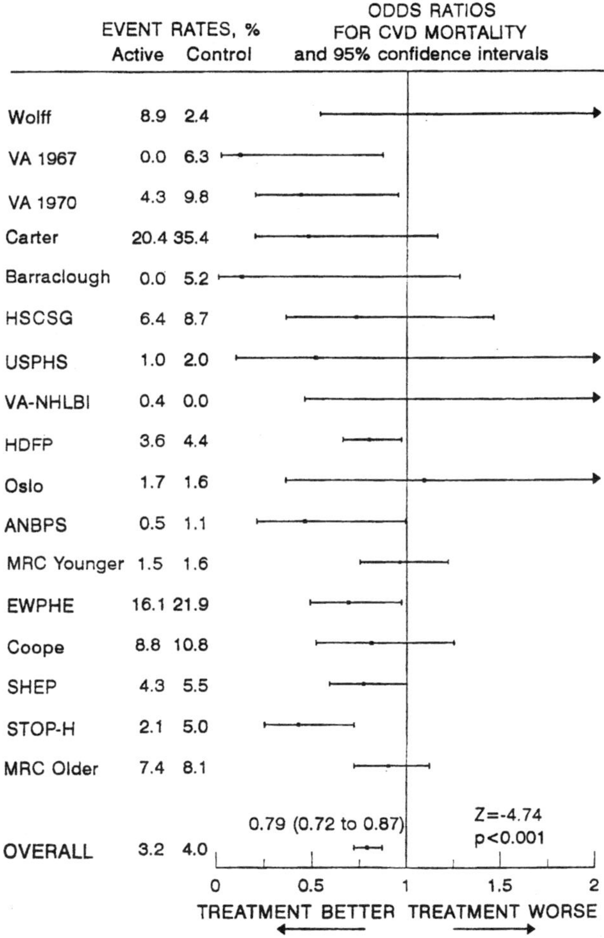

FIGURE 11 Odds ratios and 95% confidence intervals for cardiovascular mortality related to antihypertensive drug treatment.

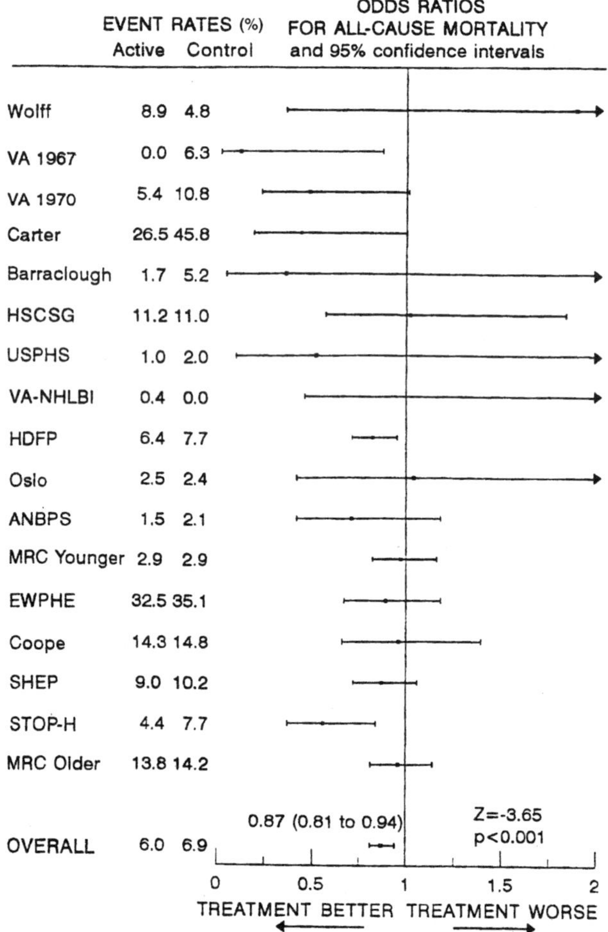

FIGURE 12 Odds ratios and 95% confidence intervals for all-cause mortality related to antihypertensive drug treatment.

CONCLUSION

Prospective cohort studies have repeatedly demonstrated that elevated blood pressure level is the most important modifiable risk factor for coronary heart disease, stroke, congestive heart failure, and end-stage renal disease. These studies have also indicated that systolic blood pressure is a stronger predictor for cardiovascular disease risk compared to diastolic blood pressure. Randomized controlled trials have documented that an average reduction

TABLE 3 Potential Effect on Mortality With Lower Average Population Systolic Pressure

	Estimated percent reduction in mortality			Potential number of lives saved per year with lower systolic BP, men and women 45 to 64 years old	
Population average systolic BP lower by	Coronary heart disease	Stroke	All causes	U.S. Population[a]	England and Wales population[b]
-2 mmHg	-4%	-6%	-3%	11,800	2,900
-3 mmHg	-5%	-8%	-4%	15,800	3,900
-5 mmHg	-9%	-14%	-7%	27,600	6,800

Based on averaged multivariate coefficients for systolic blood pressure and mortality from five large longitudinal population studies: Framingham, Chicago Heart Association, Whitehall, Western Electric, and the Multiple Risk Factor Intervention Trial (MRFIT) screenees cohort. The MRFIT study was the largest (347,936 men), and the others ranged in size from 1900 to 17,000 middle-aged persons. The Framingham and Chicago Heart Association studies included men and women; the remainder included men only.

[a] Based on all-causes mortality, 1985 US men and women, 45 to 64 years old. Rounded to nearest 100. Population 45 to 64 years old, 45,000,000.

[b] All-cause mortality, England and Wales, men and women, 45 to 64 years old, rounded to nearest 100; population 45 to 64 years old, 11,000,000.

of 5 to 6 mmHg in diastolic pressure over 4 to 5 years of follow-up is associated with a 16% reduction in coronary heart disease, a 38% reduction in stroke, a 21% reduction in cardiovascular mortality, and a 13% reduction in all-cause mortality.

To achieve the primary goal of eliminating all blood pressure-related vascular disease in the community, detection and treatment of established hypertension must be combined with equally energetic approaches directed at primary prevention of hypertension. Without primary prevention, the problem of hypertension would never be solved; efforts would rely solely on detection and treatment of existing hypertension. Primary prevention provides an attractive opportunity to interrupt and prevent the continuing costly cycle of managing hypertension and its complications.

A small downward shift in the entire distribution of blood pressure in the general population will not only reduce the incidence of hypertension, but will also substantially diminish the burden of blood pressure-related diseases in the general population (Table 3) [67], therefore an effective populationwide strategy to prevent blood pressure rise with age and to reduce overall blood pressure levels, even by a little, would affect overall cardiovascular morbidity and mortality as much as, or more than, treating only those with established disease [68]. Such a populationwide approach has been proposed. It is based on lifestyle modifications that have been shown to prevent or delay the expected rise in blood pressure with age in susceptible people.

Lifestyle modifications that are of known value in the treatment of established hypertension could have an even greater impact on disease prevention and should be recommended to the entire population. Lifestyle modifications offer the potential for preventing hypertension, have been shown to be effective in lowering blood pressure, and can reduce other cardiovascular risk factors at little cost and with minimal risk. Lifestyle modification should be a very important component in the effort to eliminate blood pressure–related vascular disease in population.

REFERENCES

1. Joint National Committee on Prevention, Detection, Evaluation, and Treatment of High Blood Pressure. The sixth report of the Joint National Committee on prevention, detection, evaluation, and treatment of high blood pressure. Arch Int Med. 1997; 157:2413–2446.
2. Stamler J, Stamler R, Neaton JD. Blood pressure, systolic and diastolic, and cardiovascular risks: US population data. Arch Int Med 1993; 153:598–615.
3. Whelton PK, He J. Blood pressure reduction. In: Hennekens C, Buring J, Furberg C, Manson J, eds. Clinical Trials in Cardiovascular Disease. Philadelphia: Saunders, 1999: 341–359.

4. He J, Whelton PK. Systolic blood pressure and risk of cardiovascular and renal disease: an overview of evidence from observational epidemiologic studies and randomized controlled trials. Am Heart J 1999;138:S211–S219.
5. MacMahon S, Peto R, Cutler J, Collins R, Sorlie P, Neaton J, Abbott R, Godwin J, Dyer A, Stamler J. Blood pressure, stroke, and coronary heart disease. part 1. prolonged differences in blood pressure: prospective observational studies corrected for the regression dilution bias. Lancet 1990; 335:765–774.
6. Prospective Studies Collaboration. Cholesterol, diastolic blood pressure, and stroke: 13,000 strokes in 450,000 people in 45 prospective cohorts. Lancet 1995;346:1647–1653.
7. Eastern Stroke and Coronary Heart Disease Collaborative Research Group. Blood pressure, cholesterol, and stroke in eastern Asia. Lancet 1998; 352: 1801–1807.
8. American Heart Association. 2002 Heart and Stroke Statistical Update. Dallas, TX: American Heart Association, 2002.
9. Stokes J III, Kannel WB, Wolf PA, D'Agostino RB, Cupples LA. Blood pressure as a risk factor for cardiovascular disease. The Framingham Study—30 years of follow-up. Hypertension 1989; 13 (suppl. 1): I13–I18.
10. Menotti A, Farchi G, Seccareccia F. The prediction of coronary heart disease mortality as a function of major risk factors in over 30 000 men in the Italian RIFLE pooling project. A comparison with the MRFIT primary screenees. The RIFLE research group. J Cardiovasc Risk 1994; 263–270.
11. Psaty BM, Furberg CD, Kuller LH, Cushman M, Savage PJ, Levine D, O'Leary DH, Bryan RN, Anderson M, Lumley T. Association between blood pressure level and the risk of myocardial infarction, stroke, and total mortality: Cardiovascular Health Study. Arch Int Med. 2001; 161:1183–1192.
12. van den Hoogen PC, Feskens EJ, Nagelkerke NJ, Menotti A, Nissinen A, Kromhout D. The relation between blood pressure and mortality due to coronary heart disease among men in different parts of the world. Seven Countries Study Research Group. N Eng J Med. 2000;342:1–8.
13. He J, Whelton PK. Epidemiology of end-stage renal disease. In: Brenner BM, Kurokawa K, eds. International Handbook of Renal Disease. London: Hoechst Marion Roussel, 1999:1–14.
14. Klag MJ, Whelton PK, Randall RL, Neaton JD, Brancati FL, Ford CE, Shulman NB, Stamler J. Blood pressure and end-stage renal disease in men. N Engl J Med. 1996;334:13–18.
15. Perry HM Jr, Miller JP, Fornoff JR, Baty JD, Sambhi MP, Rutan G, Moskowitz DW, Carmody SE. Early predictors of 15-year end-stage renal disease in hypertensive patients. Hypertension. 1995;25:687–94.
16. Iseki K, Ikemiya Y, Fukiyama K. Blood pressure and risk of end-stage renal disease in a screened cohort. Kidney Intern. 1996;55:S67–S71.
17. Ghali JK, Cooper R, Ford E. Trends in hospitalization rates for heart failure in the United States 1973–1986. Evidence for increasing population prevalence. Arch Int Med 1990; 150:769–73.

18. Gillum RF. Epidemiology of heart failure in the United States. Am Heart J 1993; 126:1042–1047.
19. Kannel WB, D'Agostino RB, Silbershatz H, Belanger AJ, Wilson PW, Levy D. Profile for estimating risk of heart failure. Arch Int Med. 1999; 159: 1197–204.
20. Levy D, Larson MG, Vasan RS, Kannel WB, Ho KK. The progression from hypertension to congestive heart failure. JAMA 1996; 275: 1557–1562.
21. Chen YT, Vaccarino V, Williams CS, Butler J, Berkman LF, Krumholz HM. Risk factors for heart failure in the elderly: a prospective community-based study. Am J Med 1999; 106:605–612.
22. Chae CU, Pfeffer MA, Glynn RJ, Mitchell GF, Taylor JO, Hennekens CH. Increased pulse pressure and risk of heart failure in the elderly. JAMA 1999; 281:634–639.
23. He J, Ogden LG, Bazzano LA, Vupputuri S, Loria C, Whelton PK. Risk factors for congestive heart failure in US men and women: NHANES I epidemiologic follow-up study. Arch Int Med. 2001; 161:996–1002.
24. Collins R, Peto R, MacMahon S, Hebert P, Fiebach NH, Eberlein KA, Godwin J, Qizilbash N, Taylor JO, Hennekens CH. Blood pressure, stroke, and coronary heart disease. part 2. short-term reductions in blood pressure: overview of randomised drug trials in their epidemiological context. Lancet 1990; 335:827–838.
25. Hebert PR, Moser M, Mayer J, Glynn RJ, Hennekens CH. Recent evidence on drug therapy of mild to moderate hypertension and decreased risk of CHD. Arch Int Med 1993; 153:578–581.
26. Kagan A, Yano K, Reed DM, MacLean CJ. Predictors of sudden cardiac death among Hawaiian-Japanese men. Am J Epidem 1989; 130:268–277.
27. Onat A, Dursunoglu D, Sansoy V. Relatively high coronary death and event rates in Turkish women. Relation to three major risk factors in five-year follow-up of cohort. Int J Cardiol 1997; 1:69–77.
28. Gagnon F, Dagenais GR, Robitaille NM, Lupien PJ. Impact of systolic and diastolic blood pressure on ischemic vascular diseases in French-Canadian men from 1974 to 1990. Can J Cardiol 1994; 10: 97–105.
29. Tomas-Abadal, L, Varas-Lorenzo C, Bernades-Bernat E, Balaguer-Vintro I. Coronary risk factors and a 20-year incidence of coronary heart disease and mortality in a Mediterranean industrial population: the Manresa Study, Spain. Eur Heart J 1994; 15:1028–1036.
30. Sesso HD, Stampfer MJ, Rosner B, Hennekens CH, Gaziano JM, Manson JE, Glynn RJ. Systolic and diastolic blood pressure, pulse pressure, and mean arterial pressure as predictors of cardiovascular disease risk in men. Hypertension 2000; 36: 801–807.
31. Lindenstrom E, Boysen G, Nyboe J. Influence of systolic and diastolic blood pressure on stroke risk: a prospective observational study. Am J Epidem. 1995;142:1279–1290.
32. Glynn RJ, Chae CU, Guralnik JM, Taylor JO, Hennekens CH. Pulse pressure and mortality in older people. Arch Int Med 2000;160:2765–2772.

33. Chae CU, Pfeffer MA, Glynn RJ, Mitchell GF, Taylor JO, Hennekens CH. Increased pulse pressure and risk of heart failure in the elderly. JAMA 1999; 281:634–639.
34. Blacher J, Staessen JA, Girerd X, Gasowski J, Thijs L, Liu L, Wang JG, Fagard RH, Safar ME. Pulse pressure not mean pressure determines cardiovascular risk in older hypertensive patients. Arch Int Med 2000;160: 1085–1089.
35. Domanski M, Mitchell G, Pfeffer M, Neaton JD, Norman J, Svendsen K, Grimm R, Cohen J, Stamler J for the MRFIT Research Group. Pulse pressure and cardiovascular disease-related mortality: follow-up study of the Multiple Risk Factor Intervention Trial. JAMA 2002;287: 2677–2683.
36. Wilson PW, Hoeg JM, D'Agostino RB, Silbershatz H, Belanger AM, Poehlmann H, O'Leary D, Wolf PA. Cumulative effects of high cholesterol levels, high blood pressure, and cigarette smoking on carotid stenosis. N Engl J Med 1997;337:516–522.
37. Anderson KM, Wilson PWF, Odell PM, Kannel WB. An updated coronary risk profile: a statement for health professionals. Circulation 1991;83:356–362.
38. Kannel WB. Blood pressure as a cardiovascular risk factor: prevention and treatment. JAMA 1996;275:1571–1576.
39. Stamler J, Stamler R, Neaton JD, Wentworth D, Daviglus ML, Garside D, Dyer AR, Liu K, Greenland P. Low risk-factor profile and long-term cardiovascular and noncardiovascular mortality and life expectancy: findings for 5 large cohorts of young adult and middle-aged men and women. JAMA 1999;282:2012–2018.
40. Vasan RS, Larson MG, Leip EP, Evans JC, O'Donnell CJ, Kannel WB, Levy D. Impact of high-normal blood pressure on the risk of cardiovascular disease. N Eng J Med 2001; 345:1291–1297.
41. Burt VL, Whelton PK, Roccella EJ, Brown C, Cutler JA, Higgins M, Horan MJ, Labarthe D. Prevalence of hypertension in the US adult population: results from the Third National Health and Nutrition Examination Survey, 1988–1991. Hypertension. 1995;25:305–313.
42. Whelton PK, He J, Appel LJ. Treatment and prevention of hypertension. In: Manson JE, Ridker PM, Gaziano JM, and Hennekens CH, eds. Prevention of Myocardial Infarction. New York: Oxford University Press, 1996.
43. Whelton PK, He J. Blood pressure reduction. In: Hennekens CH, Buring JE, Manson JE, Ridker PM, eds. Clinical Trials in Cardiovascular Disease: A Companion to Braunwald's Heart Disease. Philadelphia: Saunders, 1999.
44. Cutler JA, MacMahon SW, Furberg CD. Controlled clinical trials of drug treatment for hypertension: a review. Hypertension. 1989;13(suppl. I):I-36–I-44.
45. Collins R, Peto R, MacMahon SW, Hebert P, Fiebach NH, Eberlein KA, Godwin J, Qizilbash N, Taylor JO, Hennekens CH. Blood pressure, stroke, and CHD. part 2. short-term reductions in blood pressure: overview of randomized drug trials in their epidemiological context. Lancet. 1990;335: 827–838.
46. Hebert PR, Moser M, Mayer J, Glynn RJ, Hennekens CH. Recent evidence on

drug therapy of mild to moderate hypertension and decreased risk of CHD. Arch Int Med. 1993;153:578–581.
47. Wolff FW, Lindeman RD. Effects of treatment in hypertension: results of a controlled study. J Chron Dis 1966; 19:227–240.
48. Veterans Administration Cooperative Group on Antihypertensive Agents. Effects of treatment on morbidity in hypertension. JAMA 1967; 202:1028–1034.
49. Veterans Administration Cooperative Group on Antihypertensive Agents. Effects of treatment on morbidity in hypertension. JAMA 1970; 213: 1143–1152.
50. Carter AB. Hypotensive therapy in stroke survivors. Lancet 1970; 1:485–489.
51. Barraclough M, Bainton D, Joy MD, et al. Control of moderately raised blood pressure: report of a co-operative randomized controlled trial. BMJ 1973; 3: 434–436.
52. Hypertension–Stroke Cooperative Study Group. Effect of antihypertensive treatment on stroke recurrence. JAMA 1974; 229:409–418.
53. Smith WM. Treatment of mild hypertension: results of a ten-year intervention trial. Circ Res 1977; 40:I98–105.
54. Perry HM Jr. Treatment of mild hypertension: preliminary results of a two-year feasibility trial. Circ Res 1977; 40: I180–1187.
55. Prepared for the Veterans Administration-National Heart, Lung, and Blood Institute Study Group for Evaluating Treatment in Mild Hypertension. Evaluation of drug treatment in mild hypertension: VA-NHLBI feasibility trial. plan and preliminary results of a two-year feasibility trial for a multicenter intervention study to evaluate the benefits versus the disadvantages of treating mild hypertension. Ann NY Acad Sci 1978; 304:267–292.
56. Hypertension Detection and Follow-up Program Cooperative Group. Five-year findings of the hypertension detection and follow-up program. I. reduction in mortality of persons with high blood pressure, including mild hypertension. JAMA 1979; 242:2562–2571.
57. Hypertension Detection and Follow-up Program Cooperative Group. Five-year findings of the hypertension detection and follow-up program. II. mortality by race-sex and age. JAMA 1979; 242:2572–2577.
58. Helgeland A. Treatment of mild hypertension: a five year controlled drug trial. the Oslo study. Am J Med 1980; 69:725–732.
59. Leren P, Helgeland A. Oslo Hypertension Study. Drugs. 1986; 31(suppl. 1): 41–45.
60. Report of the Management Committee. The Australian therapeutic trial in mild hypertension. Lancet 1980; 1:1261–1267.
61. Medical Research Council Working Party. MRC trial of treatment of mild hypertension: principal results. BMJ 1985; 291:97–104.
62. Amery A, Birkenhager W, Brixko P, Bulpitt C, Clement D, Deruyttere M, De Schaepdryver A, Dollery C, Fagard R, Forette F. Mortality and morbidity results from the European Working Party on High Blood Pressure in the Elderly trial. Lancet. 1985; I:1349–1354.
63. Coope J, Warrender TS. Randomized trial of treatment of hypertension in elderly patients in primary care. BMJ. 1986; 293:1145–1151.

64. SHEP Cooperative Research Group. Prevention of stroke by antihypertensive drug treatment in older persons with isolated systolic hypertension: final results of the Systolic Hypertension in the Elderly Program (SHEP). JAMA 1991; 265:3255-3264.
65. Dahlof B, Lindholm LH, Hansson L, Schersten B, Ekbom T, Wester PO. Morbidity and mortality in the Swedish Trial in Old Patients with Hypertension (STOP-Hypertension). Lancet. 1991; 338:1281–1285.
66. MRC Working Party. Medical Research Council trial of treatment of hypertension in older adults: principal results. BMJ. 1992;304:405–412.
67. Stamler J. The intersalt study:background, methods, findings, and implications. Am J Clin Nutr 1997; 65 (2 suppl.):626S–642S.
68. Cook NR, Cohen J, Hebert PR, Taylor JO, Hennekens CH. Implications of small reductions in diastolic blood pressure for primary prevention. Arch Int Med. 1995;155:701–709.

3

Strategies for Prevention of Adverse Blood Pressure Levels

Jeremiah Stamler
Northwestern University Medical School, Chicago, Illinois, U.S.A.

Strategies for prevention of adverse blood pressure (BP) levels have as their scientific foundations the extensive current knowledge on the nature and scope of the BP problem in the population and on preventable and remediable lifestyles related to these adverse levels.

NATURE AND SCOPE OF THE POPULATION BP PROBLEM

BP and Risks of Major Diseases and Death

As shown repeatedly by prospective population studies, the relationship between BP and disease risks is continuous, graded, strong, independent of other risk factors, predictive. It is generally judged to be etiologically significant. This relationship prevails for BP and sudden cardiac death, coronary heart disease (CHD), cerebrovascular diseases (ischemic, hemorrhagic, embolic, etc.), abdominal aortic aneurysm (AAA), peripheral vascular disease (PVD), end stage renal disease (ESRD), and all cause mortality. It prevails for American women and men, middle-aged and older, and for younger adult men as well. (Data are still scant for younger adult women.) It prevails for all U.S. ethnic and socioeconomic strata (SES), and even more severely for those of lower SES. It prevails internationally for populations from both industrialized and economically developing countries. It prevails for nonsmokers and smokers, for nondiabetic and diabetic individuals, and for persons at all levels of serum cholesterol, for those with and without a history of heart attack [1–15].

Excess risk is manifest for those at every systolic BP (SBP) or DBP stratum above optimal; that is, for all persons with SBP above 120 mmHg and/or diastolic BP above 80 mmHg. Population average BP higher by as little as 2 to 3 mmHg is associated with significant increases in risks of major diseases and death; that is, *the BP problem goes beyond high blood pressure* (HBP) *as defined clinically* (SBP ≥140 mmHg and/or DBP ≥90 mmHg). Risks are also higher for adults with BP levels in the high-normal range (SBP 130 to 139 mmHg and/or DBP 85 to 89 mmHg), and even for adults in the normal (but not optimal) range (SBP 120 to 129 and/or DBP 80 to 84 mmHg) [1–15], hence the title of this chapter—*not* "Prevention of High Blood Pressure," but "Strategies for Prevention of Adverse Blood Pressure Levels."

This relationship of SBP/DBP to risks is especially well demonstrated by the 16-year follow-up data on the extraordinarily large cohort of men ages 35 to 57 screened in 18 U.S. cities from 1973 to 1975 by the Multiple Risk Factor Intervention Trial (MRFIT) (Figs. 1, 2; Table 1) [5]. Given the large sample size and the large numbers of deaths, estimated mortality rates for each BP stratum have narrow confidence intervals (i.e., are highly precise).

Only 18% of the MRFIT cohort had optimal BP (SBP/DBP <120/<80 mmHg) (Table 2) [5], thus adverse BP levels were the rule, not the exception, involving most (82%) of this sample of U.S. men, young adult and early middle-aged, weighted toward higher SES levels. About a quarter were in the normal (not optimal) stratum. Almost another quarter (22%) had high-normal levels. About another quarter (26%), high BP stage 1, and 9%, high BP stages 2–4. Based on the multivariate-adjusted relative risk data, the estimate is that 5184 (46%) of the 11,149 CHD deaths were excess deaths attributable to adverse SBP/DBP. Of these excess CHD deaths, a majority (67%, 3474 deaths) were from the three large strata with normal (not optimal) BP, high-normal BP, or stage 1 HBP. Almost a quarter of these estimated excess deaths (24%, 1231 deaths) were from the first two of these three strata; that is, the two strata of men with "nonhypertensive"—*but not optimal*—SBP/DBP.

Trend of SBP/DBP Distribution with Age

The percentage of men with optimal BP in the MRFIT cohort decreased sequentially with age, from 22% at ages 35 to 39 to 14% at ages 55 to 57, as

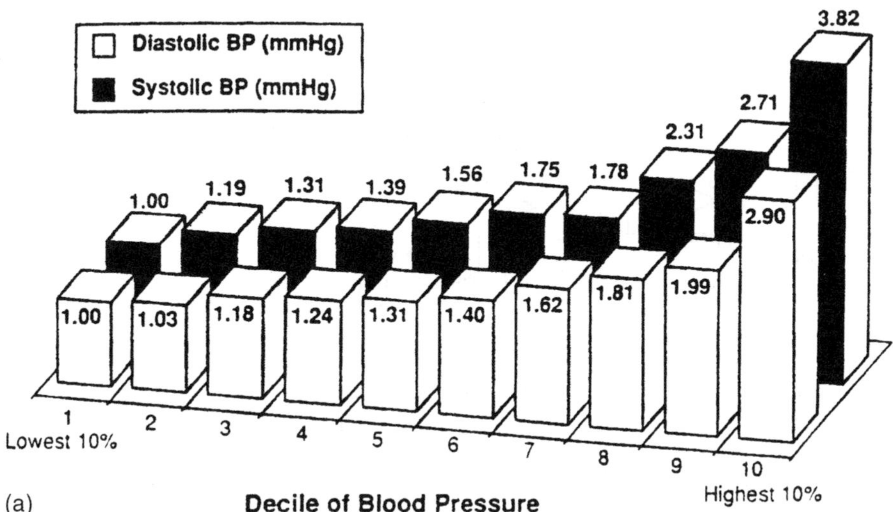

(a)

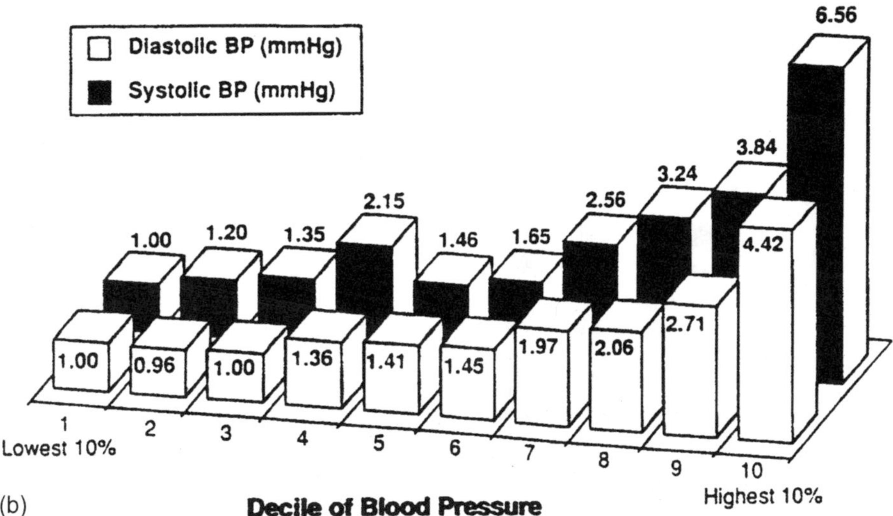

(b)

FIGURE 1 Relation of SBP and DBP decile, considered separately, to relative risk of 16-year mortality from CHD (a) and stroke (b); 347,978 men screened for MRFIT, ages 35 to 57 at baseline and without a history of hospitalization for heart attack. SBP deciles are defined by the following cutpoints: <112, 112–117, 118–120, 121–124, 125–128, 129–131, 132–136, 137–141, 142–150, >151 mmHg; DBP deciles: <71, 71–75, 76–78, 79–80, 81–83, 84–85, 86–88, 89–91, 92–97, >98 mmHg.

(a)

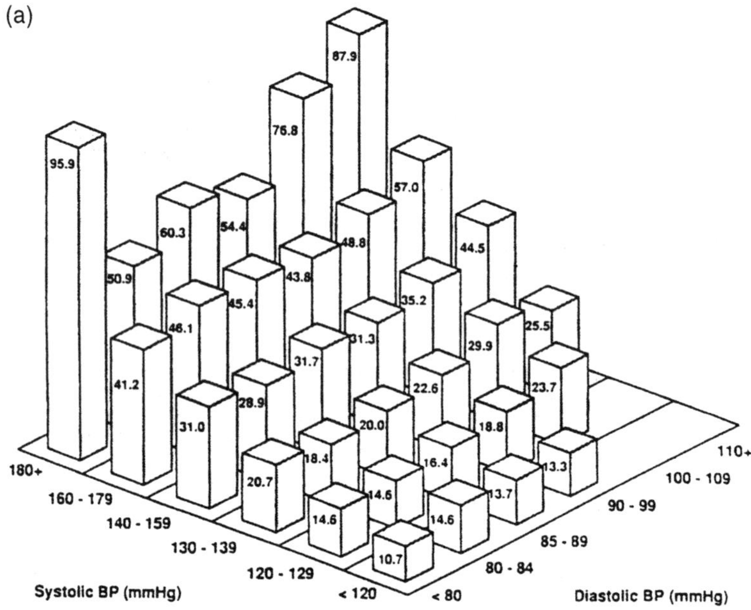

(b)

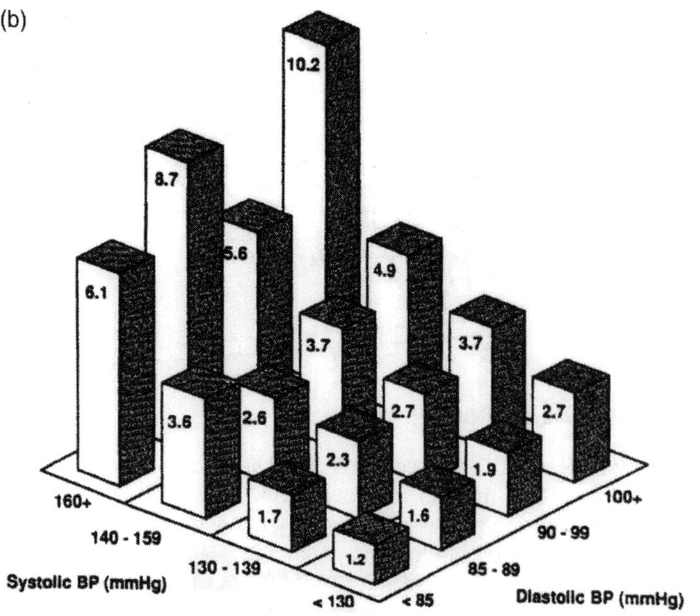

FIGURE 2 Joint effect of SBP and DBP on risk of 16-year mortality from CHD (a), stroke (b), and all causes (c); 347,978 men screened for MRFIT.

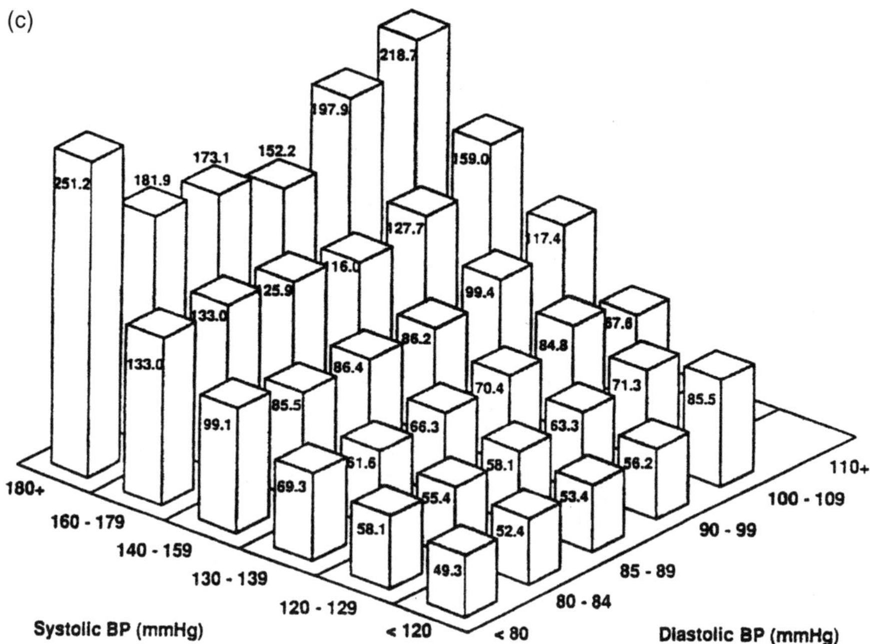

FIGURE 2 (Continued).

did the percentage with normal (but not optimal) SBP/DBP (from 28–20%) [5]. At ages 35 to 39, a bare majority were in these two strata; from ages 40 to 44 on, a minority (e.g., at ages 40 to 44, 46% and at ages 55 to 57, 33%). This trend reflected the repeatedly documented phenomenon that in most populations BP is higher with age, from youth into middle age for diastolic pressure, and over all decades of adulthood for systolic pressure, as shown repeatedly for representative samples of the U.S. population by national surveys from the early 1960s to the early 1990s (Fig. 3) [16]. Several sets of data from long-term prospective studies verify that most people experience BP increases of varying degrees during adulthood [17,18]. As a consequence, for the sample examined by the Third National Health and Nutrition Survey (NHANES III) from 1988 to 1991, prevalence of optimal SBP/DBP readings decreased for non-Hispanic white women from 78% at ages 18 to 49 to 28% at ages 50 to 69 and 12% at ages ≥70, and for non-Hispanic white men from 45% to 21% to 13% [16]. This unfavorable trend in prevalence rates of optimal SBP/DBP prevailed also for Mexican-American women and men, and was even more adverse for African-American women and men.

TABLE 1 Baseline Blood Pressure and Mortality From CHD, Stroke, All Causes: Men Screened for MRFIT

BP category[a]	Number of men	Number of deaths	Age-adjusted rate per 10,000 person years[b]	Adjusted relative risk[c]	Cumulative percentage dying[e]		
					5 years	10 years	15 years
CHD mortality							
Optimal	63,371	942	10.7	1.00	0.3	0.7	1.4
Normal but not optimal	85,273	1774	14.6	1.31[d]	0.3	1.0	1.9
High-normal	77,248	2140	18.5	1.61[d]	0.5	1.4	2.6
High							
Stage 1	90,015	3934	27.4	2.33[d]	0.7	2.1	4.1
Stage 2	24,744	1,618	39.9	3.20[d]	1.2	3.4	6.3
Stage 3	5783	550	57.3	4.64[d]	1.7	5.1	9.3
Stage 4	1544	191	83.4	6.88[d]	2.3	7.3	12.8
Stroke mortality							
Optimal	63,371	71	0.6	1.00	.02	.04	.10
Normal but not optimal	85,273	173	1.4	1.73[d]	.03	.06	.19
High-normal	77,248	208	1.8	2.14[d]	.04	.11	.24
High							
Stage 1	90,015	435	3.0	3.58[d]	.08	.22	.45

Stage 2	24,744	215	5.3	5.90[d]	.13	.40	.83
Stage 3	5783	87	9.8	9.68[d]	.37	.82	1.57
Stage 4	1544	44	19.0	19.19[d]	1.06	2.06	3.05
All cause mortality							
Optimal	63,371	4354	49.3	1.00	1.1	3.0	6.1
Normal but not optimal	85,273	6822	55.9	1.11[d]	1.2	3.5	7.2
High-normal	77,248	7281	82.9	1.23[d]	1.4	4.2	8.4
High							
Stage 1	90,015	11,489	80.1	1.55[d]	1.9	5.7	11.4
Stage 2	24,744	4431	108.9	2.04[d]	2.8	8.3	16.2
Stage 3	5,783	1447	153.0	2.77[d]	4.3	12.0	22.8
Stage 4	1,544	491	213.7	3.83[d]	5.7	16.5	29.5

[a] Classification of BP is according to Fifth Joint National Committee Report.
[b] Adjusted by the direct method to age distribution of all men screened.
[c] Estimated with use of proportional hazards regression model stratified by clinic and adjusted for age, race, income, serum cholesterol level, reported cigarettes per day, and use of medication for diabetes.
[e] Estimated by the Kaplan-Meier method.
[d] $p < 0.0001$.

TABLE 2 Percentage Distribution of SBP and DBP: Men Screened for MRFIT

	SBP (mmHg)							
DBP (mmHg)	<120	120–129	130–139	140–159	160–179	180–209	210+	Total[a]
<80	18.2	10.0	3.9	1.4	0.1	0.0	0.0	33.7
80–84	5.1	9.4	5.5	2.3	0.2	0.0	0.0	22.5
85–89	1.4	5.7	5.7	3.4	0.3	0.0	0.0	16.5
90–99	0.4	3.2	6.9	8.3	1.2	0.1	0.0	20.1
100–109	0.0	0.1	0.7	3.1	1.3	0.2	0.0	5.5
110–119	0.0	0.0	0.0	0.4	0.6	0.2	0.0	1.3
120+	0.0	0.0	0.0	0.0	0.1	0.2	0.5	0.4
Total[†]	25.1	28.4	22.8	18.9	3.8	0.8	0.1	100.0

Note: Percentages are of total number of men (347,978). The seven categories are defined by the dotted lines beginning in the upper left-hand corner: optimal, normal but not optimal, high-normal, stage 1, stage 2, stage 3, and stage 4 hypertension.
[a] Some columns do not add to totals due to rounding.

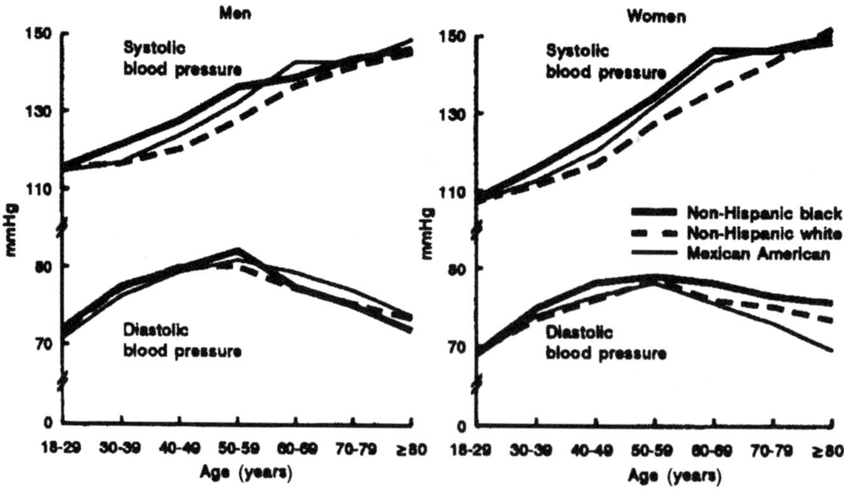

FIGURE 3 Average SBP and DBP by gender, age, ethnicity, U.S. population 18 years of age and older, National Health and Nutrition Examination Survey, 1988–1991.

These rises in SBP/DBP with age during adulthood are *not* inevitable consequences built into the human genome. This conclusion is documented by extensive data showing that these increases do not occur in a proportion of people in the United States and other populations experiencing the epidemic of adverse SBP/DBP levels [17]. It is further documented by extensive data on many isolated populations, most of them preliterate, who on average maintain optimal SBP/DBP throughout adulthood with little or no rise with age, but who, with migration and resultant changes in lifestyle to contemporary worldwide modes, then manifest increases in SBP/DBP with age like other populations, demonstrating that their prior favorable pattern was not due to exceptional population genetics, but rather to freedom from the environmental exposures leading to expression of genetic propensity (susceptibility). To paraphrase Joslin [19], *heredity loads the gun* (for profound evolutionary reasons, most of us are more or less susceptible to BP rise during adulthood), and *environmental exposures—lifestyles—pull the trigger*. Absent adverse lifestyles, there is no epidemic of adverse SBP/DBP levels.

Finally, one other aspect of the data on the nature and scope of the population BP problem needs emphasis. In contrast to ages 30 to 39 and beyond, at ages 18 to 29 the population SBP/DBP levels are on average *favorable* for women and men of all ethnicities (Fig. 3) [16]. For women, SBP/DBP average about 110/70 mmHg; for men, about 118/74; that is, are *at optimal levels*. Estimates from MRFIT and other data indicate that prevention of the age-related rise in SBP by as little as 3 mmHg would lead to lower mortality from CHD by about 6%; CVD, 7%; all causes, 4%. With age-related SBP rise reduced by 10 mmHg, these death rates would be lower by about 20%, 21%, and 14% [1–15,20].

Strategic Implications

These following facts about the nature and scope of the population BP problem critically determine the strategies needed to control and eliminate it:

1. Since the risks of major diseases and death are importantly influenced by all levels of SBP/DBP above optimal and such levels prevail for the great majority of the adult population, these strategies must have as their main and primary component the goal of achieving a progressive downward shift in population average SBP/DBP so that the percentage of people with optimal levels increases steadily over time to become the norm (rather than the exception) at all adult ages.
2. These strategies must encompass effective approaches to reduce and eliminate the present-day usual increases in SBP/DBP from youth into middle and older age.

3. These strategies must include efforts for early identification of people who already have normal (but not optimal) SBP/DBP and high-normal SBP/DBP, so that effective sustained improvements in lifestyles can be brought to bear—beyond general populationwide public health efforts—to restore them to optimal SBP/DBP levels.
4. These strategies need also to have—as a decisive policy component, influencing resource allocation year by year—explicit widespread recognition that overwhelming emphasis in practice solely on high risk strategy is not enough. However important and however massive the task, it does not suffice to focus strategy almost exclusively on detection, evaluation, and treatment of people with already established HBP. That strategy—in place since 1972 in the United States—has clearly proved to be insufficient. It is late, defensive, reactive (not proactive), incomplete (ignoring adverse SBP/DBP levels among millions and failing to achieve optimal BP levels for most patients), complex (needing to cope repeatedly with multiple drugs, their limitations, side effects, toxic effects), costly, and—above all—never-ending, i.e.; that is, needing always to be in place to deal with this year's millions of new cases. By definition it cannot put an end to the epidemic of adverse BP levels. Only primary prevention of this major risk factor can accomplish that decisive task and at one and the same time bring about a progressive large reduction in the burden of prevalent and incident cases of clinical HBP.

In this regard, the historic lessons from decades-long experiences with preceding epidemics (e.g., cholera, typhoid fever, tuberculosis, pellagra, rickets) are of incalculable importance; no epidemic is inevitable or irresistible—each and every one can be conquered. Primary prevention is essential to achieve this. The key to primary prevention is to reduce and eliminate the "disturbances of human culture" (Virchow) [21] that produced epidemic disease. All these truisms are fully applicable to the populationwide epidemic of adverse BP levels.

PREVENTABLE AND REMEDIABLE LIFESTYLES RELATED TO POPULATIONWIDE ADVERSE SBP/DBP LEVELS

Nutrition in Utero and in the First Years of Life

In recent years, evidence has been progressively accumulating that childhood and adult levels of CHD-CVD major risk factors, including SBP/DBP, are

TABLE 3 Relationship of Birth Weight and Weight at Age 4 to Age 4 SBP—Multiple Regression Analyses

Weight (kg)	Age 4 SBP difference (mmHg) per kg higher weight	95% CI
At birth	−2.8[a]	−4.1 to −1.4
At 4 years	+1.5[a]	+1.1 to +1.8

Note: 1147 children, Kent, U.K.
[a] $p<0.001$; weight at age 1 not significantly related to age 4 SBP.

determined in part by fetal intrauterine nutrient status and by dietary factors during the early postpartum years [22]. Here it suffices to cite two examples illustrative of progress in this important new ongoing research area.

Body Weight

In a study of 1147 English infants, a significant *inverse* relation of birth weight to age 4 SBP was recorded (Table 3) [23]. With 1 kg higher birth weight, age 4 SBP was lower on average by almost 3 mmHg. Further, in accordance with other data sets on young children, a significant *positive* relation was found between weight at age 4 and SBP at age 4; with 1 kg higher weight, SBP was on average higher by 1.5 mmHg.

Dietary Sodium Chloride (NaCl)

In a Rotterdam intervention trial in infants during their first 6 months of life, for the group randomized to higher (usual) NaCl intake, SBP was significantly higher by 2.1 mmHg at 6 months compared to SBP of the group randomized to lower salt intake (Table 4) [24]. At 15-year follow-up, for the group fed higher salt during the first 6 months of life, SBP (adjusted for confounders) was significantly higher by 3.6 mmHg, even though there had been no intervention since age 6 months [25].

Nutrition, Physical Activity, and Smoking in Adulthood

Body Mass (Calorie Balance), Intake of NaCl, Alcohol, Potassium

Data have been amassed over decades—by clinical, epidemiological, and interventional studies—showing direct relations between body mass and SBP/DBP [17,26]. Similarly, investigations using virtually every research methodology (the three above, along with animal experimentation, evolutionary biology, and anthropology) have produced extensive concordant findings demonstrating direct relations between dietary NaCl and SBP/DBP

TABLE 4 Higher (Usual) Versus Lower NaCl Intake and SBP in Newborns, Rotterdam Trial

Time	Adjusted SBP difference[a] (mmHg)
Baseline	—
Week 6	−0.4
Week 9	+0.4
Week 16	+0.6
Week 17	+1.2
Week 21	+1.7
Week 25	+2.1[b]

[a] SBP of higher NaCl group minus SBP of lower NaCl group, adjusted for observer, weight, length at birth, and SBP in first week; N = 245 for higher NaCl group, 231 for lower NaCl group; Na intake for higher group was three times that of lower group.
[b] $p = 0.01$ for linear trend.

[27]. It is the two ions together—Na and Cl as NaCl, derived overwhelmingly from the food additive salt [27,28]—that influence BP. Concordant evidence is also extant from many studies showing a direct relation of alcohol intake, particularly heavy drinking, to SBP/DBP [1,2,9,18,27–31]. Dietary potassium, on the other hand, apparently has an opposite effect on SBP/DBP; that is, the higher the K intake, the lower the SBP/DBP, particularly when there is considerable salt ingestion [27,29,31,32].

The large-scale high-quality data from the international cooperative INTERSALT study, done in the latter 1980s with 10,079 men and women ages 20 to 59 from 52 population samples in 32 countries worldwide, are representative in regard to the foregoing dietary traits and their independent relations to SBP/DBP. Table 5 gives overall findings for all participants considered individually [27]. Results were similar for 9343 participants from 48 samples, after exclusion of people from four remote samples, all with very low NaCl intake. Results were also similar for the relation of Na to SBP for 8344 nonhypertensive people (from all 52 samples). This latter finding indicates that "salt sensitivity" is widespread in populations; that is, it is not confined to people with high blood pressure, a conclusion supported by analyses of clinical data on salt sensitivity [27].

Since the multivariate linear regression analyses by INTERSALT indicate significant independent influences of each of the four variables on BP, the findings can be regarded as additive (Table 5) [27], thus for persons

TABLE 5 Lifestyle Traits and SBP, DBP—Five-Variable and Four-Variable Analyses, 10,074 Individuals, INTERSALT

	Systolic BP		Diastolic BP	
	Five-variable analysis	Four-variable analysis	Five-variable analysis	Four-variable analysis
24-hr urinary Na excretion 100 mmol lower (mmHg)	−3.1[b]	−6.0[b]	−0.1	−2.5[b]
24-hr urinary K excretion 50 mmol higher (mmHg)	−3.4[b]	−3.3[b]	−1.9[a]	−1.6[c]
Alcohol intake 0 vs. 1–299 ml/week (mHg)	−0.5	−0.6	−0.1	−0.2
Alcohol intake 0 vs. 300+ ml/week (mHg)	−3.5[b]	−3.2[b]	−2.1[b]	−1.8[b]
Body mass index 3 kg/m^2 lower (mmHg)	−2.2[b]	—	−1.8[b]	—

Note: Of the total (10,079 people), five were not included due to missing data on alcohol intake. Analyses were done with and without BMI since BMI and Na were significantly correlated, indicating that inclusion of BMI may represent overadjustment for the Na–BP relations, also since inclusion in the same multivariate regression analysis of a variable measured with very high reliability (BMI) along with variables measured with considerably lower reliability (Na, K, alcohol) may result in underestimation of the strength of the relation of the latter variables to BP. Coefficients multivariate adjusted for regression dilution bias.

[a] $p < 0.01$.

[b] $p < 0.001$, for unadjusted coefficients.

[c] $Z = -1.933$.

with Na intake of 150 mmol/day and K 50 mmol/day (values common in the population), improvement to levels of Na 50 and K 100 can be expected to reduce SBP/DBP by about 9/4 mmHg on average. For heavy drinkers, cessation of alcohol intake plus the foregoing two dietary modifications can be expected to lower SBP/DBP by about 12/6 mmHg on average.

The INTERSALT study also did cross-population (ecologic) analyses (N = 52 samples) related to five prior hypotheses on salt and BP (Table 6) [27]. All yielded positive significant findings. In multivariate adjusted analyses, sample median Na intake of 100 mmol/day higher was thus associated with a higher upward slope of SBP/DBP with age—higher by 10/6 mmHg from age 25 to age 55 (or age 20 to 50, or age 30 to 60). These data are concordant with the inference that high habitual salt intake is a key environmental exposure leading to BP rise with age from youth through middle age.

TABLE 6 Twenty-four-Hour Median Na Excretion and BP—Tests of INTERSALT 52-Sample Prior Ecologic (Cross-Population) Hypotheses

	Multiple linear regression coefficient	
Dependent BP variable	Age-sex standardized	Age-sex-BMI-alcohol standardized
SBP slope with age mmHg/30 yr[a]/100 mmol	9.00[e]	10.20[e]
DBP slope with age mmHg/30 yr[a]/100 mmol	6.30[e]	6.30[e]
Median SBP mmHg/100 mmol	7.09[e]	4.46[d]
Median DBP mmHg/100 mmol	3.79[d]	2.26[c]
Hypertension[b] prevalence 100 mmol	6.25[d]	4.77[c]

[a] e.g., from age 25 to age 55 (since the INTERSALT participants were ages 20 to 59).
[b] SBP ≥140 or DBP ≥90 mmHg or on antihypertensive drug.
[c] $p \leq 0.05$.
[d] $p \leq 0.01$.
[e] $p \leq 0.001$.

The extensive data available, particularly on BMI, salt, alcohol, and BP, were in the late 1980s and 1990s repeatedly assessed by independent expert groups as indicative of etiologically significant relationships [1,2,9,12,27,28]. They became the scientific basis for the landmark 1993 *Report on the Primary Prevention of Hypertension*, the first of its kind in the world [2].

Macronutrients. In a second round of analyses, INTERSALT recorded an independent inverse relation to SBP/DBP of dietary total protein intake (measured by 24-hr urinary total nitrogen or urea nitrogen) [33,34]. Similar results were reported for ones 11,000 middle-aged men randomized into the Multiple Risk Factor Intervention Trial (MRFIT), based on analyses of average dietary data from four to five annual 24-hr recalls done for each man and his average annual SBP and DBP during the 6 trial years [31,35]. Evidence from other studies is also available indicating an inverse relation of dietary protein to BP [36,37].

The analyses for men in the MRFIT cohort also showed a direct relation of dietary cholesterol or Keys 3-factor dietary lipid score to BP, independent of age, ethnicity, education, BMI, reported Na, K, protein, and alcohol intake [31,35].

Most of the reported epidemiologic analyses on diet and BP have been cross-sectional, not prospective. The Chicago Western Electric Study has reported prospective data on diet and BP for a cohort of over 1700 men who underwent two in-depth nutrition surveys at years 0 and 1 (1957 to 1958 and 1958 to 1959), and were followed annually for 9 years [18]. Data were not available on Na and K intake by these men. In multivariate analyses, dietary vegetable protein—but not total or animal protein—was inversely related to 9-year BP trend. Dietary cholesterol or Keys score, heavy alcohol intake, and 9-year weight gain were directly related to 9-year BP change.

Cross-sectional data also showing a significant inverse relation between vegetable protein and BP, but not animal or total protein and BP, have recently been reported from the international cooperative INTERMAP study of 4680 men and women ages 40 to 59 from 17 population samples in China, Japan, the United Kingdom, and the United States [38]. To assess diet, BP, and other variables, participants were seen at four visits, four 24-hr in-depth dietary recalls were done, and two timed 24-hr urine specimens collected. INTERMAP data presented to date on macronutrients also indicate an independent inverse relation of dietary omega-3 fatty acids to BP [39].

The observational epidemiologic data on dietary vegetable protein and BP from the Western Electric and INTERMAP studies are concordant with findings from a set of short-term intervention trials indicating that an increase in vegetable protein intake from soy protein produces significant BP reduction [40–42].

Micronutrients, Fiber, and Foods

In the prospective analyses of the Western Electric Study, there was a significant independent inverse relation to average annual BP change of a combined antioxidant score based on beta-carotene and vitamin C intake [18]. Also, there was a significant independent inverse relation to BP change of intake of fruits and of vegetables [43]. Correspondingly, data are available indicating an inverse relation of dietary fiber to BP [37,40].

The Two DASH Feeding Trials

Both DASH feeding trials included adult men and women—African American and non-Hispanic white—with normal (but not optimal), high-normal, and HBP (stage 1) [44,45]. Eligible participants were consumers of little or no alcohol and on average were overweight. Based on recent findings indicating that multiple dietary factors influence BP, both trials assessed effects on BP of a "combination diet" compared to the usual American diet. The combination diet was increased in fruits, vegetables, and fat-free and low-fat dairy products. It included whole grains, poultry, fish, and nuts and was reduced in fats, red meats, sweets, and sugar-containing beverages [44–46]. It was thus different from usual American fare in regard to many macro- and micronutrients—higher in total and vegetable protein, complex carbohydrates, fiber, potassium, magnesium, phosphorus, calcium, and antioxidant and other vitamins, and lower in total fat, saturated fat, cholesterol, and sucrose. In both DASH-1 and DASH-2, very high level adherence was achieved to randomly assigned diets mainly by making all foods available to participants throughout the several trial weeks; that is, they were nutritional intervention trials of the feeding—not the counseling—type. Both were isocaloric by design; that is, the energy content of supplied foods was serially adjusted to minimize loss or gain of weight. In the first trial, NaCl intake was deliberately maintained constant across groups at about 7.5 g/day (slightly below population average), so that this food additive—known to influence BP—would not be a trial confounder [44]. In the second trial [45], participants randomized to both groups (usual U.S. diet and combination diet) were also randomly fed three levels of salt, designed to supply Na at 150, 100, and 50 mmol/day—8.7, 5.8, and 2.9 g/day NaCl; that is, the usual U.S. intake, moderate reduction, and more marked reduction (physiologic need is 10 mmol/day Na, 0.58 g/day NaCl) [28].

Effects of the combination diet on SBP/DBP were similar in the two trials—reductions overall of about 6/3 mmHg (with NaCl at or near the usual U.S. average level) [44,45]. It was effective in all subgroups, defined by gender, age, income, education, ethnicity, body mass, and physical activity. Significant SBP/DBP declines were registered in response to the combination diet for both nonhypertensive (SBP/DBP 120–139/80–89 mmHg) and hypertensive participants, about 4–5/2–3 mmHg and 12/5 mmHg, respectively (Table 7) [44,45], including a net fall in SBP of 11 mmHg for a subgroup with isolated systolic hypertension (ISH) [47].

For participants on both usual U.S. and DASH combination diets, lower compared to higher salt intake substantially reduced SBP/DBP (e.g., by about 7/4 mmHg overall for those on usual American fare); SBP was decreased about 5 mmHg for nonhypertensive and 9 mmHg for hypertensive participants (Table 7) [45]. Influence on BP was greater with reduction of NaCl from intermediate to lower level than from higher to intermediate level. The overall reduction of about 7/4 mmHg with Na lower by about 90 mmol/day in the DASH-NaCl trial is quantitatively concordant with the INTERSALT estimated effect of 6.0/2.5 mmHg with 100 mmol/day lower Na intake by individuals (Table 5) [27].

The effects of the combination diet and of salt reduction were additive (partially, not completely), thus for the group on combination diet plus lower salt intake, SBP/DBP net reduction overall (compared to the group on usual U.S. fare with higher salt intake) was about 9/6 mmHg; SBP was lowered 7

TABLE 7 DASH-NaCl Feeding Trial—Effects on SBP/DBP of DASH Combination Diet (vs. Usual U.S. Diet) and of Higher (vs. Lower) NaCl Intake

BP variable	Group	DASH combination diet vs. usual U.S. diet (NaCl intake higher)	Lower NaCl[c] vs. higher NaCl[d] (usual U.S. diet)	DASH combination diet with lower NaCl[c] vs. usual U.S. diet with higher NaCl[d]
Systolic BP (mmHg)	All participants	−5.9[f]	−6.7[f]	−8.9[f] (−11.1 to −6.7[b])
	Nonhypertensive participants	Not reported[b]	about −5[f]	−7.1[f]
	Hypertensive participants	Not reported[b]	about −8[f]	−11.5[f]
Diastolic BP (mmHg)	All participants	−2.9[f]	−3.5[f]	−4.5 (−5.9 to −3.1[b])
	Nonhypertensive participants	Not reported[b]	Not reported	Not reported
	Hypertensive participants	Not reported[b]	Not reported	Not reported

[a]95% confidence interval.

[b] In the first DASH trial (NEJM 1997;336:1117–1124), SBP/DBP of nonhypertensive participants were lower by −3.5/−2.1 mmHg and −11.4/−5.5 mmHg for hypertensive participants.

[c] Based on measurement of Na in 24-hour urine collections, observed Na intake was about 65 mmol/day.

[d] Based on measurement of Na in 24-hour urine collections, observed Na intake was about 142 mmol/day.

[e]$p < 0.01$.

[f] $p < 0.001$.

mmHg for nonhypertensive participants and 12 mmHg for hypertensive participants (Table 7) [45].

Physical Activity

By the early 1990s, several research reports were extant from observational studies and intervention trials indicating that regular, frequent, moderate isotonic exercise lowered BP independent of its possible influence on body weight [2]. These served as the scientific basis for inclusion of a recommendation on exercise in the 1993 *Report on the Primary Prevention of Hypertension* [2]. In the intervening years, further concordant evidence has accrued [48–50].

Smoking

Smoking, especially cigarette smoking, is an established major risk for cardiovascular and other serious diseases, all cause mortality, and shortened life expectancy. As multiple prospective cohort studies have massively documented, including—with exquisite precision—MRFIT [4,5,10–12], at every level of BP (and at every level of serum cholesterol as well), risks are greater by twofold or more for smokers compared to nonsmokers. The force of this etiological relationship as reflected in levels of relative risk is apparently even stronger for women than men.

As to prospective data on smoking and BP, the evidence is limited. The Western Electric study reported a direct relation of smoking to postbaseline annual BP change during 9-year follow-up [18].

Conclusions

Multiple aspects of nutrition influence BP from conception on, as do habitual exercise habits and probably smoking as well. Recent advances, particularly in regard to additive effects of multiple foods-nutrients on BP culminating in the results of the two DASH feeding trials, serve as the basis for a fundamental conclusion: *The scientific foundation is now in hand to end the epidemic of population-adverse BP levels.* Research advances in this area have—so to speak—caught up with knowledge on the diet-dyslipidemia relationship, in which key evidence to solve the populationwide problem was already in hand by the 1960s [4,17,51]. During the last four decades, successes in the general application of this latter knowledge have produced progressive decline in average serum cholesterol levels of the adult population, from about 235 to 240 mg/dl in the 1950s to about 200 mg/dl in the latter 1990s—a national health goal achieved. This achievement is mainly attributable to improved nutrient composition of the diet (and has been registered despite a serial increase in weight of the population). A similar advance in regard to BP levels is now entirely possible based on the scientific knowledge now in hand on the influences of lifestyles—especially multiple dietary factors—on BP.

STRATEGIES FOR THE PREVENTION OF ADVERSE BP LEVELS

General Strategy

The *general strategy* is to effectively implement national public policy to encourage serial improvement in populationwide eating patterns per the DASH combination diet with lower salt intake, plus prevention and control of overweight-obesity and heavy alcohol consumption, populationwide improvement in leisure-time physical activity, and continued progress in achieving prevention and cessation of smoking. Serial progress in the implementation of this general strategy can be anticipated to result in lower average SBP/DBP among teenagers and young adults, substantially smaller increases in SBP/DBP during the decades of adulthood, progressively higher prevalence rates in the population of optimal SBP/DBP, and lower prevalence rates of high-normal and high BP, culminating over the years ahead in an end to the epidemic of adverse SBP/DBP levels. These advances can also be anticipated to accomplish further increases in population prevalence rates of favorable serum lipid levels (e.g., serum total cholesterol <200 mg/dl) and of nonsmoking; that is, higher and higher percentages of the adult population will be at low risk (SBP/DBP $\leq 120/\leq 80$ mmHg, serum cholesterol <200 mg/dl) because they are not smoking, not overweight (BMI <25.0), and are not diabetic, and are thus freed of the threat of epidemic CHD-CVD (attributable at the 90% level to adverse findings for one or more, especially two or more, of the foregoing major risk factors) (Table 8) [52].

Specific Strategies

From Conception on

Since intrauterine nutrition can influence adult SBP/DBP, there is a need to extend and enhance prenatal care from conception on to maximize favorable nutritional patterns and lifestyles for all pregnant women.

From Birth and Weaning on

Since dietary composition and weight gain pattern can influence childhood, teenage, and adult SBP/DBP, there is a need to enhance approaches to achieve improved nutrition from birth and weaning on. This area of strategy has a special importance since it relates to the ages of primary habit

TABLE 8 Mortality from CHD, CVD, Cancers, All Causes, Low-Risk Subcohorts and Others; Estimated Greater Life Expectancy, Low-Risk Subcohorts vs. Others

Cohort[c]	Number of people		Number of deaths and death rate[d]		Age-Adjusted RR (95% CI), low-risk subcohort vs. others	Estimated greater life expectancy, low-risk subcohort vs. others
			Low-Risk Subcohort	Others		
CHD mortality[d]						
MRFIT men ages 35 to 39	7,163[a]	64,981[b]	11 (0.2)	735 (1.5)	0.14 (0.08–0.25)	—
CHA men ages 18 to 39	942	9083	1 (0.6)	126 (5.9)	0.08 (0.01–0.61)	—
MRFIT men ages 40 to 57	16,302	254,369	126 (4.4)	9578 (19.9)	0.22 (0.18–0.26)	—
CHA men ages 40 to 59	358	7132	6 (8.8)	516 (38.1)	0.23 (0.10–0.51)	—
CHA women ages 40 to 59	421	5808	2 (3.5)	181 (14.5)	0.21 (0.05–0.84)	—
CVD mortality[d]						
MRFIT men ages 35 to 39	7,163[a]	64,981[b]	16 (0.3)	1022 (2.1)	0.15 (0.09–0.24)	—
CHA men ages 18 to 39	942	9083	3 (1.4)	163 (7.7)	0.20 (0.06–0.62)	—
MRFIT men ages 40 to 57	16,302	254,369	190 (6.7)	13,247 (27.5)	0.24 (0.21–0.28)	—
CHA men ages 40 to 59	358	7132	10 (15.8)	714 (53.1)	0.28 (0.15–0.52)	—

CHA women ages 40 to 59	421	5808	4 (5.3)	281 (22.6)	0.27 (0.10–0.72)	—
Cancer mortality[d]						
MRFIT men ages 35 to 39	7163[a]	64,981[b]	36 (0.7)	758 (1.5)	0.44 (0.32–0.62)	—
CHA men ages 18 to 39	942	9083	7 (7.9)	140 (13.7)	0.56 (0.26–1.19)	—
MRFIT men ages 40 to 57	16,302	254,369	393 (13.5)	11,579 (24.0)	0.56 (0.51–0.62)	—
CHA men ages 40 to 59	358	7,132	16 (50.7)	653 (95.6)	0.48 (0.29–0.79)	—
CHA women ages 40 to 59	421	5808	22 (45.8)	409 (69.2)	0.83 (0.54–1.28)	—
All causes mortality[d]						
MRFIT men ages 35 to 39	7163[a]	64,981[b]	139 (2.5)	2574 (5.2)	0.50 (0.42–0.59)	6.3
CHA men ages 18 to 39	942	9083	20 (10.2)	479 (23.5)	0.43 (0.28–0.68)	9.5
MRFIT men ages 40 to 57	16,302	254,369	848 (29.2)	31,034 (64.4)	0.45 (0.42–0.48)	5.9
CHA men ages 40 to 59	358	7132	36 (54.6)	1684 (124.9)	0.42 (0.30–0.58)	6.0
CHA women ages 40 to 59	421	5808	30 (36.1)	843 (68.4)	0.60 (0.42–0.87)	5.6

[a] Low risk subcohort.
[b] Others.
[c] Ages are baseline ages; follow-up averaged 16 years in the MRFIT study and 22 years in the CHA study.
[d] Data presented as number of deaths (age-adjusted mortality rate per 10,000 person years).

formation, and it is easier to establish favorable lifestyle habits from the beginning than to decondition unfavorable habits later on.

For Teenagers and Young Adults

Since it is well established that adverse levels of SBP/DBP and other major risk factors in teenagers and young adults are already predictive of increased risk of CHD-CVD and shortened life expectancy, there is a need to apply systematically the general strategy to this population stratum. This is especially important since these are years of transition in lifestyles, with a high potential for unfavorable evolution of major risk factors. For the sizable proportion of teenagers and young adults who already have SBP/DBP above optimal, special measures are needed at the clinical level (i.e., beyond general populationwide public health measures) to improve lifestyles and restore SBP/DBP to optimal levels.

For Middle-Aged and Older Adults

Since for most people SBP/DBP levels become progressively higher at these stages of the life span so that by early middle age only a minority have optimal SBP/DBP, and since CHD-CVD are epidemic during these years, major strategic emphasis is needed on the primary prevention of the SBP/DBP rises of these years. These need to include detection and care of less severe adverse SBP/DBP levels in middle-aged and older adults as an ongoing clinical effort; that is, "early" detection and care not only of people with HBP, but also those with normal (but not optimal) and high-normal levels. Care for all such people needs to have as a major ongoing component effective improvement of eating, drinking, exercise, and smoking habits, as well as antihypertensive drug therapy when indicated.

For Persons From Lower Socioeconomic Strata of all Ethnicities

The lower SES of the population have even more adverse SBP/DBP levels than others. Since these are associated with even greater risks of CHD-CVD and shortened life expectancy and the circumstances of these strata produce multiple special challenges in terms of lifestyle improvement, particular attention is needed to develop sustained effective approaches for application of the general and specific strategies throughout the life span for the lower SES strata.

PERSPECTIVE

Viewed as a set of strategic challenges for effective ongoing implementation, sustained and progressive during the next years and decades, the foregoing "tall order" is entirely realistic and achievable. The validity of this judgment is documented by the substantial progress during the last four decades in improving diet composition to lower populationwide serum cholesterol levels, by the progressive reduction in the prevalence of smoking and by the evidence already in hand that SBP/DBP levels have begun to decline, independent of antihypertensive drug influences [16]. The efforts needed are substantial, at the levels of public health, medical care, and beyond. They include neutralizing the adverse role of special commercial interests who oppose the whole undertaking. They also encompass positive involvement of the food and communications industries, essential to accomplish populationwide improvements in eating patterns. Since the goal—ending this epidemic—is about as big and exciting as any ever set for improvement of human health, the multifaceted efforts and the societal investments are undoubtedly worthwhile.

REFERENCES

1. National High Blood Pressure Education Program. The Fifth Report of the Joint National Committee on Detection, Evaluation, and Treatment of High Blood Pressure (JNC-V). Arch Int Med. 1993;154–183.
2. National High Blood Pressure Education Program Working Group. National High Blood Pressure Education Program working group report on primary prevention of hypertension. Arch Int Med. 1993;153:186–208.
3. Stamler J, Stamler R, Neaton JD. Blood pressure, systolic and diastolic, and cardiovascular risks: U.S. population data. Arch Int Med 1993;153;598–615.
4. Stamler J, Dyer AR, Shekelle RB, Neaton J, Stamler R. Relationship of baseline major risk factors to coronary and all-cause mortality, and to longevity: findings from long-term follow-up of Chicago cohorts. Cardiology. 1993;82:191–222.
5. Neaton JD, Kuller L, Stamler J, Wentworth DN. Chapter 9: impact of systolic and diastolic blood pressure on cardiovascular mortality. In: Laragh JH, Brenner BM, eds. Hypertension: Physiology, Diagnosis, and Management. 2d ed. New York: Raven, 1994.
6. Klag MJ, Whelton PK, Randall BL, Neaton JD, Brancati FL, Ford CE, Shulman NB, Stamler J. Blood pressure and end-stage renal disease in men. N Eng J Med. 1996;334:13–18.
7. Stamler J, Hazuda HP. Executive summary. In: Report of the Conference on Socioeconomic Status and Cardiovascular Health and Disease: 1995 Nov. 6–7. National Institutes of Health, National Heart, Lung, and Blood Institute, 1996: 3–10.
8. Stamler J, Stamler R, Garside D, Greenlund K, Archer S, Neaton JD, Wentworth DN. Socioeconomic status, cardiovascular risk factors, and cardiovascular disease: findings on U.S. working populations. In: Report of the Conference on Socioeconomic Status and Cardiovascular Health and

Disease: 1995 Nov. 6–7, National Institutes of Health, National Heart, Lung, and Blood Institute, 1996: 109–118.

9. National High Blood Pressure Education Program. The Sixth Report of the Joint National Committee on Detection, Evaluation, and Treatment of High Blood Pressure (JNC-VI). Arch Int Med. 1997;157:2413–2446.
10. Stamler J, Greenland P, Neaton JD. The established major risk factors underlying epidemic coronary and cardiovascular disease. CVD Prevent. 1998;1:82–97.
11. Lowe LP, Greenland P, Ruth KJ, Dyer AR, Stamler R, Stamler J. Impact of major cardiovascular disease risk factors, particularly in combination, on 22-year mortality in women and men. Arch Int Med. 1998;158:2007–2014.
12. The International Task Force for Prevention of Coronary Heart Disease in cooperation with the International Atherosclerosis Society. Coronary Heart Disease: reducing the risk. The scientific background for primary and secondary prevention of coronary heart disease. Nutr Metab Cardio Disease. 1998;8:205–271.
13. Cooper R, Cutler J, Desvigne-Nickens P, Fortmann SP, Friedman L, Havlik R, Hogelin G, Marler J, McGovern P, Morosco G, Mosca L, Pearson T, Stamler J, Stryer D, Thom T. Trends and disparities in coronary heart disease, stroke, and other cardiovascular diseases in the United States: findings of the National Conference on Cardiovascular Disease Prevention. Circulation. 2000;102:3137–3147.
14. Miura K, Daviglus ML, Dyer AR, Liu K, Garside DB, Stamler J, Greenland P. Relationship of blood pressure to 25-year mortality due to coronary heart disease, cardiovascular diseases, and all causes in young adult men: the Chicago Heart Association Detection Project in Industry. Arch Int Med. 2001;161:1501–1508.
15. Rodin MB, Daviglus ML, Wong GC, Liu K, Garside DB, Greenland P, Stamler J. Major cardiovascular risk factors in middle age and abdominal aortic aneurysm in older age: the Chicago Heart Association Detection Project in Industry Study. In press.
16. Burt VL, Whelton P, Roccella EJ, Brown C, Cutler JA, Higgins M, Horan MJ, Labarthe D. Prevalence of hypertension in the U.S. adult population. results from the Third National Health and Nutrition Examination Survey, 1988–1991. Hypertension 1995;25:305–313.
17. Stamler J. Lectures on Preventive Cardiology. New York: Grune and Stratton, 1967.
18. Stamler J, Liu K, Ruth KJ, Pryer J, Greenland P. Eight-year blood pressure change in middle-aged men: relationship to macronutrients, micronutrients, and other dietary factors—the Chicago Western Electric Study. In press.
19. Joslin EP. In: Walker A. Diabetes in Europe and beyond. Br Med J. 1991;302:1231.
20. Stamler R. The primary prevention of hypertension and the population blood pressures problem. In: Marmot M, Elliott P, eds. Coronary Heart Disease

Epidemiology: From Aetiology to Public Health. New York: Oxford University Press, 1992: 35–66.
21. Ackerknecht EH. Rudolf Virchow—Doctor, Statesman, Anthropologist. Madison: University of Wisconsin Press, 1953.
22. Barker DJP. Mothers, babies, and health in later life. Edinburgh: Churchill Livingstone, 1998.
23. Law CM, de Swiet M, Osmond C, Fayers PM, Barker DJ, Cruddas AM, Fall CH. Initiation of hypertension in utero and its amplification throughout life. Br Med J. 1993;306:24–27.
24. Hofman A, Hazebroek A, Valkenburg HA. A randomized trial of sodium intake and blood pressure in newborn infants. JAMA. 1983;250:370–373.
25. Geleijnse JM, Hofman A, Witteman JC, Hazebroek AA, Valkenburg HA, Grobbee DE. Long-term effects of neonatal sodium restriction on blood pressure. Hypertension 1997;29:913–917.
26. Stamler J. Epidemiologic findings on body mass and blood pressure in adults. Ann Epidem 1991;1:347–362.
27. Stamler J. The INTERSALT Study: background, methods, findings, and implications. Am J Clin Nutr. 1997;65 (2 suppl.):626S–642S.
28. National Research Council, Committee on Diet and Health, Food and Nutrition Board, Commission on Life Sciences. Diet and Health: Implications for Reducing Chronic Disease Risk. Washington, DC: National Academy Press, 1989.
29. INTERSALT Cooperative Research Group. INTERSALT: an international study of electrolyte excretion and blood pressure. Results for 24-hour urinary sodium and potassium excretion. Br Med J. 1988;297:319–328.
30. Marmot MG, Elliott P, Dyer AR, Shipley MJ, Ueshima H, Beevers DG, Stamler R, Kesteloot H, Rose G, Stamler J. Alcohol and blood pressure: the INTERSALT study. Br Med J. 1994;308:1263–1267.
31. Stamler J, Caggiula AW, Grandits GA. Relation of body mass and alcohol, nutrient, fiber, and caffeine intakes to blood pressure in the special intervention and usual care groups in the Multiple Risk Factor Intervention Trial. Am J Clin Nutr. 1997;65 (1 suppl.):338S–365S.
32. Whelton PK, He J, Cutler JA, Brancati FL, Appel LJ, Follmann D, Klag MJ. Effects of oral potassium on blood pressure: meta-analysis of randomized controlled clinical trials. JAMA. 1997;277:1624–1632.
33. Stamler J, Elliott P, Kesteloot H, Nichols R, Claeys G, Dyer AR, Stamler R, for the INTERSALT Cooperative Research Group. Inverse relation of dietary protein markers with blood pressure: findings for 10,020 men and women in the INTERSALT study. Circulation. 1996;94:1629–1634.
34. Dyer AR, Elliott P, Chee D, Stamler J. Urinary biochemical markers of dietary intake in the INTERSALT study. Am J Clin Nutr. 1997;65 (suppl.): 1246S–1253S.
35. Stamler J, Caggiula A, Grandits GA, Kjelsberg M, Cutler JA, for the MRFIT Research Group. Relationship to blood pressure of combinations of dietary

macronutrients: findings of the Multiple Risk Factor Intervention Trial (MRFIT). Circulation. 1996;94:2417–2423.
36. Obarzanek E, Velletri PA, Cutler JA. Dietary protein and blood pressure. JAMA. 1996;274:1598–1603.
37. He J, Whelton PK. Effect of dietary fiber and protein intake on blood pressure: a review of epidemiologic evidence. Clin Exp Hypertens 1999;21: 785–796.
38. Elliott P, for the INTERMAP Cooperative Research Group. Dietary protein and blood pressure: findings from the INTERMAP study. presented at the Symposium on the INTERMAP Study, Fifth International Conference on Preventive Cardiology, Osaka, Japan, May 29, 2001.
39. Ueshima H, for the INTERMAP Cooperative Research Group. Dietary lipids and blood pressure: findings from the INTERMAP study. presented at the Symposium on the INTERMAP Study, Fifth International Conference on Preventive Cardiology, Osaka, Japan, May 29, 2001.
40. Burke V, Hodgson JM, Beilin LJ, Giangiulioi N, Rogers P, Puddey IB. Dietary protein and soluble fiber reduce ambulatory blood pressure in treated hypertensives. Hypertension. 2001;38:821–826.
41. He J, Wu X, Gu D, Duan X, Whelton PK. Soybean protein supplementation and blood pressure: a randomized controlled clinical trial. presented at the 40th Annual Conference on Cardiovascular Disease Epidemiology and Prevention, American Heart Association, La Jolla, CA, March 2000.
42. Teede HJ, Dalais FS, Kotsopoulos D. Phytoestrogen dietary supplementation improves lipid profiles and blood pressure: a double blind, randomized, placebo-controlled study in men and postmenopausal women. Climacteric. 1999;2 (suppl. 1):127 (abstract).
43. Miura K, Stamler J, Daviglus ML, Liu K, Nakagawa H, Greenland P. Relationship of vegetable, fruit, and meat intake to 7-year blood pressure change in middle-aged men: the Western Electric Study. In press.
44. Appel LJ, Moore TJ, Obarzanek E, Vollmer WM, Svetkey LP, Sacks FM, Bray GA, Vogt TM, Cutler JA, Windhauser MM, Lin PH, Karanja N, for the DASH Collaborative Research Group. A clinical trial of the effects of dietary patterns on blood pressure. New Eng J Med. 1997;336:1117–1124.
45. Sacks FM, Svetkey LP, Vollmer WM, Appel LJ, Bray GA, Harsha D, Obarzanek E, Conlin PR, Miller ER 3rd, Simons-Morton DG, Karanja N, Lin PH, for the DASH-Sodium Collaborative Research Group. Effects on blood pressure of reduced sodium and the Dietary Approaches to Stop Hypertension (DASH) diet. New Eng J Med. 2001;344:3–10.
46. National Heart, Lung, and Blood Institute. The DASH Diet. U.S. Department of Health and Human Services, Public Health Service, National Institutes of Health. National Heart, Lung, and Blood Institute, 1998: NIH Publication No. 01-4082.
47. Moore TJ, Conlin PR, Ard J, Svetkey LP, for the DASH Collaborative Research Group. DASH (Dietary Approaches to Stop Hypertension) diet is

effective treatment for stage 1 isolated systolic hypertension. Hypertension. 2001;38:155–158.
48. Fagard RH. The role of exercise in blood pressure control: supportive evidence. J Hypertens. 1995;13:1223–1227.
49. Puddey IB, Cox K. Exercise lowers blood pressure—sometimes? Or did Pheidippides have hypertension? J Hypertens. 1995;13:1229–1233.
50. Arakawa K. Exercise, a measure to lower blood pressure and reduce other risks. Clin Exp Hypertens 1999;21:797–803.
51. Stamler J. Potential for prevention of major adult cardiovascular disease. In: Toshima H, Koga Y, Blackburn HJ, Keys A, eds. Lessons for Science from the Seven Countries Study: a 35-year collaborative experience in cardiovascular disease epidemiology. Tokyo: Springer-Verlag, 1995: 195–235.
52. Stamler J, Stamler R, Neaton JD, Wentworth D, Daviglus ML, Garside D, Dyer AR, Greenland P, Liu K. Relationship of baseline low risk factor profile to long-term cardiovascular and non-cardiovascular mortality and to life expectancy: findings for five large cohorts of young adult and middle-aged men and women. JAMA. 1999;282:2012–2018.

4

Strategies for Treatment of Hypertension

Norman M. Kaplan
The University of Texas Southwestern Medical School, Dallas, Texas, U.S.A.

INTRODUCTION

As noted in previous chapters, hypertension is a major risk factor for cardiovascular disease. Despite the enthusiasm for preventive measures described in the previous chapter, it is unlikely that most hypertension can be prevented in view of the steady deterioration of healthier lifestyles seen in all industrialized societies. As the population grows fatter, in large part from physical inactivity, more and more hypertension (and diabetes, dyslipidemia, and coronary disease) will develop. Furthermore, as life expectancy is prolonged, more people will survive to beyond age 65, by which time over 50% will have hypertension.

Unfortunately, current strategies to treat hypertension adequately have been largely unsuccessful [1], therefore better strategies are clearly needed. These strategies should include the following:

- More careful measurement of out-of-the-office blood pressure (BP) levels to ensure the usual presence of hypertension
- Assessment of other cardiovascular risk factors to determine both the need for and the type of antihypertensive therapy
- Implementation of appropriate lifestyle modifications as will be covered in subsequent chapters

Determination of the choices of drug therapy based upon evidence of randomized controlled trials (RCTs) in the overall hypertensive population and in various subgroups with coexisting conditions
Application of rational maneuvers to improve continuity of patients' adherence to therapy
Recognition of the need to provide enough medication to achieve the appropriate goals of therapy

The implementation of these strategies will not be easy, but they can be achieved even in patients with significant hypertension and other risk factors when a well-designed and coordinated approach is implemented [2,3]. These strategies will be considered in sequence.

MEASUREMENT OF OUT-OF-OFFICE BLOOD PRESSURE

Although most of the data on the risks of hypertension and the benefits of its treatment have been based on relatively few office measurements, increasingly strong evidence documents the greater validity of out-of-the-office measurements for ascertainment of both the risks of hypertension [4] and the benefits of therapy [5].

The BP measured in the office setting is usually higher than that measured out of the office, either by ambulatory monitoring or by semi automatic devices for self-use [6]. If out-of-office readings are not obtained, the 20–30% of patients who have "white-coat" or "isolated" office hypertension will be misdiagnosed [7]. Although the evidence is not conclusive, more and more follow-up data for as long as 10 years document the relative benignity of white-coat hypertension [4,8], therefore many patients who would be considered in need of antihypertensive drug therapy on the basis of office readings could be safely managed by lifestyle modifications and careful surveillance.

Out-of-office measurements are a more valid predictor of the presence of current hypertension-induced target organ damage [9] and subsequent cardiovascular risk [4,8]. Moreover, their use is associated with improved control of hypertension, likely by providing feedback that encourages appropriate changes in therapy [10].

ASSESSMENT OF OVERALL CARDIOVASCULAR RISK STATUS

Hypertension obviously is only one of the major cardiovascular risk factors (Table 1). In addition, as shown in Table 1, the presence of target

TABLE 1 Components of Cardiovascular Risk Stratification in Patients with Hypertension

Major risk factors	Target organ damage/clinical cardiovascular disease
Smoking	Heart diseases
Dyslipidemia	Left ventricular hypertrophy
Diabetes mellitus	Angina or prior myocardial infarction
Age >60 years	Prior coronary revascularization
Sex (men and postmenopausal women)	Heart failure
Family history of cardiovascular disease:	Stroke or transient ischemic failure
women <65 years or men <55 years	Nephropathy
	Peripheral arterial disease
	Retinopathy

organ damage or overt cardiovascular disease also indicates a higher degree of risk.

Based on the components shown in Table 1, the sixth report of the Joint National Committee (JNC-6) provided a simple stratification of cardiovascular risk [11]. As seen in Table 2, the three risk categories, A, B, and C, were then used along with various levels of BP to provide an overall set of recommendations for either lifestyle modifications and/or antihypertensive drug therapy.

The subsequently published guidelines from expert committees of the World Health Organization and International Society of Hypertension (WHO-ISH) [12] and the British Hypertension Society [13] used similar models for stratification and assessment of overall cardiovascular risk as guides to the need for therapy.

More recently, a simple delineation of the varying contributions of the major risk factors has been provided [14] so that each patient's relative risk status can easily be computed and translated into a single estimate of risk (Tables 3, 4).

IMPLEMENTATION OF LIFESTYLE MODIFICATIONS

Lifestyle modifications will be described in the following 10 chapters, so no additional coverage is needed beyond an iteration of the importance of effective implementation, whether they are used with or without concomitant drug therapy.

TABLE 2 Risk Stratification and Treatment

Blood pressure stages (mmHg)	Risk group A (no risk factors; no TOD/CCD)[a]	Risk group B (at least only risk factor, not including diabetes; no TOD/CCD)	Risk group C (TOD/CCD and/or diabetes, with or without other risk factors)
High-normal (130–139/85–89)	Lifestyle modification	Lifestyle modification	Drug therapy[c]
Stage 1 (140–159/90–99)	Lifestyle modification (up to 12 months)	Lifestyle modification[b] (up to 6 months)	Drug therapy
Stages 2 and 3 (160/100)	Drug therapy	Drug therapy	Drug therapy

Note: For example, a patient with diabetes and a blood pressure of 142/94 mmHg plus left ventricular hypertrophy should be classified as having stage 1 hypertension with target organ disease (left ventricular hypertrophy) and with another major risk factor (diabetes). This patient should be categorized as "stage 1, risk group C," and recommended for immediate initiation of pharmacologic treatment. Lifestyle modification should be adjunctive therapy for all patients recommended for pharmacologic therapy.

[a] TOD/CCD indicates target organ disease/clinical cardiovascular disease. (See Table 1.)

[b] For those with heart failure, renal insufficiency, or diabetes.

[c] For patients with multiple risk factors, clinicians should consider drugs as initial therapy plus lifestyle modifications.

CHOICES OF THERAPY

Beyond the need for appropriate lifestyle changes, the majority of hypertensive patients will require antihypertensive drug therapy. The choice of initial and subsequent therapy should be based on evidence from RCTs, both in the overall hypertensive population and in various subgroups with coexisting conditions.

OVERALL HYPERTENSIVE POPULATION

Relative Antihypertensive Efficacy

The choice of drug is often based on perceived differences in efficacy in lowering BP and the likelihood of side effects. In fact, overall antihypertensive efficacy varies little between the various available drugs. To gain Food and Drug Administration (FDA) approval for marketing in the United States, the drug must have been shown to be effective in reducing the BP in a large portion of the 1500 or more patients given the drug during its clinical investigation. Moreover, the dose and formulation of drug are chosen so as not to lower the BP too much or too fast to avoid hypotensive side effects. Virtually all oral drugs are designed to do the same thing: lower the BP at least 10% in the majority of patients with mild to moderate hypertension [15].

Not only must each new drug be shown to be effective in large numbers of hypertensive patients, but the drug also must have been tested against currently available agents to show at least equal efficacy. When comparisons between various drugs are made, they almost always come out close to one another. The best such comparison was performed in the Treatment of Mild Hypertension Study (TOMHS) [16]. The TOMHS involved random allocation of five drugs: the diuretic chlorthalidone, the β-blocker acebutolol, the α-blocker doxazosin, the calcium-channel blocker amlodipine, and the angiotensin-converting enzyme inhibitor (ACEI) enalapril. Each drug was given to almost 200 mild hypertensives, while another group took a placebo and all patients remained on a nutritional-hygienic program. The overall antihypertensive efficacy of the five drugs over 4 years was virtually equal [16].

Despite the fairly equal overall efficacy of various antihypertensive drugs, individual patients may vary considerably in their response to different drugs. Some of this variability can be accounted for by patient characteristics, including age and race. This was seen in a Veterans Administration (VA) cooperative 1-year trial in which 1292 men were randomly given one of six drugs from each major class. Overall and in the black patients, the calcium channel blocker (CCB) was most effective, but the ACEI was best in younger whites, and the β-blocker was best in older whites [17]. Similarly, in a randomized crossover trial of elderly patients with isolated systolic hyper-

TABLE 3 Estimate of 10-Year Risk for Men and Women Using Framingham Risk Scoring

Men: Age (years)	Men: Points	Women: Age (years)	Women: Points
20–34	−9	20–34	−7
35–39	−4	35–39	−3
40–44	0	40–44	0
45–49	3	45–49	3
50–54	6	50–54	6
55–59	8	55–59	8
60–64	10	60–64	10
65–69	11	65–69	12
70–74	12	70–74	14
75–79	13	75–79	16

Men

Total cholesterol (mg/dl)	Points: Age 20–39	Age 40–49	Age 50–59	Age 60–69	Age 70–70
<160	0	0	0	0	0
160–199	4	3	2	1	0
200–239	7	5	3	1	0
240–279	9	6	4	2	1
280	11	8	5	3	1

Women

Total cholesterol (mg/dl)	Points: Age 20–39	Age 40–49	Age 50–59	Age 60–69	Age 70–70
<160	0	0	0	0	0
160–199	4	3	2	1	1
200–239	8	6	4	2	1
240–279	11	8	5	3	2
280	13	10	7	4	2

	Points				
	Age 20–39	Age 40–49	Age 50–59	Age 60–69	Age 70–70
Nonsmoker	0	0	0	0	0
Smoker	8	5	3	1	1

HDL (mg/dL)	Points
60	−1
50–59	0
40–49	1
<40	2

Systolic BP (mmHg)	Untreated	Treated
<120	0	0
120–129	0	1
130–139	1	2
140–159	1	2
160	2	3

	Points				
	Age 20–39	Age 40–49	Age 50–59	Age 60–69	Age 70–70
Nonsmoker	0	0	0	0	0
Smoker	9	7	4	2	1

HDL (mg/dL)	Points
60	−1
50–59	0
40–49	1
<40	2

Systolic BP (mmHg)	Untreated	Treated
<120	0	0
120–129	1	3
130–139	2	4
140–159	3	5
160	4	6

Source: Modified from Ref. 14.

TABLE 4 Estimate of 10-Year Risk for Men and Women Using Framingham Risk Scoring

Men		Women	
Point total	10-year risk (%)	Point total	10-year risk (%)
<0	<1	<9	<1
0	1	9	1
1	1	19	1
2	1	11	1
3	1	12	1
4	1	13	2
5	2	14	2
6	2	15	3
7	3	16	4
8	4	17	5
9	5	18	6
10	6	19	8
11	8	20	11
12	10	21	14
13	12	22	17
14	16	23	22
15	20	24	27
16	25	25	30
17	30		

Source: Modified from Ref. 14.

tension given a representative drug from four major classes—ACEI, β-blocker, CCB, and diuretic—each for 1 month, diuretic and CCB were more effective than β-blocker or ACEI [18]. In a similarly designed trial of younger patients with combined systolic and diastolic hypertension, the ACEI and β-blocker were more effective than the CCB or diuretic [19].

The critical issue is not efficacy in lowering BP but effectiveness in reducing morbidity and mortality. All major classes of antihypertensive drugs save α-blockers have been shown to reduce mortality and morbidity in large RCTs, and there are few differences among them [20,21].

Diuretics or β-blockers were used in all of the 18 RCTs completed before 1995 [19] (Table 5). The major conclusion of the meta-analysis of the data from these 18 RCTs is that low-dose diuretic therapy (12.5 to 25 mg of hydrochlorothiazide or its equivalent) provided excellent protection against coronary disease, whereas neither high doses of diuretic nor β-blocker-based therapies did so, although all provided protection against stroke and congestive heart failure. On the basis of these RCTs, the JNC-6 report indicated

TABLE 5 Randomized Controlled Trials Prior to 1995: First Drug Therapy

	Relative risk vs. placebo			
	Stroke	Coronary heart disease	Congestive heart failure	Cardiovascular mortality
High-dose diuretic (50–100 mg)	0.49	0.99	0.17	0.78
Low-dose diuretic (12.5–25 mg)	0.66	0.72	0.58	0.76
Beta-blocker	0.71	0.93	0.58	0.89

Source: Adapted from Ref. 20.

"If there are no specific indications for another type of drug, a diuretic or β-blocker should be chosen" [11].

In the eight RCTs completed between 1995 and 2000, ACEIs or CCBs were compared either against a diuretic ± β-blocker or against one another [21]. As seen in Table 6, one conclusion from these more recent trials seems obvious: neither ACEI-based nor CCB-based therapies are better than diuretics ± β-blocker-based therapies. CCB therapy did protect better against stroke and less well against CHD and CHF, but ACEIs and CCBs provided identical effects on overall morbidity and mortality.

The bottom line of Table 6 shows data from the two trials, ABCD and STOP-2, that directly compared an ACEI to a CCB. The ABCD trial [22] had 470 patients. The STOP-2 [23] had 4401 taking either an ACEI or a CCB, so obviously most of the results are derived from STOP-2. Although there is apparently lesser protection against CHD and CHF with the CCB than with the ACEI, the words of the principal investigators of STOP-2 should be heeded: "Our results should be interpreted with some caution, since 48 statistical comparisons were done. Calcium antagonists were not, however, less effective in any other way in the prevention of cardiovascular events than conventional drugs or ACEIs, which accords with current opinion about safety of calcium antagonists when used appropriately" [23].

The results of the eight comparative trials completed since 1995 are by no means definitive. As He and Whelton [24] note: "Most of the uncertainties related to selection of initial antihypertensive drug therapy will be resolved by trials in progress and by the pooling of the findings from these trials." Fortunately, a large number of trials are in progress so that before long we should have more definitive data to guide our choices in therapy. These data will include outcome studies with angiotensin II-receptor blockers (ARBs).

Of course, the playing field keeps growing. By the time we know if ARBs are as good as ACEIs, neutral endopeptidase inhibitors will likely be

TABLE 6 Prospective Overview of Randomized Trials for Hypertension

	Relative risks (confidence interval)					
	Stroke	CHD	CHF	Major CV event	CV death	Total mortality
ACEI vs placebo (4 trials; 12,124 pts.)	.70 (.57–.85)	.80 (.72–.89)	.84 (.68–1.04)	.79 (.73–.86)	.74 (.64–.85)	.84 (.76–.94)
CCB vs placebo (2 trials; 5520 pts.)	.61 (.44–.85)	.79 (.59–1.06)	.72 (.48–1.07)	.72 (.59–.87)	.72 (.52–.98)	.87 (.70–1.09)
ACEI vs D/βB (3 trials; 16,161 pts.)	1.05 (092–1.19)	1.00 (.88–.14)	.92 (.77–1.09)	1.00 (.93–1.08)	1.00 (.87–1.15)	1.03 (.93–1.14)
CCE vs D/βB (5 trials; 23,454 pts.)	.87 (.77–98)	1.12 (1.0–1.26)	1.12 (.95–1.33)	1.02 (.95–1.10)	1.05 (.92–1.2)	1.01 (.92–1.11)
ACEI vs CCB (2 trials; 4871 pts)	1.02 (.85–1.21)	.81 (.68–.97)	.82 (.67–1.0)	.92 (.83–1.01)	1.04 (.87–1.24)	1.03 (.91–1.18)

available, so the process of finding out what's best will likely never end. In one sense, the process is irrelevant. As the need to achieve lower goals of therapy has become obvious, so has the need to use more than one drug in the majority of hypertensives. This is nowhere better seen than among diabetic patients with hypertension. The best combination of agents, almost always to include a low dose of diuretic, therefore will be a more pertinent object of trials in the future.

Differences in Adverse Effects

As to the issue of differences in adverse effects among different agents, two points are obvious. First, no drug that causes dangerous adverse effects beyond a rare idiosyncratic reaction when given in usual doses will remain on the market, even if it slips by the approval process, as witnessed by the CCB mibefradil. Second, drugs that cause frequent bothersome though not dangerous adverse effects, such as guanethidine, will likely no longer be used now that so many other choices are available.

The various antihypertensive agents vary significantly, both in the frequency of adverse effects, and to an even greater degree in their nature. The only currently available comparisons of a representative drug from all major classes given as monotherapy to sizable numbers of patients are TOMHS [16] and the VA Cooperative Study [17]. Side effects differed among the drugs, but no one drug was markedly more or less acceptable than the others. The differences may include sexual dysfunction. Impotence was twice as common in men in the TOMHS trial given the diuretic chlorthalidone than those given a placebo, whereas less impotence was seen among those given the α-blocker doxazosin [25].

Effects on Quality of Life

Over the past 25 years, a number of studies have examined the side effects of antihypertensive agents on the quality of life (QOL) using various questionnaires and scales [26]. The results of these studies confirm the general impression; although 10–20% of patients will experience bothersome adverse effects from virtually any and every antihypertensive drug, the overall impact of therapies on QOL over 2 to 6 months of observation is positive [27,28]. Different drugs do have different profiles of side effects, however and only by careful observations can subtle differences be detected, as with sexual dysfunction in the TOMHS trial [25].

More Serious Adverse Effects

More serious problems have been blamed on various classes of antihypertensive drugs. Virtually all of these claims have come from uncontrolled, often retrospective, observational case-control studies, and most of them have been subsequently proven to be wrong.

Cancer from Reserpine, CCBs, and Diuretics

The first and perhaps most egregious claim was that the use of reserpine was associated with a twofold to fourfold increased risk of breast cancer in women, a claim made in three simultaneously published papers from outstanding investigators [29–31]. As subsequently shown by Feinstein [32], these studies were all contaminated by the bias of excluding women at high risk for cancer from the control groups. Multiple subsequently published perspective studies showed no association [33].

More recently, Pahor et al. [34,35] reported a twofold greater risk for cancer in elderly patients taking short-acting CCBs compared to users of β-blockers. Unfortunately, they made no ascertainment of drug use after the original observation that the subjects had the respective drugs in their possession, so that the actual intake of drugs is totally unknown. Multiple subsequent reports of much larger populations in which drug use was appropriately ascertained have found *no increase* in cancer among users of CCBs. In their review of 14 case-control and cohort studies, Kizer and Kimmel [36] concluded that "the ensuing clinical evidence has failed to substantiate an elevation in cancer risk, overall or site specific." Moreover, in the large placebo-controlled Syst-Eur trial in the elderly, the incidence of cancer was 31% *less* in those taking the CCB than in those on placebo [37].

On the other hand, there may be an association between diuretic use and cancers arising in renal cells [38] or the colon [39]. The association with renal cell cancers has been repeatedly observed and could reflect conversion of thiazides to mutagenic nitroso derivatives in the stomach. As noted by Hamet [40], however, these claims must all be balanced against the multiple observations that the rates of cancer are increased among untreated hypertensives as well as obese patients [41]. Even if the association is true, the incidence is nonetheless so low as to be far overshadowed by the known benefits of diuretic therapy [42].

Coronary Disease from CCBs and β-Blockers

Psaty et al. [43] reported a 60% increase in the risk of acute myocardial infarction (MI) among patients taking short-acting CCBs. This report coincided with republication of a meta-analysis of the adverse effects of high doses of short-acting CCBs in the immediate post-MI period [44]. The two publications received tremendous press coverage claiming that CCBs could endanger over 6 million hypertensives in the United States alone, leading to major disruptions in the management of patients with both angina and hypertension who were receiving these agents.

Psaty et al. [43] and Furberg et al. [44] strongly suggested that their claims against short-acting CCBs (which had never been approved for the treatment of hypertension) also carried over to the longer-acting agents (which are approved for the treatment of hypertension). As Epstein [45] and I [46] pointed out, there are significant differences in the hemodynamic and hormonal responses to short-acting versus long-acting CCBs, so that the faults of the former should not be assumed to apply to the latter. For example, in the case-control study by Alderman et al. [47], patients receiving short-acting CCBs were found to have a 3.9-fold increased risk for coronary disease compared to hypertensives taking a β-blocker, whereas those receiving long-acting CCBs actually had a lesser risk (0.76).

Whereas some additional cohort observational studies have shown a higher mortality rate among CCB users than other drugs [48,49], no such increased mortality risk for CCB users was found among the 3539 subjects in the Framingham Heart Study [50]. As Michels et al. [48] conclude: "Whether the observed elevated risk [in CCB users] is real, or a result of residual confounding by indication, or chance, or a combination of the above cannot be evaluated with certainty on the basis of these observational data." The probability that confounding was a major factor in these associations is supported by the finding that among 77,000 patients the likelihood of being prescribed a CCB rather than other antihypertensives was significantly higher for patients with coexisting coronary disease (7.8-fold) or diabetes (1.5-fold) [50].

As reviewed by Kizer and Kimmel [36], prospective, controlled data show no increase in coronary disease among users of long-acting CCBs. In the Syst-Eur RCT of elderly patients with systolic hypertension, less morbidity and mortality from coronary disease was seen in those on the CCB than in those on placebo [37].

As seen in Table 6, in the comparative trials of CCBs versus diuretic/β-blocker therapy, the slight increase in coronary events seen with CCBs was balanced by a lower risk of strokes in the CCB-treated patients, with no differences in mortality between different classes [21]. As previously noted, data from ongoing large comparative trials will settle the issue.

GROUPS WITH COEXISTING CONDITIONS

Whereas a diuretic or a β-blocker is recommended in JNC-6 for initial therapy in those with no specific indications for another type of drug, the report subsequently details a number of other factors to be considered in selecting drugs, including "demographic characteristics, concomitant diseases that may be beneficially or adversely affected by the antihypertensive agent chosen, quality of life, cost, and the use of other drugs that may lead to drug interactions" [11]. These additional factors will translate into a continuation of current trends—the use of various classes, and the specific drug chosen on the basis of multiple considerations, an approach best described as individualized [52].

Individualized Therapy

The individualized approach is predicated on the following three major principles:

The first choice may be one of a variety of antihypertensives from any of the major classes of drugs.

The choice can be logically based on the characteristics of the patients, in particular the presence of concomitant diseases.

Rather than proceeding with a second drug if the first is not effective or if side effects ensue, a substitution approach is used—stop the first drug and try another from a different class.

Characteristics of the Drugs

Each class of drugs has different features that make its members more or less attractive.

Diuretics

In the past, diuretics were almost always chosen first, particularly since reactive fluid retention with other drugs used without a diuretic often blunted their effect. Recognition of the "hidden" side effects and costs of diuretics, however, along with the lesser protection from coronary mortality in the initial trials wherein they were used in high doses, caused many investigators to doubt the wisdom of routine use of diuretics. At the least these factors have led to the more widespread use of lower doses of diuretics and their combinations with potassium-sparing agents. Low-dose diuretic-based therapy is clearly protective, and as seen in Table 6, has now been shown to be as protective as either ACEI- or CCB-based therapies.

β-Blockers

In the 1970s and 1980s, β-blockers became increasingly popular. Contraindications to their use and recognition of their potential for altering lipids adversely dampened their popularity, however. The failure to find primary protection against coronary disease in trials with a β-blocker, particularly in the elderly, further weakened the argument for their use. Their ability to provide secondary cardioprotection and to treat heart failure has recently embellished their status, however.

Indirect Vasodilators

Drugs that act primarily as indirect vasodilators—α-blockers, ACEIs, and CCBs—are being more widely advocated for initial therapy. There seems to be an inherent logic in using drugs that induce vasodilation, since an elevated peripheral resistance is the hemodynamic fault of established hypertension.

Characteristics of the Patient

Demographic Features

Individual patients' characteristics may affect the likelihood of a good response to various classes of drugs. As shown in crossover rotations of the four major classes [18,19], younger and white patients will usually respond better to either an ACEI or a β-blocker, perhaps because they tend to have higher renin levels, whereas older and black patients will respond better to diuretics and CCBs, perhaps because they have lower renin levels and their hypertension is more "volume"-mediated. These differences apply to monotherapy; with a low-dose of a diuretic as part of the regimen, responses to all other agents are largely equalized. Moreover, for the individual patient, any drug may work well or poorly, and there is no set formula that can be used to predict certain success without side effects.

Concomitant Conditions

Patients with hypertension, particularly the elderly, often have other medical problems, some related to their hypertension, others coincidental. All of the recent guidelines have listed specific choices of drugs for a variety of "compelling indications." Table 7 is the listing in the WHO-ISH report [12]. There is evidence of additional value to the use of these choices in various subgroups of hypertensives. A hypertensive patient with angina would thus logically be given a β-blocker or a CCB; a patient with CHF, an ACEI and a diuretic. Alpha-blockers, CCBs, and ACEIs are attractive choices for those in whom a diuretic or β-blocker may pose particular problems, such as diabetics or hyperlipidemic patients. In an elderly hypertensive man with benign prostatic hypertrophy, an α-blocker would be a logical choice. In view of the benefits of adding the ACEI ramipril to the therapy of high-risk patients shown in the HOPE trial [53], it would be appropriate to use an ACEI in all suitable patients at high risk for atherothrombotic cardiovascular events.

TABLE 7 Guidelines for Selecting Drug Treatment of Hypertension

Class of drug	Compeling Indications	Possible indications
Diuretics	Heart failure Elderly patients Systolic hypertension	Diabetes
β-blockers	Angina After myocardial infarct Tachyarrhythmias	Heart failure Pregnancy Diabetes
ACE inhibitors	Heart failure Left ventricular dysfunction After myocardial infarct Diabetic nephropathy	
Calcium antagonists	Angina Elderly patients Systolic hypertension	Peripheral vascular disease
α-blockers	Prostatic hypertrophy	Glucose intolerance Dyslipidemia
Angiotensin II antagonists	ACE inhibitor cough	Heart failure

Substitution Rather Than Addition

If the first choice, even if based on all reasonable criteria, does not lower the BP much or is associated with persistent, bothersome side effects, that drug should be stopped and one from another class should be tried, thereby the least number of drugs should be needed to achieve the desired fall in BP with the fewest side effects.

Patients with milder hypertension will often need only one drug, therefore substitution should work for them. For those with more severe hypertension, the first drug may do all that is expected and still not be enough. The addition of a second or, if needed, a third drug added in a stepwise manner therefore is logical.

RESISTANT HYPERTENSION

Resistance to therapy may occur for many reasons (Table 8). The most likely is volume overload caused by either excessive sodium intake or inadequate diuretic. In one series of 91 patients whose BPs remained above 140/90 mmHg despite use of three antihypertensive agents, the mechanisms were suboptimal drug regimen (mainly inadequate diuretic) in 43%, intolerance to medications in 22%, noncompliance in 10%, and secondary hypertension in 11% [54]. In a disadvantaged minority population, uncontrolled hypertension is most

TABLE 8 Causes of Inadequate Responsiveness to Therapy

- Pseudo-resistance
  - White coat or office elevations
  - Pseudohypertension in the elderly
- Nonadherence to therapy
  - Side effects or costs of medication
  - Lack of consistent and continuous primary care
  - Inconvenient and chaotic dosing schedules
  - Instructions not understood
  - Organic brain syndrome (e.g., memory deficit)
- Drug-related causes
  - Doses too low
  - Inappropriate combinations
  - Rapid inactivation (e.g., hydralazine)
  - Drug actions and interactions
    - Sympathomimetics
      - Nasal decongestants
      - Appetite suppressants
      - Cocaine and other street drugs
      - Caffeine
    - Oral contraceptives
- Adrenal steroids
- Licorice (as may be found in chewing tobacco)
- Cyclosporine, tacrolimus
- Erythropoietin
- NSAIDS
- Associated conditions
  - Smoking
  - Increased obesity
  - Sleep apnea
  - Insulin resistance or hyperinsulinemia
  - Ethanol intake more than 1 oz a day
  - Anxiety-induced hyperventilation or panic attacks
  - Chronic pain
  - Intense vasoconstriction (Raynaud phenomenon, arteritis)
- Identifiable causes of hypertension
- Volume overload
  - Excess sodium intake
  - Progressive renal damage (nephrosclerosis)
  - Fluid retention from reduction of blood pressure
  - Inadequate diuretic therapy

Source: From Ref. 11.

closely related to limited access to care, noncompliance with therapy, and alcohol-related problems [55].

Before starting a workup for identifiable causes and altering drug therapy, BPs should be checked out of the office setting, since as many as half of resistant patients turn out to have controlled hypertension [56]. Recall as well the evidence that patients may appear to be resistant only because their physicians simply do not keep increasing their therapy [57].

MANEUVERS TO IMPROVE ADHERENCE TO THERAPY

Causes of Poor Adherence

Obviously, physicians and their assistants must be willing to provide whatever therapy is needed to control hypertension. The patient is the most important contributor to the success or failure of therapy, however. The most careful physician prescribing the most effective therapy will not control hypertension unless the patient is willing and able to take the pills and modify his or her lifestyle as needed.

Hypertensive patients have special problems related to the nature of their disease. Many are largely unaware of the definition, possible causes, sequelae, and therapeutic needs of hypertension. Being asymptomatic, patients may have little motivation to seek or follow treatment. Many are found to have high BP at the age (late 30s and early 40s) when the threat of a loss of vigor and vitality is insidiously beginning, and the recognition of hypertension often provokes a strong denial reaction. Moreover, the diagnosis carries considerable economic and social threats—loss of job, insurance, and sexual potency—that may further inhibit people from accepting the diagnosis and dealing with the problem.

Additional barriers may preclude long-term management in the steadily increasing number of uninsured people in the United States who often receive only episodic care at public hospitals and who may not be able to afford their medications [58].

Moreover, the therapy of hypertension has all the wrong characteristics for compliance, requiring daily, continuous, lifelong modification with no obvious benefit to the patient but often bothersome side effects and considerable expense. The problems are often compounded by clinical practices such as the use of multiple daily doses of medications.

Ways to Improve Pill Taking

In their review of more than 1500 citations about ways to improve pill taking, Haynes et al. [59] concluded that

> The interventions that were effective were complex, including various combinations of more convenient care, information, counseling, reminders, self-monitoring, reinforcement, family therapy, and other forms of additional supervision or attention. Even the most effective interventions did not lead to substantial improvements in adherence.

Nonetheless, reasonable and likely helpful ways to increase maintenance of therapy are available [60,61], as summarized in Table 9. A few deserve additional comment.

Compared to physicians, nurses using detailed clinical protocols can provide more efficient follow-up care [62] with comparable patients' outcomes [63].

To reduce costs, the minimum effective doses should be prescribed, generic brands should be used, and larger doses of tablets that are not specially designed for slow release should be broken in half with readily available pill cutters.

More and more once-a-day formulations are available so that fewer tablets are needed.

The use of less expensive medications is being emphasized in an attempt to reduce the costs of health care and to ensure that the uninsured indigent are not denied needed medications whenever there is no safety net in place to ensure care for the poor. Although the indigent can often be provided medications through pharmaceutical company programs, the cost of therapy remains a barrier to the management of hypertension [58].

On the other hand, simplistic comparisons of costs based purely on the costs per tablet may be misleading. For example, in a survey of hypertensive patients in South Carolina, the experiences of 947 who were given three 60-mg doses of short-acting generic diltiazem per day were compared to the experiences of 301 given one 180-mg dose of the more expensive brand of long-acting diltiazem per day [64]. Those on the once-a-day dose required fewer concomitant antihypertensive drugs, adhered more closely to therapy, and required less expenditures for physician and hospital services. Although their drug costs were higher, their total costs of health care were less.

THE NEED TO REACH THE GOAL OF THERAPY

The optimal goal of antihypertensive therapy in most patients with combined systolic and diastolic hypertension who were not at high risk is a BP of below 140/90 mmHg. The greatest benefit is likely derived from lowering the diastolic pressure to 80 to 85 mmHg. Not only is there no proven benefit

TABLE 9 Guidelines to Improve Maintenance of Antihypertensive Therapy

Be aware of the problem and be alert to signs of inadequate intake of medications
- Recognize and manage depression

Articulate the goal of therapy: to reduce blood pressure to near normotension with few or no side effects

Educate the patient about the disease and its treatment
- Provide individual assessments of current risks and potential benefits of control
- Involve the patient in decision making
- Provide written instructions
- Encourage family support

Maintain contact with the patient
- Encourage visits and calls to allied health personnel
- Allow the pharmacist to monitor therapy
- Give feedback to the patient via home BP readings
- Make contact with patients who do not return

Keep care inexpensive and simple
- Do the least workup needed to rule out secondary causes
- Obtain follow-up laboratory data only yearly unless indicated more often
- Use home blood pressure readings
- Use nondrug, low-cost therapies
- Use once-daily doses of long-acting drugs
- Use generic drugs and break larger doses of tablets in half
- If appropriate, use combination tablets
- Use calendar blister packs (if and when they are marketed)
- Tailor medication to daily routines
- Use detailed clinical protocols monitored by nurses and assistants

Prescribe according to pharmacological principles
- Add one drug at a time
- Start with small doses, aiming for 5- to 10-mmHg reductions at each step
- Have medication taken immediately on awakening in the morning or after 4 a.m. if patient awakens to void

Be willing to stop unsuccessful therapy and try a different approach

Anticipate and address side effects
- Adjust therapy to ameliorate side effects that do not spontaneously disappear

Continue to add effective and tolerated drugs, stepwise, in sufficient doses to achieve the goal of therapy

Provide feedback and validation of success

with more intensive control, but also there is added cost and the potential for more side effects associated with more intensive antihypertensive therapy.

In elderly patients with ISH, the goal should be a systolic BP of 140 to145 mmHg since that was the level reached in the RCTs in which benefit was shown. Caution is advised if diastolic pressures inadvertently fall below 65 mmHg. In such an event, less than ideal reductions in systolic levels need to be balanced against the potential of harm if diastolic levels fall below that level [65].

In patients who start with a diastolic pressure between 90 and 94 mmHg, lowering the BP by about 10 mmHg appears to provide optimal cardiovascular protection [66].

More intensive therapy to attain a diastolic pressure of 80 mmHg or lower may be desirable in some groups, including the following:

Black patients, who are at greater risk for hypertensive complications and who may continue to have progressive renal damage despite a diastolic pressure of 85 to 90 mmHg.

Patients with diabetes mellitus, in whom a BP below 130/85 mm Hg reduces the incidence of cardiovascular events [2]. In the United Kingdom Prospective Diabetes Study (UKPDS) population of 3642 type 2 diabetic hypertensives, no threshold of risk for systolic pressure was noted; the lower the systolic BP down to 110 mmHg, the lower the risk of both micro- and macrovascular complications related to diabetes [67].

Patients with slowly progressive chronic renal disease excreting more than 1 to 2 g of protein per day, in whom reducing the BP to 125/75 may slow the rate of loss of renal function [68].

Despite the concerns over a J curve if BP is lowered below the level needed to maintain perfusion to the heart and brain, we should not lose sight of the fact that the reason for the lesser protection found among most treated hypertensives reflects undertreatment, not overtreatment. Clearly, it is essential that all patients have their systolic BP brought down at least to 140 and diastolic BP to the 85 to 90 range to provide the demonstrated benefits of therapy.

CONCLUSION

When all of the previously described strategies for improved treatment of hypertension are considered, an even simpler approach than that recommended in current guidelines can be envisioned, namely

Start therapy in virtually all patients who are in need of antihypertensive drugs with a low dose of a once-a-day thiazide diuretic, (e.g., 12.5 mg of hydrochlorothiazide). The only exceptions would be patients allergic to thiazides and those in whom prior low-dose thiazide therapy has been found to precipitate bothersome adverse effects such as gout or erectile dysfunction. The rationale for starting with a low-dose of a diuretic is that such inexpensive therapy has been shown to be equally effective as other classes, particularly in the elderly, and the efficacy of all other classes is enhanced in the presence of a diuretic.

Even with low doses, diuretics may cause potassium wastage so that a combination with a potassium-sparing agent should usually be prescribed. Although triamterene has been the usual choice, the evidence of additional cardioprotective effects of spironolactone [69] make that an attractive alternative for a thiazide + potassium sparer combination.

For those with a compelling indication for another drug, as listed in Table 7, start with a low dose of that agent in addition in addition to the low dose of the diuretic. In those with high-normal (130–139/85–89) or stage 1 hypertension (140–149/90–99), the dose of diuretic may be reduced further if either a β-blocker or an ACEI is indicated since combination tablets with only 6.25 mg of HCTZ are available with those classes.

It may be prudent to start only with the agent needed for the "compelling" indication if the BP is minimally elevated or if there are concerns about lowering BP too quickly, as in frail, elderly patients with orthostatic hypotension.

If the BP does not reach the goal of therapy with the combination of a low-dose diuretic plus the agent needed for a "compelling" indication, a third drug should be added. Most likely, the third drug should be either an ACEI/ARB or a CCB, depending upon whether one or the other has been chosen as the second drug.

It is likely preferable to add additional drugs rather than increase the dose of initial choices to high levels, thereby avoiding dose-dependent adverse effects. This is particularly true for diuretics in which little additional antihypertensive effect is likely for doses of HCTZ beyond 12.5 mg/day unless very large amounts of sodium are ingested or renal insufficiency is present.

Whether or not this simpler approach is used, the blood pressure in virtually all hypertensive patients can be reduced to the appropriate goal of therapy. It may take considerable time, effort, and expense to reach the goal, but the effort is clearly worthwhile.

REFERENCES

1. Kaplan NM. Hypertension in the population at large. In: *Clinical Hypertension*. 8th ed. Baltimore: Williams & Wilkins, 2002.
2. Hannson L, Zanchetti A, Carruthers SG, et al. Effects of intensive blood-pressure lowering and low-dose aspirin in patients with hypertension. *Lancet*. 1998;351:1755–1762.
3. Singer GM, Odama U, Robin JC, Black HR. How well does a specialist clinic

compared to managed care organizations for hypertension control? *Am J Hypertens*. 2001;14:3A (abstract).

4. Verdecchia P. Prognostic value of ambulatory blood pressure. *Hypertension*. 2000;35:844–851.
5. Staessen JA, Thijs L, Fagard R, et al. Predicting cardiovascular risk using conventional vs. ambulatory blood pressure in older patients with systolic hypertension. *JAMA*. 1999;282:539–546.
6. Kaplan NM. Measurement of blood pressure. In: *Clinical Hypertension*. 8th ed. Baltimore: Williams & Wilkins, 2002.
7. McAlister FA, Straus SE. Measurement of blood pressure: an evidence based review. *Br Med J*. 2001;322:908–911.
8. Schwartz JE, Verdecchia P, Pickering TG, Lapuerta P. Ambulatory vs. clinic blood pressure as a predictor of cardiovascular morbidity incidence. *Am J Hypertens*. 2001;14:22A (abstract).
9. Bjorklund K, Lind L, Andrén B, Lithell H. White-coat hypertension is related to insulin resistance, but not increased left ventricular mass in elderly men. *Am J Hypertens*. 2001;14:5A (abstract).
10. Rogers MAM, Small D, Buchan DA, Butch CA, Stewart CM, Krenzer BE, Husovsky HL. Home monitoring service improves mean arterial pressure in patients with essential hypertension: a randomized, controlled trial. *Ann Int Med*. 2001;134:1024–1032.
11. Joint National Committee. The sixth report of the Joint National Committee on Detection, Evaluation, and Treatment of High Blood Pressure (JNC VI). *Arch Int Med* 1997;157:2413–2446.
12. Guidelines Subcommittee. 1999 World Health Organization–International Society of Hypertension guidelines for the management of hypertension. *J Hypertens*. 1999;17:151–183.
13. Ramsay LE, Williams B, Johnston GD, et al. Guidelines for management of hypertension. *J Human Hypertens*. 1999;13:569–592.
14. Expert Panel. Executive summary of the third report of the National Cholesterol Education Program (NCEP) expert panel on detection, evaluation, and treatment of high blood cholesterol in adults (adult treatment panel III). *JAMA*. 2001;285:2486–2497.
15. Kaplan NM. The appropriate goals of antihypertensive therapy. *Ann Int Med*. 1992;116:686–690.
16. Neaton JD, Grimm RH Jr, Prineas RJ, et al. Treatment of mild hypertension study (TOMHS). *JAMA*. 1993;270:713–724.
17. Materson BJ, Reda DJ, Cushman WC. Department of Veterans Affairs single-drug therapy of hypertension study. *Am J Hypertens*. 1995;8: 189–192.
18. Morgan TO, Anderson AIE, MacInnis RJ. ACE inhibitors, beta-blockers, calcium blockers, and diuretics for the control of systolic hypertension. *Am J Hypertens*. 2001;14:241–247.
19. Dickerson JEC, Hingorani AD, Ashby MJ, et al. Optimisation of antihypertensive treatment by crossover rotation of four major classes. *Lancet*. 1999;353:2008–2013.

20. Psaty BM, Smith NL, Siscovick DS, et al. Health outcomes associated with antihypertensive therapies used as first-line agents. *JAMA*. 1997;277: 739–745.
21. Blood Pressure Lowering Treatment Trialists' Collaboration. Effects of ACE inhibitors, calcium antagonists, and other blood-pressure-lowering drugs. *Lancet*. 2000;355:1955–1964.
22. Schrier RW, Estacio RO. Additional follow-up from the ABCD trial in patients with type 2 diabetes and hypertension. *N Engl J Med*. 2000;343:1969.
23. Hansson L, Lindholm LH, Ekbom T, et al. Randomised trial of old and new antihypertensive drugs in elderly patients. *Lancet*. 1999;354:1751–1756.
24. He J, Whelton PK. Selection of initial antihypertensive drug therapy. *Lancet*. 2000;356:1942–1943.
25. Grimm RH Jr, Grandits GA, Prineas RJ, et al. Long-term effects on sexual function of five antihypertensive drugs and nutritional hygienic treatment of hypertensive men and women. *Hypertension*. 1997;29:8–14.
26. Testa MA. Methods and applications of quality-of-life measurement during antihypertensive therapy. *Curr Hypertens Rep*. 2000;2:530–537.
27. Weir MR, Prisant LM, Papademetriou V, et al. Antihypertensive therapy and quality of life. *Am J Hypertens*. 1996;9:854–859.
28. Wiklund I, Halling K, Ryden-Bergsten T, et al. What is the effect of lowering the blood pressure on quality of life? *Arch Mal Couer Vaiss*. 1999; 92:1079–1082.
29. Armstrong B, Stevens N, Doll R. Retrospective study of the association between use of rauwolfia derivatives and breast cancer in English women. *Lancet*. 1974;21;672–675.
30. Boston Collaborative Drug Surveillance Program. Reserpine and breast cancer. Lancet. 1974;2:669–671.
31. Heinonen OP, Shapiro S, Tuomenen L, Turunen MI. Reserpine use in relation to breast cancer. *Lancet*. 1974;2:674–677.
32. Feinstein AR. Scientific standards in epidemiologic studies of the menace of daily life. *Science*. 1988;242:1257–1263.
33. Mayes LC, Horwitz R, Feinstein AR. A collection of 56 topics with contradictory results in case-control research. *Int J Epidemiol*. 1988;17: 680–685.
34. Pahor M, Guralnik JM, Ferrucci L, et al. Calcium-channel blockade and incidence of cancer in aged populations. *Lancet*. 1996;348:493–497.
35. Pahor M, Guralnik JM, Salive ME, et al. Do calcium channel blockers increase the risk of cancer? *Am J Hypertens*. 1996;9:694–699.
36. Kizer JR, Kimmel SE. Epidemiologic review of the calcium channel blocker drugs: an up-to-date perspective on the proposed hazards. *Arch Int Med*. 2001;161:1145–1158.
37. Staessen JA, Fagard R, Thijs L, et al. Randomised double-blind comparison of placebo and active treatment for older patients with isolated systolic hypertension. *Lancet*. 1997;350:757–764.
38. Grossman E, Messerli FH, Goldbourt U. Does diuretic therapy increase the risk of renal cell carcinoma? *Am J Cardiol*. 1999;83:1090–1093.

39. Tenenbaum A, Motro M, Jones M, et al. Is diuretic therapy associated with an increased risk of colon cancer? *Am J Med.* 2001;110:143–145.
40. Hamet P. Cancer and hypertension. *Hypertension.* 1996;28:321–324.
41. Yuan J-M, Castelao JE, Gago-Dominguez M, et al. Hypertension, obesity and their medications in relation to renal cell carcinoma. *Br J Cancer.* 1998;77:1508–1513.
42. Lip GYH, Ferner RE. Diuretic therapy for hypertension: a cancer risk? *J Human Hypertens.* 1999;13:421–423.
43. Psaty BM, Heckbert SR, Koepsell TD, et al. The risk of myocardial infarction associated with antihypertensive drug therapies. *JAMA.* 1995;274: 620–625.
44. Furberg CD, Psaty BM, Meyer JV. Nifedipine: dose-related increase in mortality in patients with coronary heart disease. *Circulation.* 1995;92: 1326–1331.
45. Epstein M. Calcium antagonists. *Am J Hypertens.* 1996;9:110–121.
46. Kaplan NM. Do calcium antagonist cause death, gastrointestinal bleeding, and cancer? *Am J Cardiol.* 1996;78:932–933.
47. Alderman MH, Cohen H, Roque R, Madhavan S. Effect of long-acting and short-acting calcium antagonists on cardiovascular outcomes in hypertensive patients. *Lancet.* 1997;349:594–598.
48. Michels KB, Rosner BA, Manson JE, et al. Prospective study of calcium channel blocker use, cardiovascular disease, and total mortality among hypertensive women. *Circulation.* 1998;97:1540–1548.
49. McInnes G, Hole D, Lever A, et al. Outcome differences between ACE inhibitor and calcium channel blocker treated hypertensive patients. *J Hypertens.* 2000;18(suppl. 4):S155 (abstract)
50. Abascal VM, Larson MG, Evans JC, et al. Calcium antagonists and mortality risk in men and women with hypertension in the Framingham heart study. *Arch Int Med.* 1998;158:1882–1886.
51. Leader S, Mallick R, Roht L. Using medication history to measure confounding by indication in assessing calcium channel blockers and other antihypertensive therapy. *J Human Hypertens.* 2001;15:153–159.
52. Pignone M, Mulrow CD. Using cardiovascular risk profiles to individualise hypertensive treatment. *Br Med J.* 2001;322:1164–1166.
53. Yusuf S. Clinical, public health, and research implications of the Heart Outcomes Prevention Evaluation (HOPE) study. *Eur Heart J.* 2001;22: 103–104.
54. Yakovlevitch M, Black HR. Resistant hypertension in a tertiary care clinic. *Arch Int Med.* 1991;151:1786–1792.
55. Shea S, Misra D, Ehrlich MH, et al. Predisposing factors for severe, uncontrolled hypertension in an inner-city minority population. *N Eng J Med.* 1992;327:776–781.
56. Redon J, Campos C, Narciso ML, et al. Prognostic value of ambulatory blood pressure monitoring in refratory hypertension. *Hypertension.* 1998;31: 712–718.

57. Berlowitz DR, Ash AS, Hickey EC, et al. Inadequate management of blood pressure in a hypertensive population. *N Eng J Med* 1998;339:1957–1963.
58. Tamblyn R, Laprise R, Hanley JA, et al. Adverse events associated with prescription drug cost-sharing among poor and elderly persons. *JAMA*. 2001;285:421–429.
59. Haynes RB, McKibbon KA, Kanani R. Systemic review of randomised trials of interventions to assist patients to follow prescriptions for medications. *Lancet*. 1996;348:383–386.
60. Miller NH, Hill M, Kottke T, Ockene IS. The multilevel compliance challenge. *Circulation*. 1997;95:1085–1090.
61. Freis ED. Improving treatment effectiveness in hypertension. *Arch Int Med* 1999;159:2517–2521.
62. DeBusk RF, West JA, Miller NH, Baylor CB. Treating the patient with disease(s) vs treating disease(s) in the patient. *Arch Int Med*. 1999;159: 2739–2742.
63. Mundinger MO, Kane RL, Lenz ER, et al. Primary care outcomes in patients treated by nurse practitioners or physicians. *JAMA*. 2000;283:59–68.
64. Sclar DA, Tessier GC, Skaer TL, et al. Effect of pharmaceutical formulation of diltiazem on the utilization of Medicaid and health maintenance organization services. *Curr Ther Res*. 1994;55:1136–1149.
65. Kaplan NM. What is goal pressure for the treatment of hypertension? *Arch Int Med*. 2001;161:1480–1482.
66. Cooper SP, Hardy RJ, Labarthe DR, et al. The relation between degree of blood pressure reduction and mortality among hypertensives in the Hypertension Detection and Follow-Up Program. *Am J Epidemiol*. 1988; 127:387–392.
67. Adler AI, Stratton IM, Neil HAW, et al. Association of systolic blood pressure with macrovascular and microvascular complications of type 2 diabetes (UKPDS 36). *Br Med J*. 2000;321:412–419.
68. Lazarus JM, Bourgoignie JJ, Buckalew VM, et al. Achievement and safety of a low blood pressure goal in chronic renal disease. *Hypertension* 1997;29: 641–650.
69. Pitt B, Zannad F, Remme WJ, et al. The effect of spironolactone on morbidity and mortality in patients with severe heart failure. *N Eng J Med*. 1999;341:709–717.

5

Weight Reduction

Shiriki Kumanyika and Nayyar Iqbal
University of Pennsylvania School of Medicine,
Philadelphia, Pennsylvania, U.S.A.

INTRODUCTION

Of the various lifestyle risk factors for hypertension, body weight is perhaps the one most readily and strongly linked to blood pressure levels [1]. The Sixth Report of the Joint National Committee on the Prevention, Detection, Evaluation and Treatment of High Blood Pressure (JNC VI) [2] notes the consistent correlation of excess body weight with increased blood pressure, the increased risk of hypertension and other cardiovascular (CVD) risk factors with increased abdominal fat, the probable reduction of blood pressure in most overweight persons with hypertension with a weight loss of as little as 4.5 kg, and the ability of weight loss to enhance the blood pressure-lowering effect of antihypertensive medications. "Lose weight if overweight" is the first listed of the JNC VI lifestyle modification recommendations for hypertension prevention and management. The primary prevention of hypertension—that is, decreasing the likelihood that individuals will develop hypertension—is also facilitated by weight reduction [3]. The National Heart, Lung, and Blood Institute (NHLBI) expert panel on the identification, evaluation, and treatment of overweight and obesity in adults [4] has reaffirmed that improved blood pressure control is one of the potential benefits of modest weight reduction. In addition, because obesity is also associated with numerous other health problems and has increased dramatically in prevalence in recent decades, weight reduction and prevention of inappropriate weight gain have become public health priorities generally [5].

This chapter reviews the evidence supporting recommendations for weight reduction as a blood pressure control strategy, focusing particularly on lifestyle intervention studies. Evidence from trials of weight reduction involving antiobesity drugs or obesity surgery is included to provide a complete picture of relevant issues. As background we describe epidemiologic observations of associations between body weight and blood pressure levels in population data. Following the review of weight reduction studies we summarize current thinking on the mechanisms whereby weight and blood pressure are interrelated. We conclude with comments about implications for public health programs and clinical practice in general, and particularly for African Americans, in whom obesity is even more prevalent than in the U.S. population overall.

EPIDEMIOLOGIC DATA ON BODY WEIGHT AND BLOOD PRESSURE

Comparisons Across Populations

The positive association between weight and blood pressure has been documented in men and women both within and across populations that are diverse with respect to ethnicity, region of residence, body weight levels, and hypertension prevalence [1,6]. The INTERSALT study collected standardized data from samples of 20- to 59-year-old men and women in 52 centers around the world. Relative weight [either body mass index (BMI, calculated as weight in kg divided by the square of height in meters) or weight adjusted for height] was positively associated with both systolic blood pressure (SBP) and diastolic blood pressure (DBP) in almost all of the INTERSALT study populations after adjustment for age, alcohol intake, and sodium and potassium excretion, and the association was statistically significant in a substantial number of these populations [6,7]. Mean SBP and DBP increased, respectively, by 0.91 and 0.75 mmHg for men and 0.72 and 0.50 mmHg, respectively, for women per unit of BMI [6]. The magnitude of the dose response of blood pressure increase with increasing body weight is relatively modest; that is a correlation in the range of .20 [7]. The association, however, is extremely reproducible, is independent of other lifestyle influences on blood pressure, is relatively consistent across sex and age, and is of sufficient magnitude to have important implications for the distribution of blood pressure within any given population. On average, in the INTERSALT population a 10-kg difference in body weight was associated with a SBP/DBP difference of 3.0/2.2 mmHg [6]. On a population basis, blood pressure differences of this magnitude are associated with substantial differences in the rates of mortality from stroke and coronary heart disease [8].

Complementary to the INTERSALT data are data reported by the International Collaborative Study on Hypertension in Blacks (ICSHIB). The ICSHIB studied the association of body weight with blood pressure within and across populations of African descent but living in societies with different degrees of westernization (i.e., in Nigeria, Cameroon, Caribbean countries, and Maywood, Illinois, near Chicago) [9]. In this sample of more than 9000 men and women ages 25 to 74 years, the prevalence of obesity (defined as BMI $\geq$ 31.1 for men and $\geq$ 32.2 for women) ranged from 1–20% in men and from 5–36% in women. Hypertension was approximately three times more prevalent in Maywood (30% and 35% for men and women, respectively) compared to rural Africa (12% and 14% for men and women, respectively). Within each of the ICSHIB sites, the association of obesity with hypertension—estimated from the ratio of the age-adjusted prevalence of hypertension in the obese vs. the nonobese—was relatively consistent, in the range of 1.28 to 2.25, with the exception of the African men from rural farm and urban poor communities (ratios of .74 and .96, respectively). Similar results were reported when the weight variable used was "overweight" (defined as BMI $\geq$ 27.8 for men and $\geq$ 27.3 for women) [9].

Cross-Sectional U.S. Data

The cross-sectional association of BMI with blood pressure and hypertension prevalence in U.S. adults has been described by Brown et al. [10] based on detailed analyses of data from the 1988–1994 National Health and Nutrition Examination Survey (NHANES III). Both DBP and SBP increase across BMI categories in such a way that there is a 10 to 11 mmHg higher SBP and 6 to 7 mmHg higher DBP in those with BMI of 30 or greater compared to those with BMI less than 25 [10]. The difference in hypertension prevalence across BMI categories in the NHANES III data is shown in Fig. 1 by age or by ethnicity. The prevalence of hypertension increases with age, but within each category it also increases across BMI categories. For example, among 20- to 59-year-old men and women, those with a BMI of 30 or greater are 4.5 to 7.8 times as likely to have hypertension as their same-sex counterparts with BMI $<$ 25 [10]. The gradient is less consistent and less striking at ages 60 and older, but the highest prevalence of

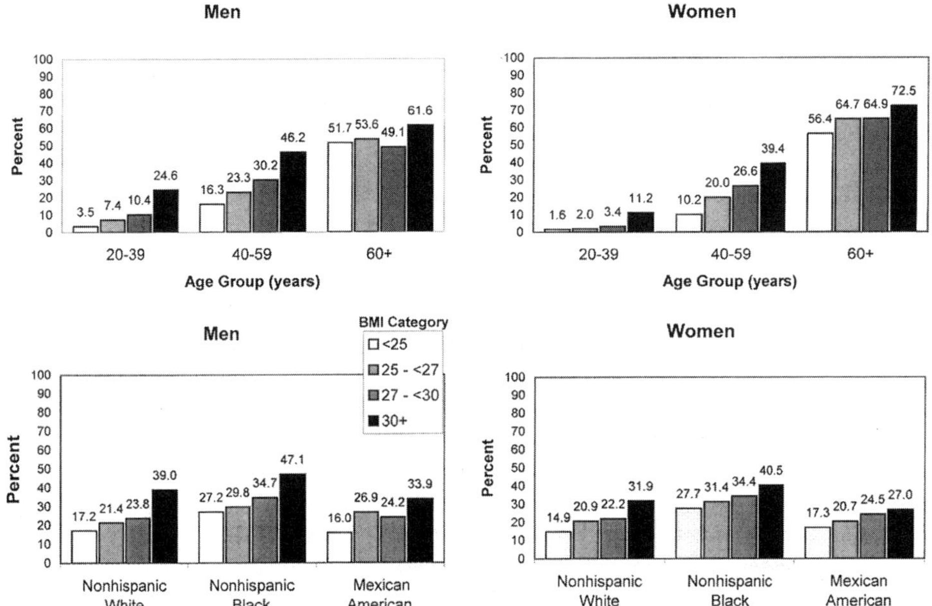

FIGURE 1 Association of body mass index (BMI) category with hypertension prevalence within sex and by age group or ethnicity in U.S. adults ages 20 years and older. Data are from the 1988–1994 National Health and Nutrition Examination Survey (NHANES III). *Source*: Adapted from Ref. 10.

hypertension is still observed in those with BMI of 30 or greater. Figure 1 also shows that the positive gradient in hypertension prevalence across BMI categories applies to non-Hispanic whites and blacks and to Mexican Americans. Within sex, non-Hispanic black men and women have the highest prevalence of hypertension in every BMI category.

Longitudinal Data

The association of excess weight and weight gain over time with the development of hypertension is evident in longitudinal data for diverse populations [1], including data from several recent or ongoing prospective studies. In 7-year follow-up data from the Coronary Artery Risk in Young Adults study (CARDIA)—which involved more than 5000 men and women ages 18 to 30 years at enrollment—both baseline BMI and change in BMI were significantly associated with SBP and DBP in blacks and whites of both sexes [11]. In addition, together with other lifestyle risk factors, obesity appeared to explain a substantial proportion of the increasing black–white differences in blood pressure that emerged in this young adult sample during the follow-up period. The average baseline BMI levels in the CARDIA study population were between 24 and 26; that is, below or in the lower end of the range that is now considered overweight [4]. Mean SBP and DBP were in the desirable range (66 to 71 mmHg systolic and 105 to 116 mmHg diastolic), and fewer than 1% were taking antihypertensive medication, suggesting that preventing weight gain in this age group might prevent the age-related rise in blood pressure and subsequent hypertension [11].

Additional longitudinal analyses of the association of relative weight and the development of hypertension over a 10-year period are available from two large prospective studies of primarily white U.S. male and female health professionals: the Nurses' Health Study, which in 1976 began biennial follow-up of 121,701 female registered nurses, aged 30 to 55 years, and the Health Professionals Study, which in 1986 began following 51,529 men, aged 40 to 75 years in 1986 [12]. In analyses limited to the period between 1986 and 1996 that included approximately 78,000 women and 46,000 men, 16.5% of the women and 19.2% of the men were newly diagnosed as having high blood pressure. As shown in Fig. 2, there was a three- to fourfold risk gradient for developing hypertension from the lowest to the highest BMI category over the 10-year observation period. In a prior analysis of 4-year follow-up data from the Nurses' Health Study (from 1989 to 1993), Field et al. [13] reported an association of weight gain but not weight cycling ("severe" and "mild" weight cycling were defined, respectively, as having intentionally lost ≥9 kg or ≥4.5 kg three or more times during the follow-up period) with the development of hypertension. The risk of developing hypertension increased 20% for each 4.5 kg weight gain, but only an insignificant association was observed for weight cycling, by either definition, after adjustment for baseline BMI and weight gain [13]. Other examples of populations in which the longitudinal association of BMI and weight change with blood pressure change has been documented include the Tromsø Study in Norway [14] and the San Antonio Heart Study of Mexican Americans in Texas [15].

Body Fat and Body Fat Distribution

As will be discussed, the mechanism whereby excess weight causes blood pressure elevations is still uncertain. There have been attempts, however, to determine whether the association with BMI reflects an effect of fat mass vs. lean body mass or of abdominal or upper body fat. Based on their review of studies published through the mid-1980s, MacMahon et al. [16] concluded

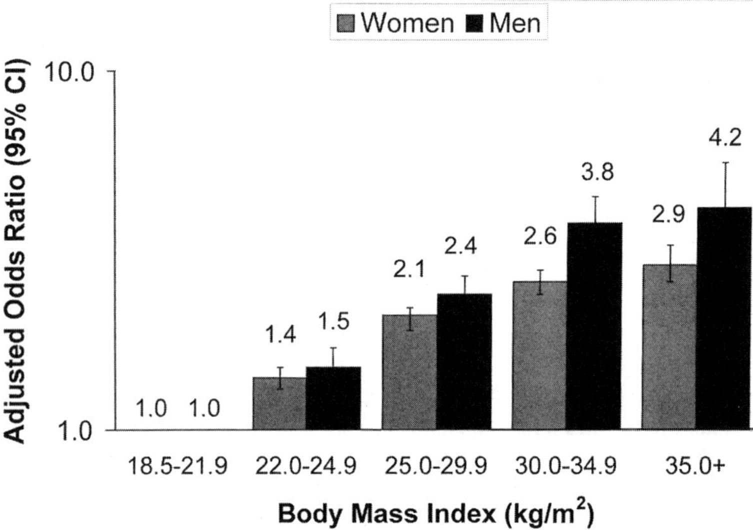

FIGURE 2 Risk of developing hypertension over 10 years of follow-up (1986–1996) according to initial BMI level for female (Nurses' Health Study) and male (Health Professionals Study) health professionals, adjusted for age, smoking status, and race. CI = confidence interval. *Source*: Adapted from Ref. 12.

that while there was some evidence of a specific influence of total fat mass vs. lean body mass on blood pressure levels there was also evidence in the opposite direction (e.g., an undifferentiated effect of excess weight or a primary effect of lean body mass as such). Discrepancies in this respect are difficult to reconcile because of the high correlation of body weight with total body fatness in overweight and obese individuals (e.g., most excess weight is excess fat). In addition, most of the weight lost by obese individuals is body fat.

With respect to body fat distribution, MacMahon et al. found the evidence more consistent in suggesting an association of abdominal or upper body fat with elevated blood pressure, in spite of the differing approaches to assessing and defining these fat distribution variables across studies [16]. This impression is supported by more recent studies. For example, Sakurai et al. [17] demonstrated this association using the waist-to-hip circumference ratio (WHR) on SBP and DBP levels in a cross-sectional study of over 2200 middle-aged (49 to 55 years) Japanese men who were self-defense officials and, on average, relatively lean (mean BMI was 23.8). Similarly, Harris et al. [18] demonstrated gradients of hypertension prevalence, independent of BMI level, across quintiles of WHR, waist circumference, and waist/height index in the large multicenter Atherosclerosis Risk in Communities Study cohort of more than 15,000 adults initially ages 45 to 64 years. Gillum et al. [19] evaluated the 10-year prospective association of body fat distribution in data for 25- to 74-year-old men and women in the National Health and Nutrition Examination Survey (NHANES) I Epidemiologic Follow-up Study using the ratio to subscapular to triceps skinfold thickness as a measure of truncal obesity. A significant association of subscapular skinfold with hypertension was observed in white women and white men and in black women with low BMI.

BLOOD PRESSURE RESPONSE TO WEIGHT REDUCTION

Overview

There is consistent and convincing evidence that weight reduction has a favorable effect on blood pressure control across the continuum from prevention to treatment [4,16,20–24]. The NHLBI Expert Panel on the Identification, Evaluation, and Treatment of Overweight and Obesity [4] identified 76 potentially informative randomized controlled trials (RCTs) relating to the influence of weight reduction on blood pressure, including 60 lifestyle interventions and 16 studies of antiobesity drugs, in literature published between 1980 and 1997. Of these, 35 studies were considered acceptable for the formal evidence review, and some permitted evaluation of the specific effects of weight reduction on blood pressure apart from other concurrent lifestyle changes, such as sodium reduction or decreased alcohol intake. Sixteen of these studies involved hypertensive patients and 19 involved individuals with normal blood pressure or blood pressure at the higher end of the normal range. This panel gave the highest rating (category A) to evidence based on "substantial number of studies involving substantial numbers of participants" and based on the "endpoints of well-designed RCTs (or trials that depart only minimally from randomization) that provide a consistent pattern of findings in the population for which the recommendation is made" [4]. After reviewing the eligible studies related to blood pressure, the panel concluded that there was category A evidence that "weight loss produced by lifestyle modifications reduces blood pressure in overweight hypertensive patients ... and in overweight non-hypertensive individuals."

Following are highlights from six of the most recent, relatively long-term trials that were designed at least in part to specifically evaluate the effects of weight reduction on blood pressure [25–34]. These trials, which are listed in Tables 1 and 2, were conducted in diverse populations and settings and used different types of blood pressure endpoints.

TABLE 1 Randomized Trials of Lifestyle Weight Reduction to Prevent Hypertension

Study	Sample size[a]	Demographic characteristics: Mean age	Male (%)	White (%)	Components of weight loss intervention	Follow-up	Average initial BMI (kg/m^2) range and blood pressure (mmHg): BMI	SBP	DBP	Average net (active control) effect, Change in weight (kg) and BP (mmHg): Weight	SBP	DBP
Hypertension Prevention trial (HPT) [25]	380	38	68	80	Reduced calorie intake	36 months	29.0	125.0	83.2	−3.5	−2.4	−1.8
		39	62	82	Reduced calorie and sodium intake		29.0	124.5	82.9	−2.0	−1.0	−1.3
Trials of Hypertension Prevention, phase I, (TOHP I) [26,27]	564	43	72	79	Reduced calorie intake and increased physical activity	18 months	29.5	124.4	83.8	−3.9	−2.9	−2.3
Trials of Hypertension Prevention, phase II (TOHP II) [28,29]	1788	43	63	78	Reduced calorie intake and increased physical activity	36 to 48 months	31.0	127.6	86.0	−1.9	−1.3	−0.9
		44	69	78	Reduced calorie intake, increased physical activity, and reduced sodium intake		31.0	127.4	86.0	−2.1	−1.1	−0.6

Note: BMI = body mass index, SBP = systolic blood pressure, DBP = diastolic blood pressure.
[a] Overweight strata only and including only those assigned to a weight loss intervention or to usual care.
Source: Adapted from Ref. 3, Table 3.

Lifestyle Weight Reduction in Hypertension Prevention

Primary prevention of hypertension involves two complementary strategies: (1) creating a downward shift in the entire distribution of blood pressure in the population, and (2) lowering blood pressure levels in the subset of individuals who are at high risk of developing hypertension [3]. The actual blood pressure changes associated with either of these strategies (e.g., 1 to 3 mmHg may seem small if viewed as clinical outcomes for any given individual. From a public health perspective, however, these small average changes represent downward shifts in the aggregate SBP or DBP distributions that can be extremely important from a public health perspective. Although those in the upper tail of the distribution are at highest risk, large numbers of events arise from lower in the distribution, thus even small downward shifts in the distribution reduce the size of the pool of persons at risk. Cook et al. [8] have estimated based on combined data from the Framingham study and NHANES that a 2-mm reduction in DBP would result in a 17% decrease in the prevalence of hypertension, as well as a 6% reduction in the risk of CHD and a 15% reduction in the risk of stroke and transient ischemic attacks. In addition, as will be discussed, there is dose response of blood pressure change on weight change even within the normotensive blood pressure range.

Table 1 gives pertinent findings from three U.S. multicenter trials of hypertension prevention that have involved weight loss interventions. In two of the trials weight loss was evaluated alone (without dietary changes other than calorie and fat restriction) and also in combination with reductions in sodium intake or sodium/potassium intake ratio.

The Hypertension Prevention Trial (HPT) enrolled 25- to 49-year-old women in four U.S. cities in a set of 3-year parallel trials to evaluate reduction of sodium intake, increased potassium intake, calorie restriction for weight reduction, and combinations of these approaches as measures to prevent increases in blood pressure, with 36 months of follow-up [25]. Eligible participants had DBPs between 78 and 89 mmHg. Relevant here are results for the 380 participants with "high BMI" ($\geq$23–25kg/m^2) who were randomly assigned to interventions involving caloric restriction only (with the objective of a 5% average reduction in mean body weight) or caloric restriction combined with sodium reduction (5% reduction in mean body weight and 50% reduction in mean urinary sodium excretion) or usual care (no caloric reduction or sodium reduction). Lifestyle counseling was conducted in groups by specially trained personnel on a weekly basis for the first 10 weeks, and decreased to monthly for the duration of follow-up. Follow-up rates for measurements were in the 80–90% range, and 60–70% of participants attended all 12 of the initial dietary counseling sessions. Among the HPT participants assigned to caloric restriction, the net average weight loss of 5.76

TABLE 2 Randomized Trials of Lifestyle Weight Reduction Adjunctive or Alternative to Drug Treatment of Hypertension

Study	Sample size[a]	Demographic characteristics			Drug treatment conditions	Components of weight loss intervention	Follow-up	Average initial BMI (kg/m^2) range and BP (mmHg)			Findings
		Mean age	Male (%)	White (%)				BMI	SBP	DBP	
Trial of Nonpharmacologic Interventions in the Elderly (TONE) [30 31 32]	441	66	48	72	Withdrawal of BP medication attempted ~90 days after randomization	Reduced calorie intake and increased physical activity, or reduced calorie intake and increased physical activity and reduced sodium intake	Median 29 months	31	129	72	The relative hazard of having an endpoint (elevated BP; return to BP medication, or a CVD event) compared to usual care was 0.64 for weight loss ($p = .002$) and 0.47 for combined weight loss–sodium reduction ($p < .001$).
Trial of Antihypertensive	587	48	56	67	Placebo, chlorthalidone	Reduced calorie intake, or	Mean 4.5 years		143	93	The reduction in the 5-year incidence

Interventions and Management (TAIM) [33]					(25 mg), or atenolol (50 mg)	reduced calorie intake, reduced sodium intake, increased potassium intake					of treatment failure (DBP >90 requiring additional drug treatment) associated with weight loss vs. usual diet was .27, .32, and .12, respectively in those assigned to placebo, chlortalidone, and atenolol and .23 overall.
Hypertension Optimal Treatment (HOT) substudy [34]	102	58	48	60% white	Protocol-driven stepped treatment with felodipine, enalapril, metropolol or atenolol, and HCTZ	Counseling to reduce dietary total calories and fat vs. usual care	30 months	34	166	105	Blood pressure control was similar for weight intervention and control participants but was achieved with fewer drugs (2.92 vs. 3.47 steps of drug therapy, $p = .03$).

Note: BMI = body mass index, SBP = systolic blood pressure, DBP = diastolic blood pressure, HCTZ = hydrochlorothiazide.
[a] Overweight strata only and including only those assigned to a weight loss intervention or to usual care.

kg by 6 months was associated with net SBP and DBP decreases of −5.1 and −2.8 mmHg, respectively. As shown in Table 1, the net weight loss at the end of 3 years was somewhat smaller than at 6 months—3.49 kg, also associated with smaller SBP and DBP decreases (2.4 and 1.8 mmHg, respectively).

The Trials of Hypertension Prevention, phase I (TOHP I) included weight reduction as one of seven nonpharmacologic interventions tested to prevent blood pressure elevations in individuals with high-normal blood pressure at baseline [26]. Participants were men and women initially ages 30 to 54 years who were not being treated with antihypertensive medications, were within 165% of desirable body weight according to the 1983 Metropolitan Life Insurance Company criteria (BMI $\leq$ 36.1 kg/m^2), and whose average DBP was between 80 and 89 mmHg during the screening period. Across TOHP I centers in six of the clinical centers, a total of 564 enrollees who were approximately 115% or more above desirable weight (BMI $\geq$ 26.1 and 24.3 kg/m^2 for men and women, respectively) were randomly assigned to weight reduction (n = 308) or to no lifestyle intervention (usual care, n = 256) [27]. The treatment goal was a loss of at least 4.5 kg during the first 6 months of the program, with maintenance of this weight loss during the subsequent year of follow-up. Treatment consisted of 14 weekly group meetings, with the remaining contact through monthly meetings and opportunities for interim weigh-ins. Counseling focused on achieving gradual weight loss of up to 0.9 kg per week through dietary change (reduction in energy intake and fat intake) and exercising (primarily walking) 4 to 5 days per week with between 30 and 45 min of exercise per session, and emphasized the use of behavioral self-management techniques. Follow-up data were obtained for more than 90% of enrollees. Attendance at intervention contacts remained at nearly 90% throughout when makeup contacts were included. The 6-month net (active intervention minus control) weight loss was 5.7 kg, associated with a decrease of 3.8/2.5 mmHg, respectively, in SBP and DBP [26,27]. The 18-month net weight loss was 3.9 kg, associated with a net decrease of 2.9/2.3 mmHg, respectively, in SBP and DBP [26]. Regression analyses indicated that a decrease in weight of 1 kg was associated with decreases of .43 mmHg and .33 mmHg, respectively, in SBP and DBP. Adjusting for change in frequency of regular exercise had no effect on the regression coefficient for DBP and only a minimal effect on that for SBP [27].

A second phase of TOHP [28, 29], involving clinical centers in nine U.S. cities, enrolled 2382 men and women ages 30 to 54 years who were not taking antihypertensive medication, who had high-normal blood pressure (average DBP between 83 and 89 mmHg and SBP < 140 mmHg during screening), and who all were overweight (BMI 26.1 to 37.4 kg/m^2 for men and 24.4 to 37.4 kg/m^2 for women). Follow-up in TOHP lasted for 36 to 48 months, depending on enrollment date. Similar to the HPT, TOHP II tested weight loss both alone and in combination with sodium reduction vs. no weight intervention or no sodium intervention. The weight loss intervention goals, approach, and results with respect to attendance and completeness of follow-up were similar to those described for TOHP I, except that the 14 weekly meetings were followed by six biweekly group meetings before decreasing to monthly contact.

In the weight loss arm (compared to usual care), the 6-month weight change was 4.5 kg, associated with a decrease of 3.7/2.7 mmHg, respectively, in SBP and DBP [28]. The 36-month net weight loss in this arm was 1.9 kg, associated with a net decrease of 1.3/0.9 mmHg, respectively, in SBP and DBP. In the arm with combined weight loss and sodium reduction (compared to usual care), the 6-month weight change was 4.3 kg, associated with a decrease of 4.8/2.0 mmHg, respectively, in SBP and DBP. The 36-month net weight loss in this arm was 2.1 kg, associated with a net decrease of 1.1/0.6 mmHg, respectively, in SBP and DBP. The effect on DBP at 36 months was not statistically significant [28]. The combined weight-sodium intervention in TOHP resulted in weight loss and blood pressure changes that were similar to those observed for the weight-reduction only condition. (See Table 1.) Weight reduction and sodium reduction appeared to interact with respect to behavioral goal achievement. Apparently, a simultaneous focus on these two lifestyle changes results in a lesser achievement of one or both of the intervention goals [25,28,30,35].

The overall mean changes in blood pressure shown in Table 1 understate the effect for individuals who achieved substantial weight losses. For example, in TOHP I, at 18 months those in the highest quintile of weight loss ($\geq$ 9.5 kg) had a mean SBP/DBP decrease of 8.4/9.4 mmHg compared to a decrease of 1.4/3.3 in those with a gain of 1.0 kg or more [27]. The dose response of blood pressure change by level of weight change in pooled data for the 1191 TOHP II participants assigned to weight loss only or usual care is shown in Fig. 3 [36]. Figure 4 addresses the issue of blood pressure change when the weight lost is regained vs. maintained [36]. As shown, those who were initially successful in losing weight had the largest blood pressure decreases, but only those who were able to maintain the weight loss sustained the decrease in blood pressure. The subgroup differences shown in Fig. 3 were statistically significant for both SBP and DBP ($p = 0.04$ and .007, respectively).

The efficacy of weight reduction in preventing the development of hypertension in TOHP I and II is shown in Fig. 5. In TOHP I the reduction was 51% and was significant (RR = .49; 95% confidence intervals .29, 0.83) [37]. The reduction in hypertension incidence attributable to weight reduction or combined weight-sodium reduction over the 36-month follow-up in TOHP II was of a smaller magnitude—16–19%—but was statistically significant ($p = .009$ and .02 for weight loss and combined, respcctively, vs. usual care)

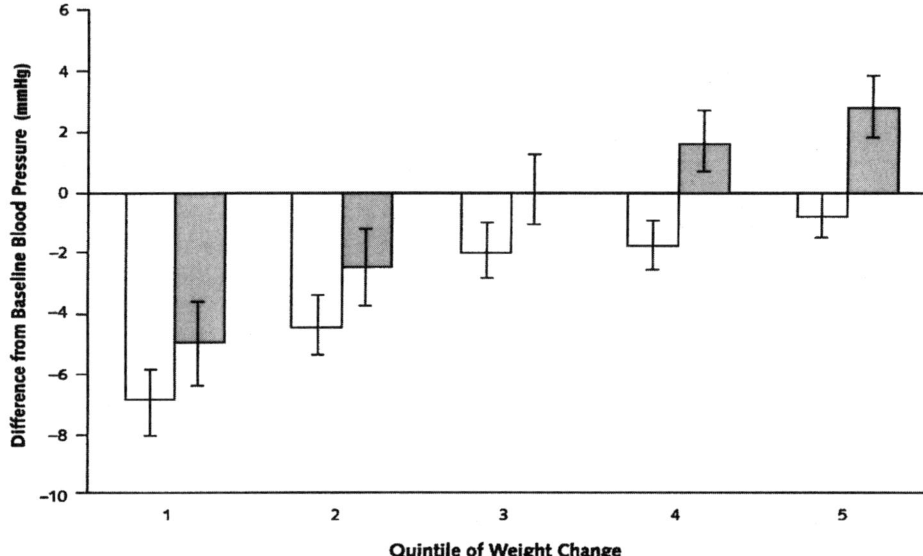

FIGURE 3 Dose response of blood pressure change by level of weight change in pooled data for Trials of Hypertension phase II participants assigned to weight loss only or usual care. Error bars show 95% confidence intervals. Open bars are diastolic blood pressure and shaded bars are systolic blood pressure. *Source*: From Ref. 36.

[28]. TOHP II also collected 48-month follow-up data for the subsample of participants enrolled early in the trial. Based on life table analysis using all follow-up data available, hypertension incidence was reduced at 48 months by 13% (RR = .87; p = .06) and 15% (RR = .85; p = .02), respectively, for the weight loss and combined weight-sodium interventions [28].

The Johns Hopkins TOHP I center in Baltimore collected follow-up data on 87% of the original participants from that study center approximately 7 years after the initial enrollment period—53 of 60 weight loss intervention participants and 42 of the 49 overweight usual care controls [38]. In the absence of intervention during the period after the TOHP study, the overall 7-year weight changes were nearly identical in the active intervention and usual care groups (a gain of 4.9 and 4.5 kg from baseline, respectively, p = .75). The proportion of participants who reported vigorous physical activity at least once per week was also similar at the posttrial follow-up (77% and 71% for weight loss vs. usual care, p = .54), although this was higher than the proportion who reported this level of activity at baseline (62%). Blood pressure was lower, but not significantly, in the active intervention group

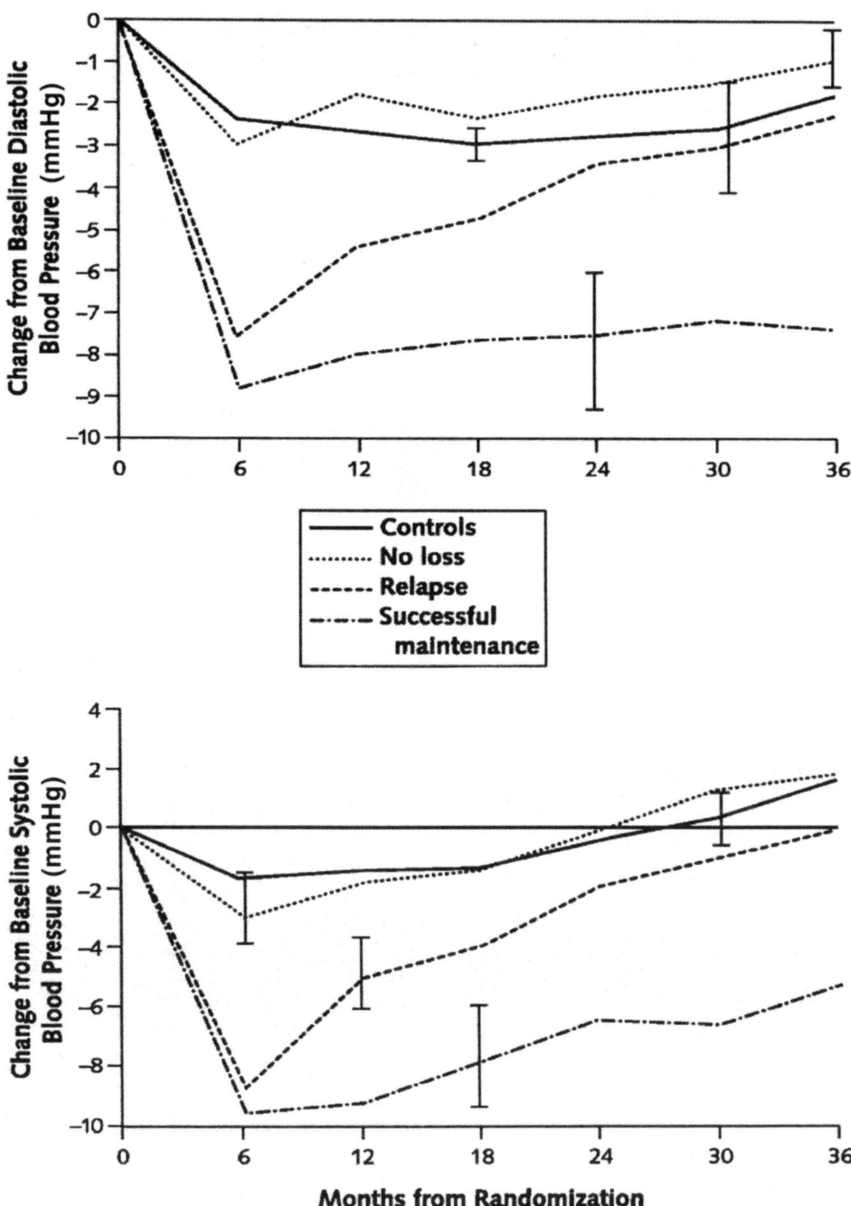

Figure 4 Blood pressure change in usual care participants and subgroups of active weight loss intervention participants according to initial weight loss success and weight loss maintenance. Error bars show 95% confidence intervals. *Source*: From Ref. 36.

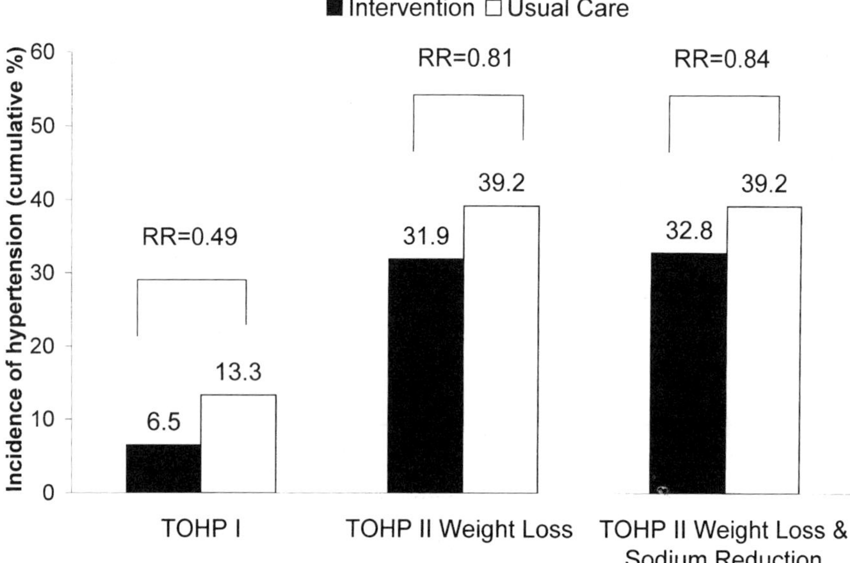

FIGURE 5 Incidence and relative risk of developing hypertension in usual care vs. active intervention participants assigned to weight loss only or combined weight loss and sodium reduction in the Trials of Hypertension Prevention, phase I (TOHP I) or phase II (TOHP II). Follow-up in TOHP I and TOHP II was 18 and 36 months, respectively. RR = relative risk. *Source*: Adapted from Ref. 37 and 28.

by 1.8 mmHg for SBP ($p = .52$) and 1.3 mmHg for DBP ($p = .42$). The difference in the proportion who were taking antihypertensive medication approached statistical significance, however; 13.2 vs. 28.6%, respectively, for those originally assigned to active intervention vs. usual care $p = .06$). In addition, even in this small sample, there was a significant difference in the cumulative incidence of hypertension (defined as taking antihypertensive medications or having a SBP $\geq$ 160 mmHg or a DBP $\geq$ 90 mmHg at the posttrial follow-up examination): 18.9% vs. 40.5% weight loss vs. usual care participants, respectively ($p = .02$).

Lifestyle Weight Reduction in Hypertension Treatment

Three trials in individuals with established hypertension are listed in Table 2 and summarized below. These studies illustrate the effects of weight reduction as an alternative to antihypertensive drug therapy e.g., the Trials of Non-pharmacologic Interventions in the Elderly—TONE [30–32] adjunctively to enhance the effects of drug therapy in patients with mild hypertension (the

Trial of Antihypertensive Interventions and Management; TAIM) [33], or to minimize the need for drug therapy in attaining goal blood pressure in patients with stage II or III hypertension (the Hypertension Optimal Treatment Study; HOT) [34].

TONE assessed whether weight loss and/or sodium reduction could successfully substitute for pharmacological treatment of hypertension among older adults whose blood pressure was well controlled on a single medication [30]. Men and women aged 60 to 79 years were recruited from four U.S. communities and followed for 15 to 36 months. Those in the overweight stratum (BMI levels between 27.8 and 33 for men and 27.3 and 37 for women) were randomly assigned to weight reduction only, sodium reduction only, combined weight and sodium reduction, or usual care (no dietary counseling). The objective for those assigned to weight interventions was to achieve and maintain a 4.5-kg weight loss with an additional goal of achieving and maintaining sodium intake ≤ 80 mEq per 24 hr for those in the combined intervention. Participants assigned to the active interventions were counseled both in groups and individually on a weekly basis for 4 months and then in decreasing frequency. Those assigned to usual care met quarterly thereafter for educational sessions unrelated to nutrition and cardiovascular disease (e.g. sleep, cancer, retirement issues). TONE participants had an average duration of antihypertensive therapy of nearly 12 years at the time of enrollment. Withdrawal of antihypertensive medications was attempted approximately 90 days after the first intervention session. The study endpoint was either reinstatement of drug therapy for hypertension or the occurrence of a cardiovascular event (e.g., myocardial infarction or stroke). Follow-up data were available for more than 90% of those initially enrolled.

The average net weight reduction in TONE participants was 4.9 and 3.9 kg, respectively, for those assigned to weight loss and combined weight-sodium compared to 0.1 kg for usual care [32]. As shown in Table 2, the relative risk of having an endpoint was significantly lower for those assigned to the weight interventions compared to usual care. For example, the proportions who were endpoint-free at 30 months of follow-up were 37% and 44% for weight and weight-sodium, respectively, versus 16% for usual care. A significant dose response trend related to the amount of weight loss was also observed. In pooled data after controlling for intervention assignment, the relative hazard (95% confidence interval) in comparison to those who lost less than 2.3 kg (i.e., less than 50% of the 4.5-kg goal) was 0.84 (0.63, 1.12) for those who lost between 2.3 and 3.6 kg and 0.68 (0.52, 0.90) for those who lost 3.6 kg or more (i.e., were within 80% of the 4.5 kg goal, p for trend = .005) [31]. The average SBP/DBP levels among participants who were still off antihypertensive medications were 133/75 mmHg for those assigned to weight loss and 130/73 mmHg for those assigned to weight-sodium.

The TAIM study investigated the long-term effects of weight loss on the ability to maintain blood pressure control either without drug therapy or while taking a low-dose diuretic or beta-blocker [33]. TAIM phase I used a randomized 3 × 3 factorial design to study the effects of chlorthalidone or atenolol vs. placebo in combination with weight loss or a diet with reduced sodium and increased potassium vs. usual diet as lifestyle therapy. That initial, 6-month phase demonstrated the superiority of weight loss vs. either usual diet or a low sodium diet for lowering blood pressure. Phase II (see Table 2) continued to follow most of the original TAIM, rerandomizing those assigned to usual diet to remain in that condition or to weight loss. Weight loss was also added to the intervention for those originally randomized to the reduced sodium/increased potassium diet. All phase II participants remained on their original blood pressure medications in a double-blind manner if they had achieved blood pressure control and were otherwise on a combination of the two study medications (atenolol or chlorthalidone) or on open label therapy with either the weight loss or the usual diet. Similar to the other studies described here, the weight loss goal was approximately 4.5 kg (or 10% of baseline weight, if greater than 4.5 kg). The weight loss intervention consisted of 10 weeks of behavioral counseling in groups followed by individual maintenance sessions held every 6 weeks. The study endpoint was the failure to maintain blood pressure control on the original drug treatment. Total follow-up from the phase I baseline through phase II was up to 6 years, with the average phase II follow-up lasting 4.5 years and an overall follow-up rate of 76% of the expected participation.

Net weight losses of 2 to 3 kg were observed at 6 months, smallest for those receiving atenolol and largest for those receiving chlorthalidone [33]. Those assigned to weight loss regained weight after 6 months. The 6-month net changes in blood pressure associated with weight loss vs. no usual diet were −4 mmHg, −2 mmHg, and −2 mmHg in the chlorthalidone, atenolol, and placebo groups, respectively. Weight loss was associated with an approximately 25% decrease in the risk of treatment failure; however, the benefits of weight loss appeared to apply primarily to the less obese. Specifically, there was a 40% reduction in risk for those between 110–129% of ideal weight and no reduction in risk for those between 129–160% of ideal weight. Treatment with chlorthalidone and atenolol markedly reduced the risk of treatment failure (by 75% and 62%, respectively). The greatest treatment success was in those assigned to weight loss and chlorthalidone; those assigned to placebo and usual diet had the least success. The chlorthalidone findings suggest a synergism between weight reduction and the action of diuretics. The finding for atenolol may reflect a broader issue of a potential effect of beta-blockers in depressing energy metabolism and either inhibiting weight loss or predisposing to small weight gain [39]. Current guidelines, however, do not mention obesity or the potential interactions with weight loss as specific considerations in the choice of drug treatment for hypertension [2].

The HOT study (see Table 2) was designed to determine the optimal approach to lowering of blood pressure in men and women ages 50 and over with DBPs over 100 mmHg [34]. Participants were randomly assigned to achieve one of three goal levels for DBP: 90, 85, or 80 mmHg, using a protocol to guide stepwise increases in the choice and dosage of selected drugs. The HOT weight loss component was a substudy to determine whether or not a dietary behavior intervention for weight loss would permit the achievement of goal blood pressure in obese participants (BMI ≥ 27) with fewer medication steps (i.e., fewer medications or lower doses of medications; see Table 5.2) in comparison to those not given this intervention. Randomization to weight loss was balanced with respect to other aspects of the HOT study design (e.g., goal blood pressure level). Participants in the weight loss arm were counseled individually by a dietitian within 10 days of randomization and 2 and 4 weeks later and were also invited to group support sessions, twice monthly for 3 months and then every 3 to 6 months through the end of follow-up. Patients were counseled to reduce calorie and fat intake but not to exercise. Patients in the control group were told to lose weight but were not provided with counseling or group support. Follow-up data were available for 102 of 112 patients initially enrolled.

Both the weight loss and control groups lost some weight at 3 months. By 6 months weight intervention participants lost significantly more weight than controls (-3.2 v -1.8 kg; $p = .05$). Weight intervention participants, however, subsequently regained weight and there was no significant difference in weight loss from baseline in the intervention and controls after 6 months. Compared to those not given the weight intervention, the weight intervention group had equivalent blood pressure control with fewer medication steps at 6 months (2.92 vs. 3.47 steps; $p = .03$) and at each follow-up visit between 6 months and 30 months, in spite of the weight regain. This was true for all three goal blood pressure strata.

Blood Pressure Response to Pharmacologically or Surgically Induced Weight Loss

The above-described studies involve weight reduction achieved through lifestyle behavior changes. People with BMI ≥ 30 or ≥ 27 with concomitant medical risk factors or diseases, however, are potential candidates for antiobesity drug therapy, and those with BMI ≥ 40 or ≥ 35 with comorbid conditions are potential candidates for obesity surgery [4]. It is thus important to ask whether the potential benefits of lifestyle weight reduction for blood pressure control also extend to pharmacologically or surgically induced weight reduction. Both pharmacological and surgical approaches to weight reduction require adjunctive lifestyle therapy in order to be effective [4], but the overall physiological effects may differ from those observed when only dietary and physical activity changes are involved. In addition, in practice, the adjunctive lifestyle change recommendations may not always be offered or adhered to.

Pharmacologically Induced Weight Loss

The difficulty of achieving long-term success in weight reduction, combined with breakthroughs in our understanding of the molecular mechanisms regulating body weight, have led to marked increases in prescriptions for antiobesity drugs [40], and this trend can be expected to continue as new drugs are developed. Drugs that suppress the appetite, alter metabolism, or alter increased energy expenditure have been used to treat obesity since the late 1800s, although progress in identifying drugs that are safe and effective has been slow [41]. Nearly every drug treatment developed for obesity has generated undesirable outcomes that have resulted in the drug's termination [42]. These outcomes have included adverse effects on the cardiovascular system [43]. Of the numerous antiobesity drugs that have been studied, only two drugs—sibutramine and orlistat—are currently approved by the Food and Drug Administration (FDA) for obesity treatment [42]. Sibutramine, a sympathomimetic drug, acts to suppress appetite and therefore food intake by blocking of reuptake of both norepinephrine and 5 hydroxytryptophan. Orlistat inhibits gastrointestinal (GI) lipases, is minimally absorbed, and works nonsystemically to decrease by about 30% the proportion of ingested fat that is absorbed [44]. The adverse effects of consuming a large high-fat meal after taking orlistat (e.g., oily and loose stools due to partial fat malabsorption) presumably provide negative feedback that results in modified food intake behavior. Both of these drugs require continued use for continued effectiveness [42].

In the NHLBI expert panel review, 10 of 16 identified obesity pharmacology studies with blood pressure data were considered eligible as evidence. The overall quality of the evidence with respect to drug therapy for obesity was rated category B, however, reflecting RCT evidence of limited overall quality because of such methodological issues as an insufficient number of studies, small sample size, post hoc or subgroup analyses, or inconsistent results across studies [4]. Most of the trials reviewed were short-term (i.e., 6 months or less) and had been conducted in white women. All were placebo-controlled trials in which both the active drug and placebo groups received dietary counseling, thus the weight loss attributable to drug treatment in these studies was in comparison to that achieved by dietary counseling only.

The NHLBI panel concluded that "weight loss produced by most weight loss medications (except for sibutramine) and adjuvant lifestyle modifications is accompanied by reductions in blood pressure" (4, p. 84S). The exception for sibutramine relates to the observation that small increases in blood pressure and heart rate are common side effects of this drug, thus for sibutramine (as well as for other sympathomimetic drugs likely to be used to aid weight loss; see Ref. 45 for a comprehensive review) the relevant questions relate to the risk: benefit ratio associated with chronic use. For example, is the drug contraindicated for long-term use in individuals with uncontrolled hypertension or for whom concurrent use of sibutramine increases the required dose of antihypertensive medication? Is its use potentially justified by improvements in cardiovascular risk other than blood pressure (e.g., lipid profile or glucose tolerance) or in quality of life even where there is some negative effect on hypertension management?

Wadden et al. [46] reported blood pressure data from a randomized trial of the effect of sibutramine on weight loss with and without adjunctive lifestyle modifications. Initial participants were 53 women with a mean age of 47 years and mean BMI of 37.7 kg/m^2 at enrollment. Among the 43 participants who completed the study, the mean weight loss was equivalent to 10% or more of their initial body weight. This weight loss was associated with significant improvements in lipid profiles (e.g., a decrease in the ratio of total cholesterol to high-density lipoprotein cholesterol from 3.8 to 3.3), but also with significant elevations in blood pressure (5 to 6 mmHg increase in SBP and DBP). The authors comment that these blood pressure elevations would have been higher if the drug had not been withdrawn or reduced in dose due to blood pressure elevations in some women during the course of the study. All women had controlled blood pressure at the beginning of the study, including four who were taking antihypertensive medications. One additional woman was taking antihypertensive medication by the end of the study. The absence of an untreated control group limits the interpretation of these findings, but the opposing direction of the effects on lipids and blood pressure is nevertheless noteworthy.

MacMahon et al. [47] conducted a study to specifically address the efficacy and safety of sibutramine use in obese patients with hypertension. Participants (64% white and 36% black; mean age 53 years; mean BMI 34) included men and women with a history of hypertension that was controlled with a calcium channel blocker (with or without concomitant treatment with a thiazide diuretic) who were randomized to receive sibutramine (n = 150) or placebo (n = 74). Dietary counseling about weight loss was provided briefly at the initial run-in visit only. The mean change in body weight was 3.9 kg (net of active drug minus placebo), equivalent to 4% of body weight. Significant improvements werc reported for lipid profiles, serum uric acid levels, quality of life, mobility, and activities of daily living. In follow-up data on blood pressure (reported for 142 active treatment and 69 placebo participants), the mean changes in SBP and DBP (mmHg) and pulse rate (beats per min) were +2.7, +2.0, and +4.9, respectively, for the treatment group and 1.5, −1.3, and 0.0 for the placebo group. Substantially more active treatment group participants had an increase of more than 10 mmHg in SBP or an increase in pulse rate of 10/beats per min or more at three consecutive visits compared to the placebo group. Treatment was discontinued due to hypertension for 5.3% of those receiving sibutramine (vs. 1.4 in the placebo group). All results were similar for African Americans and whites.

Orlistat facilitates weight loss through an entirely different mechanism (inhibition of gastrointestinal lipase) than sibutramine. It might be expected that orlisat would favorably influence blood lipid levels but generally have no direct effect on blood pressure. Davidson et al. [48] reported results of a two-phase RCT of orlistat (n=657) vs. placebo (n=223) for a total of 2 years conducted in 18 U.S. research centers. Participants were men and women, primarily white (14% were black and 4% were Hispanic), with a mean age of 44 years and a mean BMI of 36. About 8% had DBP ≥90 mmHg at entry. All participants received dietary counseling to reduce energy intake and consume 30% of total calories as fat and were also given a vitamin and mineral supplement to counteract the anticipated decrease in absorption of fat-soluble vitamins associated with taking orlistat. By design, some participants were randomly assigned to be taken off orlistat after 1 year or to decrease the dosage of orlistat by 50%. The following comparisons refer to the active treatment group that received orlistat at 120 mg three times a day with those who received placebo throughout the 2-year study period in the Davidson et al. study [48].

Weight losses were relatively modest, but were larger in those receiving orlistat (7.6% vs. 4.5% in the placebo group). Twice as many subjects on orlistat (34.1% vs. 17.5% of those on placebo) maintained a loss of more than 10% of initial body weight [48]. The orlistat vs. placebo differences in SBP and DBP were statistically significant ($p=.02$) at 1 year but were small (about 2 mmHg net of active minus control for both SBP and DBP). Total- and low-density lipoprotein cholesterol levels were improved (i.e., either a decrease or a lesser increase was observed) in the orlistat group compared with placebo by 11 and 8 mg/dl, respectively (both $p<.001$). Statistically significant improvements in fasting serum glucose, fasting insulin, and waist circumference were also reported. A separate study conducted in 17 primary care centers demonstrated very similar results with respect to the amount of weight loss and the size and direction of changes in blood pressure and lipid variables and fasting insulin [44].

Although orlistat does not raise the same benefit to risk issues with respect to blood pressure changes as does sibutramine, the blood pressure changes in these studies with primarily normotensive individuals are relatively modest. No long-term studies of orlistat-induced weight reduction in hypertensive patients were identified.

Surgically Induced Weight Loss

Results from the Swedish Obese Subjects Intervention Study (SOS) [49–51] provide possible insights into the effects of large and relatively well-maintained weight losses over a follow-up period of up to 8 years. This study was designed to compare surgically treated individuals with comparable individuals given conventional weight loss treatment. Although those enrolled in SOS were not randomly assigned to receive surgical treatment, the comparison group was selected from a registry of obese individuals using a computer algorithm to match on 18 variables, including sex, age, weight, height, waist circumference, hip circumference, SBP, serum cholesterol and triglycerides, smoking, diabetes, menopausal status for women, and selected psychosocial and personality variables. Baseline BMI was approximately 41, equivalent to approximately 45 kg overweight. Surgical treatment (gastric banding, vertical banded gastroplasty, or gastric bypass) was associated with weight losses of up to 31 kg, with up to 20 kg maintained after 8 years. An early report from this study [49] indicated that a mean loss of 28 kg in surgically treated patients (vs. 0.5 kg in controls) was associated with a significant dramatic reduction in the 2-year incidence of hypertension: 5.4% compared to 13.6% [unadjusted odds ratio (95% CI) 0.38 (0.22,0.65)], respectively, in patients treated with surgical intervention compared to controls. After 8 years, however, the incidence of hypertension was found to be similar in the surgically treated and control participants (26%) in spite of maintenance of most of the weight loss (mean 20-kg loss at 8 years compared to 31 kg after year 1). In contrast, the effect of the weight loss on diabetes incidence, also substantially reduced after 2 years, was apparently well maintained at 8 years. This finding is in conflict with the impression from lifestyle weight loss programs and also with the impression from previous uncontrolled studies involving the surgical treatment of obesity that had shorter follow-up periods indicating a favorable effect on hypertension [52, 53]. One possible interpretation of the SOS findings is that weight regain between years 2 and 8 contributed to blood pressure elevations even though a substantial proportion of the original weight loss was maintained. Subgroup analyses to determine whether or not those who were able to avoid weight regain had a more favorable blood pressure outcome than those who regained were not presented (e.g., the effect reported by Stevens et al. from subgroup analyses of the TOHP II data

[36]). (See Fig. 4.) Weight regain in the setting of the effects of aging on blood pressure [51, 54] may be particularly harmful. Also, it would be of interest to know whether hypertension control was achieved at a lower dose of medication among the surgery patients who maintained their weight loss in comparison to those who did not or to controls.

MECHANISMS LINKING EXCESS WEIGHT AND WEIGHT CHANGE TO HYPERTENSION

Although there is a clear association between weight gain and an increase in blood pressure, the specific mechanism whereby weight gain or chronic obesity leads to chronic elevations in blood pressure remains unclear. Following is a summary of several pathways that appear to be involved.

Obesity is known to be associated with high intravascular volume, high cardiac output and inappropriately normal peripheral resistance [55, 56]. This added stress on the heart leads to eccentric left ventricular hypertrophy, as opposed to the concentric hypertrophy that is observed in hypertension in nonobese individuals [57]. In kidneys, obese subjects have an elevated glomerular filtration rate and abnormal pressure natriuresis, which shift toward higher blood pressure [58]. This resetting of pressure natriuresis and sodium retention in obesity is primarily due to increased renal tubular reabsorption, which may also contribute to the blood pressure elevations [59]. Licata et al. [60] have shown that obese subjects have delayed urinary sodium excretion and blunted response of plasma atrial natriuretic peptide to saline load.

Obesity is also associated with an increase in insulin resistance, which is defined as a clinical state in which a normal or elevated insulin level produces an impaired biological response. Insulin causes vasodilation in lean normotensive individuals. In obesity this effect of insulin is blunted, however, and leads to an increase in peripheral vascular resistance [61] and blood pressure elevation. Landsberg [62] argued that (in obesity) while insulin causes an increase in central sympathetic outflow, it causes peripheral vascular resistance, and a combination of these two effects leads to higher blood pressure. Other investigators have disputed these findings, however, Hall et al. [63] showed that hyperinsulinemia did not increase arterial pressure in insulin-resistant subjects. Finally, there is extensive evidence that sympathetic stimulation plays a major role in causing obesity-induced hypertension [64]. This effect may be compounded by leptin, which is secreted by adipocytes and causes sympathetic activation [65].

The effect of weight loss in lowering blood pressure can be plausibly explained by these same mechanisms (e.g., reversing effects in the same

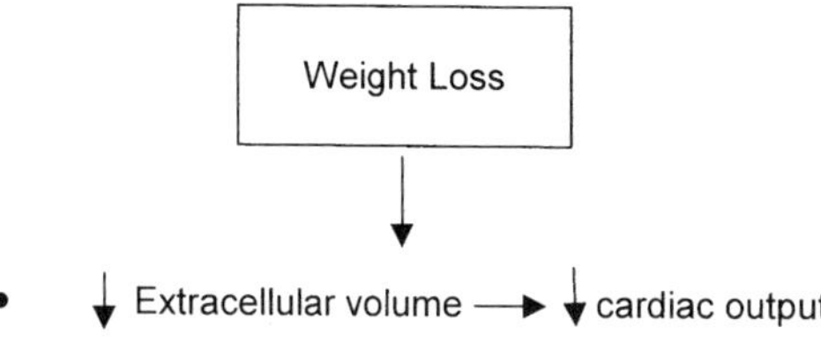

FIGURE 6 Possible mechanisms for the blood pressure-lowering effect of weight loss. *Source*: From Ref. 24.

pathways). As summarized in Fig. 6, from a review of this issue by Mertens and Van Gaal [24], weight loss leads to a reduction in insulin and leptin resistance with an increased biologic activity of natriuretic peptide. This leads to natriuresis with a concomitant reduction in cardiopulmonary volume and decreased cardiac output. The decrease in insulin resistance leads to changes in vascular responsiveness. In the kidney, the decreased sympathetic nervous system and renin-angiotensin system activity, together with improved insulin sensitivity, are thought to facilitate renal sodium excretion and thereby lead to further reduction in cardiopulmonary volume and cardiac output.

SUMMARY AND IMPLICATIONS

Weight reduction has been shown to reduce blood pressure levels or prevent blood pressure elevations in individuals with blood pressure at the higher end of the normotensive range and in individuals with established hypertension, with and without drug therapy. The evidence to this effect has withstood the scrutiny of expert panels [2,4] and led to clinical guidelines to include weight loss as a key component of hypertension control [2] and blood pressure control as a goal of obesity treatment [4]. These benefits of weight loss for blood pressure control have been demonstrated for relatively small weight losses (e.g., 4.5 kg) for periods lasting from 3 to 7 years, in both sexes, at ages ranging from 30 to 80 years and in both African Americans and whites.

Although exercise also decreases blood pressure [2], the favorable effect of weight loss on blood pressure control appears to result from caloric reduction with or without the addition of increased physical activity. In fact, the findings related to the blood pressure effects when weight loss is maintained vs. regained suggest an effect, at least in part, of caloric restriction rather than weight loss as such [66]. Also, although this aspect of the evidence was not reviewed here in detail, sodium reduction was held relatively constant in the intervention conditions that targeted only weight loss [25,26,28,30], thus the effect of weight reduction on blood pressure was demonstrated to be independent of sodium reduction. As discussed elsewhere in this book, sodium reduction has independent effects in lowering blood pressure. The apparent behavioral complexity of concurrent weight reduction and sodium reduction limits the possibilities for completely additive effects of combining these two approaches, however. Whether or not there are circumstances in which weight reduction and sodium reduction are synergistic in their effects on blood pressure is unclear from the available studies. The TAIM findings on weight reduction and chlorthalidone, however, suggest a favorable interaction between weight reduction and pharmacologically induced sodium diuresis in African Americans with mild hypertension.

As reviewed elsewhere [67,68], the weight losses achieved in these trials have generally been smaller for black than for white participants. The dose response of blood pressure change for a given amount of weight change appears to be relatively similar across ethnicity, however, as well as across gender [27,67], and the evidence from trials is supported by the epidemiologic data showing the influence of weight levels on blood pressure for both sexes and for diverse ethnic groups. Where ethnic differences have been observed in the attributable risk of obesity in hypertension (in African Americans vs. whites, e.g.), this may reflect differences across populations in risk of hypertension due to factors other than obesity (e.g., lean African Americans are at higher risk of hypertension than lean whites) [69]. The notably higher prevalence and greater severity of obesity in African American compared to white women when linked to the potential for obesity to elevate blood pressure, underscores the need for effective prevention and treatment for hypertension control in the black population. In the NHANES III data, nearly 40% of African-American women had BMI levels of 30 or greater, compared with less than 25% of white women or African-American men and white men [70]. Class III obesity (BMI levels of $\geq$ 40 kg/m^2) occurred in 8% of African-American women ages 30 to 39 and 10–11% of those ages 40 to 69, compared with 3–5% of white women in the 30-to-69-year age range [70].

This review suggests several types of research needed to further our understanding of the potential impact of weight reduction in reducing the overall burden of hypertension and, ultimately, cardiovascular diseases. For example, there is as yet limited evidence on the extent to which weight reduction also reverses the effects of chronic blood pressure elevations on the heart or kidneys and reduces related cardiovascular and cerebrovascular events. Interactions between the direct effects of weight reduction on blood pressure and those mediated through effects on glucose tolerance are of interest, given the very strong association of obesity with the development of diabetes [23]. Within the literature on weight loss and blood pressure, the current evidence is strongly supportive for a benefit of weight loss achieved through dietary and lifestyle changes, and less clear for weight loss achieved when drug therapy is included or, over the long term, for those very obese individuals who elect obesity surgery. Given that very obese individuals have been excluded from many of the trials reviewed here and together with the finding from TAIM [33] that weight reduction did not reduce the likelihood of treatment failure in the more obese individuals, more studies in very obese populations are needed.

Whatever we conclude about the *potential* impact of weight reduction in hypertension prevention and control and cardiovascular risk reduction, this potential will not be realized unless we can identify and implement effective approaches to obesity prevention and control. The epidemic of obesity is occurring worldwide, and in the United States at least, is affecting both children and adults, with particularly dramatic rises in African-American children [5,71]. Fortunately, there has already been an official call for coordinated national action on this issue [5]. It remains for us to respond effectively, however. As is evident by reference to the descriptions of the intervention approaches used in the trials listed in Tables 1 and 2, the relatively modest weight losses achieved required relatively labor-intensive and extended interventions. Feasible and cost-effective approaches to facilitating weight control in clinical settings have not yet been identified. Moreover, it is highly unlikely that any clinical or individually-oriented approaches to obesity prevention or treatment can achieve long-term effectiveness in the absence of additional environmental strategies to address the plethora of obesity-promoting societal forces [71,72].

REFERENCES

1. Stamler J. Epidemiologic findings on body mass and blood pressure. Ann Epidemiol. 1991; 347–362.
2. The Sixth Report of the Joint National Committee on Prevention, Detection, Evaluation, and Treatment of High Blood Pressure. Arch Int Med. 1997; 157:2413–2446.

3. Working Group on Primary Prevention of Hypertension. National High Blood Pressure Working Group Report on Primary Prevention of Hypertension. Arch Int Med. 1993; 153:186–208.
4. National Institutes of Health, National Heart, Lung, and Blood Institute. Clinical guidelines on the identification, evaluation, and treatment of overweight and obesity in adults: the evidence report. Obes Res 1998; 6(suppl. 2):51S–209S.
5. U.S. Department of Health and Human Services. The Surgeon General's Call to Action to Prevent and Decrease Overweight and Obesity, 2001. Rockville, MD: U.S. Department of Health and Human Services, Public Health Service. Office of the Surgeon General, 2001.
6. Dyer AR, Elliott P. The INTERSALT study. Relations of body mass index to blood pressure. INTERSALT Co-operative Research Group. J Human Hypertens. 1989; 3: 299–308.
7. Dyer AR, Elliott P, Shipley M. Body mass index versus height and weight in relation to blood pressure: findings for the 10,079 persons in the INTERSALT study. Amer J Epidemiol. 1990; 131:589–596.
8. Cook NR, Cohen J, Hebert PR, et al. Implications of small reductions in diastolic blood pressure for primary prevention. Arch Int Med. 1995; 155:701–709.
9. Kaufman JS, Durazo-Arvizu RA, Rotimi CN, McGee DL, Cooper RS, for the investigators of the International Collaborative Study on Hypertension in Blacks. Epidemiology. 1996; 7:398–405.
10. Brown CD, Higgins M, Donato K, Rohde FC, Garrison R, Obarzanek E, Ernst ND, Horan M. Body mass index and the prevalence of hypertension and dyslipidemia. Obes Res. 2000; 8:605–619.
11. Liu K, Ruth KJ, Flack JM, Jones-Webb R, Burke G, Savage PJ, Hulley SB. Blood pressure in young blacks and whites: relevance of obesity and lifestyle factors in determining differences. Circulation. 1996; 93:60–66.
12. Field AE, Coakley EH, Must A, et al. Impact of overweight on the risk of developing common chronic disease during a 10-year period. Arch Int Med. 2001; 161:1581–1586.
13. Field AE, Byers T, Hunter DJ, et al. Weight cycling, weight gain, and risk of hypertension in women. Amer J Epidemiol 1999; 150:573–579.
14. Wilsgaard T, Schirmer H, Arnesen E. Impact of body weight on blood pressure with a focus on sex-differences: the Tromsø Study, 1986–1995. Arch Int Med. 2000; 160:2847–2853.
15. Rainwater DL, Mitchell BD, Comuzzie AG, VandeBerg JL, Stern MP, MacCluer JW. Associations among 5-year changes in weight, physical activity, and cardiovascular disease risk factors in Mexican Americans. Amer J Epidemiol 2000; 152:974–982.
16. MacMahon S, Cutler J, Brittain E, Higgins M. Obesity and hypertension: epidemiological and clinical issues. Euro Heart J 1987; 8(suppl. B):57–70.
17. Sakurai Y, Kono S, Shinchi K, Honjo S, Todoroki I, Wakabayashi K, Imanishi K, Nishikawa H, Ogawa S, Katsurada M. Relation of waist-hip ratio to glucose

tolerance, blood pressure, and serum lipids in middle-aged Japanese males. Int J Obes. 11995; 19:632–637.
18. Harris MM, Stevens J, Thomas N, Schreiner P, Folsom AR. Associations of fat distribution and obesity with hypertension in a bi-ethnic population: the ARIC study. Obes Res. 2000;8:516–524.
19. Gillum RF, Mussolino ME, Madans JH. Body fat distribution and hypertension incidence in women and men: the NHANES I Epidemiologic Follow-up Study. Int J Obes Relat Matab Disord. 1998; 22:127–134.
20. Corrigan SA, Raczynski JM, Swencionis C, Jennings SG. Weight reduction in the prevention and treatment of hypertension: a review of representative clinical trials. Amer J Health Promo 1991; 5:208–214.
21. Cutler JA. Randomized clinical trials of weight reduction in non-hypertensive persons. Ann Epidemiology 1991; 1:363–370.
22. Goldstein DJ. Beneficial health effects of modest weight loss. Int J Obes 1992; 16:397–415.
23. Pi-Sunyer FX. A review of long-term studies evaluating the efficacy of weight loss in ameliorating disorders associated with obesity. Clin Ther 1996; 18:1006–1035.
24. Mertens IL, Gaal FV. Overweight, obesity and blood pressure: the effects of modest weight reduction. Obes Res 2000; 8:270–278.
25. Hypertension Prevention Trial Research Group. The Hypertension Prevention Trial: three-year effects of dietary changes on blood pressure. Arch Int Med. 1990; 150:153–162.
26. The Trials of Hypertension Prevention Cooperative Research Group. The effects of non-pharmacological interventions on blood pressure of persons with high normal levels: results of the Trials of Hypertension Prevention (phase I). JAMA. 1992; 267:1213–1220.
27. Stevens VJ, Corrigan SA, Obarzanek E et al. Weight loss intervention in phase I of the Trials of Hypertension Prevention. Arch Int Med. 1993; 153:849–858.
28. The Trials of Hypertension Prevention Collaborative Research Group. Effects of weight loss and sodium reduction intervention on blood pressure and hypertension incidence in overweight people with high normal blood pressure. Arch Int Med. 1997; 157:657–667.
29. Appel LJ, Hebert PR, Cohen JD, et al. Baseline characteristics of participants in phase II of the Trials of Hypertension Prevention (TOHP II). Ann Epidemiol 1995; 5:149–155.
30. Whelton PK, Appel L, Espeland MA, et al. Sodium reduction and weight loss in the treatment of hypertension in older persons: a randomized controlled Trial of Nonpharmacologic Interventions in the Elderly (TONE). JAMA 1998; 279:839–846.
31. Kumanyika SK, Espeland MA, Bahnson JL. Ethnic comparison of weight loss in the trial of nonpharmacologic interventions in the elderly (TONE). Obes Res 2002; 10:96–106.
32. Espeland MA, Whelton PK, Kostis JB, et al. Predictors and mediators of successful long-term withdrawal from antihypertenstive medications. Arch Fam Med. 1999; 8:228–236.

33. Davis BR, Blaufox D, Oberman A, et al. Reduction in long-term antihypertensive medication requirements: effects of weight reduction by dietary intervention in overweight persons with mild hypertension. Arch Int Med. 1993; 153:1773–1782.
34. Jones DW, Miller ME, Wofford MR, et al. The effect of weight loss intervention on antihypertensive medication requirements in the Hypertension Optimal Treatment (HOT) Study. Amer J Hypertens. 1999; 12:1175–1180.
35. Elmer PJ, Grimm RH Jr, Flack J, Laing, B. Dietary sodium reduction for hypertension prevention and treatment. Hypertension. 1991; 17:I182–1189.
36. Stevens VJ, Obarzanek E, Cook NR, et al. Long-term weight loss and changes in blood pressure: results of the Trials of Hypertension Prevention, phase II. Ann Int Med. 2001; 134:1–11.
37. Whelton PK, Kumanyika SK, Cook NR, Cutler JA, Borhani NO, Hennekens CH, Kuller LH, Langford H, Jones D, Satterfield S, Lasser NL, Cohen J. Efficacy of nonpharmacologic interventions in adults with high normal blood pressure: results from phase I of the Trials of Hypertension Prevention (TOHP). Amer J Clin Nutr 1997; 65:652S–660S.
38. He J, Whelton PK, Appel LJ, Charleston J, Klag MJ. Long-term effects of weight loss and dietary sodium reduction on incidence of hypertension. Hypertension. 2000; 35:544–549.
39. Pischon T, Sharma AM. Use of beta blockers in obesity hypertension: potential role of weight gain. Obes Rev. 2001; 2:275–280.
40. Kushner R. The treatment of obesity: a call for prudence and professionalism. Arch Int Med. 1997; 157:602–604.
41. Bray GA. A concise review on the therapeutics of obesity. Nutrition. 2000; 16:953–960.
42. Bray GA, Greenway FL. Current and potential drugs for treatment of obesity Endocr Rev 1999; 20:805.
43. Connolly HM, Cary JL, McGoon MD, et al. Valvular heart disease associated with fenfluramine-phentermine. N Eng J Med. 1997; 337:581–588.
44. Hauptman J, Lucas C, Boldrin M, Collins H, Segal K. Orlistat in the long-term treatment of obesity in primary care settings. Arch Fam Med 2000; 9:160–167.
45. Bray GA, Tartaglia LA. Medicinal strategies in the treatment of obesity. Nature 2000; 404:672–677.
46. Wadden TA, Berkowitz RI, Sarwer DB, Prus-Wisniewski R, Steinberg C. Benefits of lifestyle modification in the pharmacologic treatment of obesity. Arch Int Med. 2001; 161:218–227.
47. MacMahon FG, Fujioka K, Singh BN, et al. Efficacy and safety of sibutramine in obese white and African American patients with hypertension. Arch Int Med 2000; 160:2185–2191.
48. Davidson M, Hauptman J, DiGirolamo M, et al. Weight control and risk factor reduction in obese subjects treated for 2 years with Orlistat: a randomized control trial. JAMA 1999:281:235–242.
49. Sjöström CD, Lissner L, Wedel H, Sjöström L. Reduction in incidence of diabetes, hypertension and lipid disturbances after intentional weight loss

induced by Bariatric surgery: the SOS Intervention Study. Obes Res. 1999; 7:477–484.
50. Sjöström CD, Peltonen M, Wedel H, Sjöström L. Differentiated long term effects of intentional weight loss on diabetes and hypertension. Hypertension 2000; 36:20–25.
51. Sjöström CD, Peltonen M, Sjöström L. Blood pressure and pulse pressure during long term weight loss in the obese: the Swedish Obese Subjects (SOS) Intervention Study. Obes Res. 2001; 9:188–195.
52. Foley EF, Benotti PN, Borlase BC, et al. Impact of gastric restrictive surgery on hypertension in the morbidly obese. Am J Surg. 1992; 163:294–297.
53. Carson JL, Ruddy ME, Duff AE, et al. The effect of gastric bypass surgery on hypertension in morbidly obese patients. Arch Int Med. 1994; 154:193–200.
54. Flegal K. Obesity, overweight, hypertension, and high blood cholesterol. The importance of age. Obes Res. 2000; 8:676–677.
55. Messerli FH, Christie B, DeCarvalho JG, Aristimuno CG, Suarez DH, Dreslinski GR, Frohlich ED. Obesity and essential hypertension: hemodynamics, intravascular volume, sodium excretion and plasma renin activity. Arch Int Med 1981; 141:81–89.
56. Frohlich ED, Messerli FH, Reisin E, Dunn FG. The problem of obesity and hypertension. Hypertension. 1983; 5S71–5S78.
57. Mikhail N, Golub MS, Tuck ML. Obesity and hypertension. Prog Cardiovasc Dis. 1999; 42:39–58.
58. Simon G, Devereux RB, Roman MJ. Relation of obesity and gender to left ventricular hypertrophy in normotensive and hypertensive adults. Hypertension. 1994; 23:600–606.
59. Hall JE, Brands MW, Henegar JR, Shek EW. Abnormal kidney function as a cause and a consequence of obesity hypertension. Clin Exp Pharmacol Physiol. 1998; 25:58–64.
60. Licata G, Volpe M, Scaglione R, Rubattu S. Salt-regulating hormones in young normotensive obese subjects: effects of saline load. Hypertension 1994; 3(suppl. 1):120–124.
61. Zemel MB. Nutritional and endocrine modulation of intracellular calcium: implications in obesity, insulin resistance and hypertension. Moll Cell Biochem. 1998; 188:129–136.
62. Landsberg L. Hyperinsulinemia: possible role in obesity-induced hypertension. Hypertension 1992; 19(suppl. 1):I-61–I-66.
63. Hall JE, Brands MW, Zappe DH, et al. Cardiovascular actions of insulin: are they important in long-term blood pressure regulation? Clin Exp Pharmacol Physiol 1995; 22:689–700.
64. Julius S, Valentini M, Palatini P. Overweight and hypertension: a 2 way street? Hypertension 2000; 35:807–813.
65. Lee GH, Proenca R, Montex JM, Carroll KM, Darvishzadeh JG, Lee J, Friedman JM. Abnormal splicing of the leptin receptor in diabetic mice. Nature 1996; 379:632–635.
66. Lee, I-M, Blair SN, Allison DB, Folsom AR, Harris TB, Manson JE, Wing

RR. Epidemiologic data on the relationships of caloric intake, energy balance, and weight gain over the life span with longevity and morbidity. J Gerontol 2001; 56A (special issue IX):7–19.67.

67. Kumanyika SK. The impact of obesity on hypertension management in African Americans. J Health Care Poor Underserv. 1997; 8:352–365.
68. Kumanyika SK. Obesity Treatment in minorities. In: Wadden TA, Stunkard AJ, eds. Handbook of Obesity Treatment. New York: Guilford, 2002.
69. Kumanyika SK. The association between obesity and hypertension in blacks. Clin Cardiol. 1989; 12:IV-72–77.
70. Flegal, KM, Carroll, MD, Kuczmarski, RJ, Johnson, CL. Overweight and obesity in the United States: prevalence and trends, 1960–1994. Int J Obes. 1998; 22:39–47.
71. Kumanyika S. Minisymposium on obesity. Overview and some strategic considerations. Ann Rev Pub Health. 2001; 22:293–308.
72. French SA, Story M, Jeffery RW. Environmental influences on eating and physical activity. Ann Rev Pub Health. 2001; 22:309–335.

6

Dietary Salt Reduction

Jeffrey A. Cutler, Eva Obarzanek, and Edward J. Roccella
National Heart, Lung, and Blood Institute, Bethesda, Maryland, U.S.A.

INTRODUCTION

Dietary sodium intake is among the most important lifestyle influences on blood pressure (BP) levels in humans. There is clear evidence that reducing intake can assist in the management of hypertension, and more importantly can shift BP distributions to lower levels, thereby preventing hypertension and/or progression to more severe forms of cardiovascular disease. Information on other health effects of reducing dietary sodium is less abundant, but overall, supports policies of decreasing sodium intake.

HIGH SODIUM AS A CAUSE OF HIGH BLOOD PRESSURE

A variety of mechanisms appears to be involved in pathways from high sodium intake to chronic BP elevation, including impairment of renal handling of sodium. These processes are affected by interrelationships of the renin-angiotensin-aldosterone system activity, vascular tone, and the sympathetic nervous system. Central portions of the autonomic nervous system are also likely involved, particularly the areas of the anterior hypothalamus that regulate thirst and extracellular volume. Cellular processes of cation flux may be important, especially as they operate in vascular smooth muscle cells, with the effects of sodium flux operating through intracellular calcium. Overall, sodium balance is an essential factor for producing hypertension in most animal models, particularly inbred rodent strains [1–4].

A major landmark animal experiment regarding the causal role of sodium on BP involved 26 adult chimpanzees, the species genetically closest to humans. Half of the colony had salt (sodium chloride) added progressively to their diet over 5 months, reaching 15 g/day, which was then maintained over the next 15 months, followed by a 6-month period of salt removal [5]. Average BP (systolic/diastolic) increased by 33/10 mmHg compared to controls during salt addition. The BP increase completely reversed during salt removal. Eight of 13 animals in the salt-loaded experimental group had a increase in BP, but three of the five that did not respond had quite variable compliance with the added salt. The manipulation of salt occurred without other environmental changes; both groups continued to receive a vegetarian, high-fruit diet with very high potassium content and provision of supplementary calcium. This study is as close to a definitive experiment as is likely to be performed of salt independently causing—and its removal reversing—high BP.

Many but not all observational epidemiologic studies have reported direct associations of individual and population levels of dietary sodium and average BP or hypertension prevalence. Most of the observational studies measuring urinary sodium excretion have been cross-sectional; they have controlled variably for confounding factors [6].

The largest and most rigorous observational study of sodium and BP has been INTERSALT, a 32-country cross-sectional study with 52 centers, each with approximately 200 men and women aged 20 to 59 years (total sample size of 10,079). INTERSALT's cross-population and within-population analyses provided concordant results, substantiating the relationships of 24-h sodium and potassium excretion (directly and inversely, respectively), as well as direct associations of body mass index (BMI) and alcohol intake, with BP levels and hypertension prevalence. The first published findings from INTERSALT gave estimates for sodium's effects on systolic BP among the 10,079 individuals of +2.2 mmHg/100 mmol higher sodium, adjusting for potassium excretion, BMI, alcohol, age, sex, reliability (measurement error) of a single day's urinary excretion (by collecting a second 24-h urine from a random 8% of participants), and center effects [7]. Subsequently published estimates using more sophisticated adjustments for reliability and demographics increased the estimate to 3.1 mmHg/100 mmol sodium [8]. The relation of sodium to systolic BP (SBP) was nearly identical for the 8343 nonhypertensive participants as for the total sample; they were doubled for the older compared to the younger half of the sample, and for women compared to men. Additional regression analyses were conducted that did not adjust for BMI, because BMI and sodium excretion were significantly correlated, and BMI is measured much more reliably than sodium excretion, which could lead to some overadjustment. In these analyses, the association increases to 6 mmHg. Table 1 summarizes these findings.

The INTERSALT study also examined the influence of sodium on slope of BP with age, by relating this slope for each center to median sodium excretion for that center. Based on the linear fit across the age range of the participants and assuming that these cross-sectional data can be thought of as reflecting an aging cohort, this analysis led to the estimate of a 9 to 10 mmHg greater increase in SBP from ages 25 to 55 per 100 mmol/24 hr higher sodium excretion (Table 1). It is thus concluded that sodium intake is one of the key modifiable factors accounting for the high worldwide prevalence of hypertension in middle-aged and older adults.

TABLE 1 Relationship Between Sodium and Blood Pressure from INTERSALT Study

Reference number	Sodium difference	Mean SBP difference (mmHg)	Mean DBP difference (mmHg)	Comments
7	100 mmol	2.2	0.1	Adjusted for age, sex, BMI, alcohol, urinary potassium, and sodium reliability
8	100 mmol	3.1	0.1	Same as above plus better adjustment for sodium reliability
8	100 mmol	6.0	2.5	Same as above but not adjusted for BMI
7	100 mmol change from age 25 to 55 (cross-sectional)	9.0–10.2	4.5–6.3	Adjusted for age, sex, BMI, and alcohol intake (results from 48 centers and 52 centers)
8	100 mmol change from age 25 to 55 (cross-sectional)	10.2	6.3	Same as above plus better adjustment for sodium reliability (results from 52 centers)

Further evidence for a causal role of dietary sodium on BP level comes from randomized clinical trials, which control optimally for confounding factors. One clinical trial that provides a unique perspective on change in sodium intake producing long-lasting BP effects was conducted among infants in the Dutch town of Zoetermeer [9]. Newborns (N = 476) were randomized to a customary infant diet (control diet) or to one with 64% less sodium (experimental diet) for 6 months. By the end of this period, SBP was 2.1 mmHg ($p < .01$) lower in infants consuming less salt than those on the control diet. Fifteen years later, 167 of the children were traced and examined, and persistent differences in BP were found. With adjustment for small differences in birth size, sex, maternal and child's education level, maternal SBP, and parental antihypertensive treatment, the lower sodium diet group's BP was significantly lower than that of controls by 3.6/2.2 mmHg. There were no significant differences at follow-up in sodium or potassium excretion, BMI, or physical activity. The authors suggested that the apparent "programming" effect of higher sodium intake during early life may reflect subtle damage to organs (e.g., kidneys) involved in BP regulation [10].

CLINICAL TRIALS OF SODIUM REDUCTION IN ADULTS

Two large, long-term trials that are the most relevant to clinical and public health objectives have been reported: the Trial of Nonpharmacologic Interventions in the Elderly, or TONE [11], and the Trials of Hypertension Prevention, phase II, or TOHP-II [12].

TONE tested whether sodium reduction and/or weight loss are effective in secondary prevention of hypertension in 975 men and women, aged 60 to 80 years. At baseline the participants had well-controlled hypertension on a single antihypertensive medication. Treatment success was defined as BP control (< 150/90 mmHg) following drug withdrawal without cardiovascular events or the need to restart medication during the 30-month follow-up. Groups assigned to sodium reduction maintained average 24-hr sodium excretion at 40 and 49 mmol/day lower (depending on overweight status) than those not receiving this intervention. The rate of treatment failure was reduced by 31% ($p < .001$) compared to controls; 38% of the sodium reduction group remained free of an endpoint compared to 24% of controls. Among overweight participants, the effect of sodium reduction was about equal to the effect of the 3.5-kg weight loss in the weight-reduction group compared to controls. Also, among overweight participants, sodium reduction combined with weight loss provided as much benefit compared to weight loss alone as did sodium reduction alone compared to the usual care group in non-overweight participants. This result was seen even though the combined weight-plus-sodium-reduction group had decreased sodium intake by about 15 mmol/day less than the sodium-reduction-only group. This finding suggests a greater benefit of lowering sodium among overweight than nonoverweight persons. Although the trial was not designed to study clinical cardiovascular disease (CVD) events, the rate was lower in the sodium reduction group (44/370, or 11.9%) than in usual care controls (57/371, or 15.4%).

TOHP-II was conducted with 2382 overweight men and women, aged 30 to 54 years, who had high normal diastolic BP (DBP) (83 to 89 mmHg). Participants were randomized into four groups: sodium reduction alone, weight loss alone, combined weight and sodium reduction, and usual care. At 6 months the sodium reduction group's 24-hr urinary excretion averaged 50 mmol/day lower compared to usual care, with the difference declining to 40 mmol/day among those attending the 36-month visit. In the combined intervention group the net sodium excretion change at each visit was about 15 mmol/day less than the sodium reduction group. In both the weight loss and combined groups weight was reduced about 4.5 kg at 6 months, with the difference diminishing to about 2 kg by 36 months. At 6 months the net effects on BP (mmHg) were reductions of 2.9/1.6 with sodium reduction, 3.7/2.7 for weight loss, and 4.0/2.8 with the combined intervention (Table 2). Although BP effects diminished during follow-up, they remained significant for SBP throughout the 3 years. This attenuation was explained by moderate recidivism of the lifestyle changes and by a diluting effect caused by over 40% developing hypertension, almost half of whom started drug treatment over 3 to 4 years of follow-up. During the first 6 months, sodium reduction and weight loss as single interventions reduced hypertension incidence by 39% and 42%, respectively, and the combination by 63%, thus during this period relative risk reductions were multiplicative [(1−.39)(1−.42)=1−.63]. Over 4 years, sodium reduction alone lowered the cumulative incidence of hypertension by 14% (p=.04). The long-term effects on incidence were similar for the other active interventions.

Several meta-analyses of sodium reduction trials have been reported [13–15]. Estimates of BP effects did not differ substantially among the analyses. The report by Graudal [15] included the most trials, including short-term studies, studies in children, and studies with sodium intake not usually seen in free-living populations. The Cutler et al. meta-analysis [14] was restricted to adults and adolescents, and to intake ranges normally encountered in free-living Western populations. Cutler reported on 32 trials with outcome data for 2635 participants, and the results are summarized in Table 2. Twelve trials involved nonhypertensives. The median duration for all trials was about 1 month. With a median estimated difference in 24-hr sodium

TABLE 2 Selected Randomized Trials of Sodium Reduction and Blood Pressure

Reference number	Study population	N	Follow-up time	Mean sodium level achieved (mmol/day) in intervention group	Net mean sodium change (mmol/day)	Net mean SBP change (mmHg)	Net mean DBP change (mmHg)
12	TOHPII (all nonhypertensives)	1191	6 months	108	−78	−2.9	−1.6
			3 years	135	−51	−1.2	−0.7
14	Meta-analysis:						
	Hypertensives	1043	1–3 months (median)[a]		−77 (median)	−4.8	−2.5
	Nonhypertensives	1689	1–6 months (median)[b]	Not given	−76 (median)	−1.9	−1.1
24,25	Control (typical American) diet:						
	All participants	204	1 month	65	−77	−6.7	−3.5
	Hypertensives	83				−8.3	−4.4
	Nonhypertensives	121				−5.6	−2.8
24,25	DASH + lower sodium[c]						
	All participants	208	1 month	65	−77	−8.9	−4.5
	Hypertensives	85				−11.5	−5.7
	Nonhypertensives	123				−7.1	−3.7

[a] Median duration is 1 month for crossover trials and 3 months for parallel trials.
[b] Median duration is 1 month for crossover trials and 6 months for parallel trials.
[c] Compared with control (typical American) diet at higher sodium level (142 mmol/day).

excretion between intervention and control groups of 77 mmol, the pooled net effects on BP (mmHg) in hypertensive persons were −4.8/−2.4 mmHg, and for a similar sodium difference the BP effects in nonhypertensive persons were −1.9/−1.1 mmHg. This was the only meta-analysis to present a detailed trial-by-trial review of the possible effects of confounding variables. The authors found little influence of such confounding factors and minimal evidence for publication bias.

TRIALS TESTING OTHER NUTRIENT CHANGES

Important insights have emerged from trials targeting other nutrients along with lowering sodium intakes. Two trials that used a mineral salt reduced in sodium and increased in potassium and magnesium found substantial BP reductions in "mild to moderate" hypertensive patients [16,17]. The most plausible interpretation of these trials is to attribute much of the effect to the approximately 35 mmol/day reduction of sodium excretion, and perhaps some benefit to the increase in potassium, because with lower sodium intake potassium supplementation appears to have only a small effect. In a recently published meta-analysis of randomized trials testing potassium supplementation [18], the most striking variation in BP reduction among subgroups was seen based on average sodium excretion during the trial, with the potassium-induced effects ranging from −7.3/−4.7 mmHg for participants with sodium excretion of > 164 mmol/day to −1.2/+0.1 mmHg for participants with sodium excretion < 140 mmol/day ($p < .001$ for trend).

The Dietary Approaches to Stop Hypertension (DASH) clinical trial was an 8-week outpatient feeding study testing effects on BP of dietary patterns designed to produce changes in nonsodium cations as well as other dietary constituents [19]. The study included two intervention diets—an increased fruit and vegetable diet and a combination diet—and a control diet typical of what many Americans eat. All three diets had a sodium chloride content of about 7.5 g per day, which was 1.5 g below pretrial (and typical U.S.) levels. The increased fruit and vegetables diet and the combination diet had estimated potassium contents that were about 2.5 times more than the control diet, about 110 mmol/day, as well as increased magnesium and fiber. In addition, the combination diet had lower saturated and total fat and cholesterol content because of reduced consumption of red meats, visible fats, and oils, and increased calcium and protein content from both low- and nonfat dairy foods and fish. The BP-lowering effects of these diets were significant: −2.8/−1.1 mmHg for the fruits and vegetables diet and −5.5/−3.0 mmHg for the combination diet compared with the control diet. In hypertensive persons, the effects were −7.2/−2.8 mmHg and −11.4/−5.5 mmHg, respectively.

In a separate and subsequent outpatient feeding trial, the joint effects on BP of the DASH combination diet and changes in salt intake were examined [20]. Four hundred twelve participants were randomly assigned to either the DASH diet or the control diet for 3 months. Participants were fed their assigned diet at three levels of sodium for 30 days in random order in a crossover design. Mean urinary sodium excretion levels were 142 mmol/day for the higher sodium level (representing somewhat less than usual U.S. consumption), 107 mmol/day for the intermediate sodium (reflecting approximately the upper limit of current U.S. recommendations), and 65 mmol/day for the lower sodium level, a potentially more optimal level based on epidemiologic observations [7] and data from both small clinical studies [21,22] and a trial [23]. The results demonstrated a substantial effect of salt intake on BP (Table 2) [24]. In the control diet, a 77-mmol difference in sodium intake between the higher and lower sodium levels resulted in a BP change of −6.7/−3.5 mmHg ($p < 0.001$). A sodium-intake reduction of approximately 40 mmol/day from the intermediate sodium level reduced BP more than a similar reduction in sodium intake from the higher level ($p < 0.05$ for interaction); BP change between the higher and intermediate sodium levels was −2.1/−1.1 mmHg, while BP change between the intermediate and lower sodium levels was −4.6/−2.4 mmHg ($p < 0.001$ for all except $p < 0.01$ for DBP in the comparison between higher and intermediate sodium) (Fig. 1). Blood pressure was also reduced in the DASH diet with changes in sodium intake, although to a lesser extent than in the control diet. Overall, a 77-mmol difference in sodium intake with the DASH diet resulted in a reduction in BP of −3.0/−1.6 mmHg ($p < 0.001$ for both). The DASH diet reduced BP at every sodium level compared to the control diet: −5.9/−2.9 mmHg at the higher sodium level ($p < 0.001$); −5.0/−2.5 mmHg at the intermediate level ($p < 0.001$ for SBP and < 0.01 for DBP); and −2.2/−1.0 mmHg at the lower sodium level ($p < 0.05$ for SBP and $p < 0.10$ for DBP). The DASH diet had a greater effect on BP at the higher sodium levels than at the lower sodium level ($p < 0.001$ for interaction). The most substantial effect on BP was between the higher sodium level with the control diet versus the lower sodium level with the DASH diet: −8.9/−4.5 mmHg ($p < 0.001$ for both), an effect that was greater than sodium reduction alone or the DASH diet alone. In participants with hypertension, this combination lowered BP by −11.5/−5.7 mmHg, and in participants without hypertension by −7.1/−3.7 mmHg ($p < 0.01$ for interaction). The DASH-sodium trial [24,25] demonstrated that sodium reduction can substantially reduce BP in people both with and without hypertension. Additional analyses showed BP reduction in a wide array of subgroups, including older and younger, men and women, African-American and other races, and obese and nonobese [25].

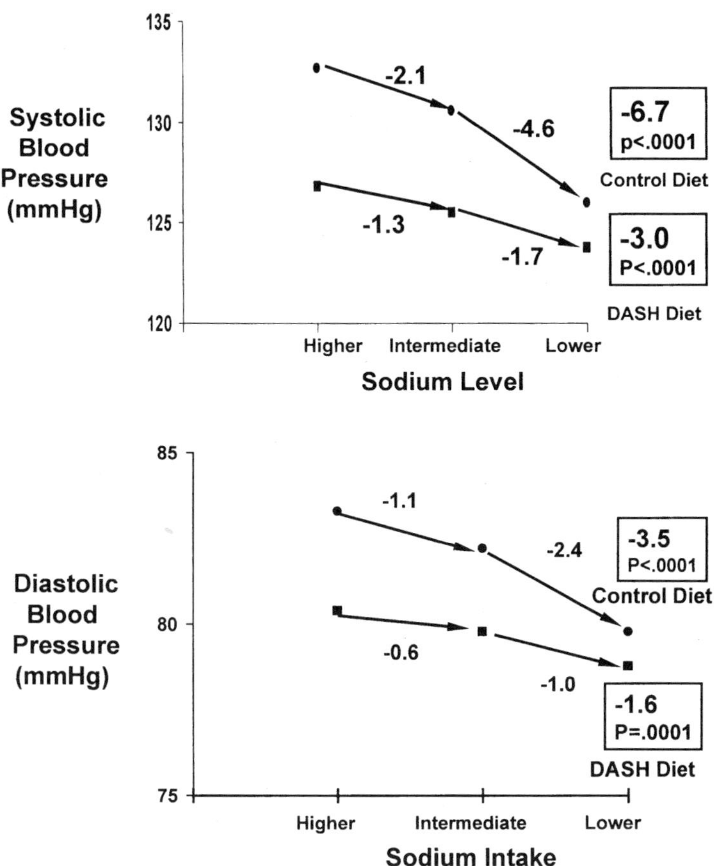

FIGURE 1 Effect of sodium level on SBP (upper panel) and DBP (lower panel). Unidirectional arrows are used for simplicity, although the order in which participants were given the sodium levels was random, with a crossover design. *Source*: Figure adapted from Ref. 24.

VARIATION IN RESPONSE TO DIETARY SODIUM CHANGES

There is considerable literature on variation in response of BP and other variables to short-term manipulation of sodium balance [26,27]. There are three principal problems with practical applications of this work. First, authors have taken what is universally acknowledged to be a continuous, approximately normal distribution of responses and applied arbitrary cutpoints based on an arbitrary magnitude of BP change such as 5 mmHg or 10%. This has led to classification of individuals as "salt-sensitive" and "salt-resistant." Although none of these studies was population-based, categories have then been extrapolated to populations of hypertensive and nonhypertensive persons to produce estimates of "prevalence of salt-sensitivity," implying that salt intake has no effect on the rest of the population. In fact, by varying the cutpoint to define "salt-sensitivity," one can obtain a variety of prevalence estimates from low to high. Second, the inference that these sodium-loading and -depletion protocols are measuring a stable characteristic of individuals rests on limited evidence [28–30], and several investigators have failed to find good evidence of reproducibility [31–33]. Although the interpretation of these data is to some extent in the eye of the beholder, it is clear that the reproducibility is far from perfect. Third, there is a question of validity: Do very short-term changes covering a period of 1 to 7 days observed under these protocols, many of which use extreme levels of salt loading and depletion, predict BP (and other) effects of long-term, gradual, and moderate changes in average intakes? This question has not been addressed by direct experimentation.

Although much of the literature on salt reduction and BP derives from relatively short-term clinical trials, there is evidence that average responses in groups are maintained over time. There is some evidence that predictors of the size of individual responses can take a long time to emerge, and may involve different mechanisms to an important degree. In a substudy from TOHP-II, an association between a polymorphism of the angiotensinogen gene and the BP response to sodium reduction (as well as weight loss) was not present at 6 months, and did not clearly emerge until the 36-month follow-up visit [34].

EFFECTS OF SODIUM INTAKE OTHER THAN ON BLOOD PRESSURE

Tobian and others have demonstrated in experimental rat models that high salt intake can cause lethal cerebrovascular lesions independent of their effects on arterial pressure [35], and limited epidemiologic data support a similar phenomenon in humans [36]. In human intervention studies, change in sodium has been associated directly with changes in left ventricular mass, a powerful CVD risk factor, independent of clinic-based BP measurements [37,38].

In the past few years evidence has been published that raises the possibility of an opposite phenomenon for dietary sodium; that is, that excessively low levels could increase cardiovascular risk. These studies have been of two types: sodium-reduction randomized trials that reported plasma levels of hormones or lipids, and observational studies of sodium intake or excretion and morbidity/mortality rates. Graudal has summarized the former studies [15], and most of the data come from very short-term studies of extremely low sodium, especially for effects on plasma cholesterol. A few of the studies reporting increases in plasma renin and aldosterone used moderate sodium reductions and durations of 4 weeks or longer [39], but these hormones are not established as CVD risk factors. In contrast with findings from the cohort of treated hypertensive patients cited below, Meade and colleagues [40] studied a cohort of 803 middle-aged men not selected based on hypertension status and found no association of plasma renin activity with risk of subsequent coronary death or nonfatal myocardial infarction (MI). In the subgroup of men with hypertension, further analysis suggested a slightly elevated but insignificant coronary risk in the upper tertile of renin level. For nonhypertensives there was no hint of increased risk associated with higher renin.

In the studies of sodium intake and morbidity and mortality, data have been reported for four U.S. cohorts [41–44] and one Finnish cohort [45]: (1) a worksite-based cohort of mostly treated hypertensive men (n = 1900) and women (n = 1037), with sodium intake based on a single 24-hr urine collected after a short drug washout period while being instructed to limit sodium intake [41]; (2) 11,696 middle-aged men followed for mortality during approximately 14 years after the end of the Multiple Risk Factor Intervention Trial (MRFIT), with sodium intake averaged for up to five annual 24-hr diet recalls during the trial [42]; (3) men (n = 4478) and women (n = 6868) followed for up to 21 years for mortality after participating in the first National Health and Nutrition Examination Survey [43] (NHANES I); (4) participants from NHANES I divided into overweight (n = 2688) and non-overweight (n = 6797) adults [44]; and (5) Finnish men (n = 1173) and women (n = 1263) followed for up to 13 years [45].

The worksite cohort [41] found a significant *inverse* association between sodium excretion and MI rate in men but not in women. No adjustment for other dietary factors could be done, as dietary and alcohol intakes were not collected. In addition, the potential existed that those with lower sodium excretion levels were in worse health than those with higher sodium excretion levels; BMI was lower, possibly indicative of coexisting illness, and creatinine clearance was lower, potentially reflecting poor renal function. In the MRFIT cohort [42] mortality rates from MI, coronary heart disease, and CVD were *higher* in the higher quintiles of baseline sodium intake than the lowest, but not significantly so when adjusted for several potentially confounding variables, the most influential one of which was total caloric intake. Similar results were observed in NHANES I [43] in that the association with CVD and all-causes mortality of baseline sodium intake was *inverse* without including total calories in the model, but *direct* when calories were considered, in the form of sodium/calorie ratio. This direct relationship was also found by He et al. [44], significant only in the overweight, with analyses adjusted for caloric intake. The one study with measures of urinary sodium found a *direct* relation with coronary heart disease (CHD) incidence and with mortality from coronary heart disease, CVD, and all causes, even when adjusted for other CHD risk factors [45]. These last two studies found the beneficial effect of lower sodium only in overweight adults [44], or stronger in overweight than nonoverweight adults [45]. Given the high prevalence of overweight in the United States and many other countries, a direct relationship between salt intake and CVD in overweight people would be a public health concern. The inverse relationship in the earlier NHANES I study was seen because higher total caloric intake was strongly associated with lower risk of death. The reason for this powerful relationship is unclear, but two possibilities are that higher caloric intake represents higher energy expenditure—that is, greater physical activity (as it must since BMI did not differ across calorie categories)—and that the group with low caloric intake included a higher percentage of people in poor health. These alternative hypotheses challenge interpretations that suggest these observational studies provide credible evidence for an adverse effect of lower sodium intake. Moreover, the study with the best objective measure of sodium intake derived from 24-h urinary excretion showed a lower incidence of CVD with lower salt intake. In addition, a study examining salt-sensitive and non-salt-sensitive people found those with salt sensitivity had twofold increased mortality, regardless of whether or not they had high BP at baseline. This study supports observational data indicating that in a salt-abundant environment, people who are salt-sensitive, likely a large percentage of the population, will have an increase in BP, particularly as they age, which will eventually shorten their life span [45a].

Finally, there is evidence from epidemiologic studies that higher salt intake is associated with higher risks of other widespread diseases, including osteoporosis and renal stones (both presumably due to increased calcium excretion), gastric cancer (the secular decline of which may reflect earlier decreases in the use of salt in food preservation), and asthma, the latter relationship supported by some intervention data as well [46].

LOWERING SALT INTAKE

There are no good estimates of the current salt intake in the population. National dietary surveys generally use 24-h dietary recalls that estimate, from nutrient databases, the sodium naturally occurring in foods and added to processed foods. Sodium added at the table is not routinely ascertained. Furthermore, portion sizes are not well estimated [47], and underreporting is common [48], which would result in underestimates of sodium intake.

Information on trends in sodium intake is also lacking. The NHANES III national survey used a different dietary ascertainment method than previous NHANES surveys, making comparisons over time problematic [49]. Despite these shortcomings, self-reported data from NHANES III indicate that adult men and women consume approximately 170 and 120 mmol/day of sodium, respectively. Higher sodium intake in men compared to women is most likely due to men's overall higher caloric intake. Only about 10% or less of adult men under age 60, and 20–30% of adult women under age 60, consumed less than 100 mmol/day of sodium [49], approximately the upper limit of sodium intake recommended by several health organizations [50,51].

In the current environment in the United States, salt is plentiful in the food supply because of its extensive and pervasive use in commercial food processing and in food preparation outside the home, particularly in restaurants, food carryouts, and fast food establishments, where a large proportion of daily meals is obtained. As a result, population levels of salt consumption are high, and acceptability of and adherence to lower salt intake are difficult to achieve. In BP trials to reduce salt intake by dietary modifications, adherence has not been optimal. Although lower salt intakes, as measured by 24-hour urinary excretion levels of sodium, have been achieved relative to baseline, intensive behavioral interventions have managed to reduce sodium intake over the long term by only about 40 to 60 mmol/day, with achieved intakes of approximately 90 to 135 mmol/day [11,12,52–55]. Average intakes thus still tended to be above the 100 mmol/day recommended limit. The range represents variations in population sample characteristics as well as degree of adherence to lower salt regimes. For example, older participants consume fewer calories and consequently less sodium, so in TONE the attained sodium level after 30 months of intervention was 95 mmol/day, a reduction of approximately 40 mmol/day [11].

Although promoting adherence to lower salt regimens has been challenging, studies have shown that preference for a salty taste decreases after about 2 to 3 months of consuming lower salt intake [56]. This increased acceptance of low-salt foods occurs mainly when discretionary salt use (salt at the table and used in cooking) is decreased, so that the direct sensory exposure to the salt taste is reduced. If salt intake is reduced by consuming foods lower in salt but allowing discretionary salt use, which results in similar sensory exposure as before the reduced salt diet, the preference for a salty taste does not change. It is therefore important to encourage people to reduce their discretionary use of salt so that their taste for salt decreases. In addition, it is important to encourage people to consume foods with lower salt content to achieve substantial reductions in salt intake, because discretionary salt use contributes only a small portion of total sodium intake [49,57].

PHYSICIAN ADVICE TO LOWER SALT INTAKE

Because there is no clinically useful way to identify individuals who are specifically salt-sensitive, all patients whose BP is greater than optimal (120/80 mmHg), which represents over 50% of the population [58], could benefit from lower sodium intake. To encourage all patients to lower their salt intake, two approaches are necessary. First, to reduce the taste for salt, patients should be advised not to add salt when cooking and preparing foods or at the table when consuming their foods. The second approach is to choose foods that are low in salt. Reading the nutrition facts label on foods is the first step to identifying which foods to choose. Among different brands of similar food items, the one with the lowest sodium content should be chosen. A general rule is to choose foods for which the percent of daily value for sodium (2400 mg) on the nutrition facts label is 5% or less. Product descriptions of sodium content per serving include sodium-free (5 mg or less), very low-sodium (35 mg or less), and low-sodium (140 mg or less), and are also useful in finding foods low in sodium. Other strategies are listed in Table 3. Many print materials and resources exist on Web sites from government and other health organizations (e.g., www.nhlbi.nih.gov/hbp/prevent/sodium/sodium.htm;

TABLE 3 Strategies to Reduce Salt and Sodium

Read and compare nutrition facts food labels.
Choose ready-to-eat breakfast cereals and breads and rolls that are lower in sodium (compare food labels).
Choose convenience foods that are lower in sodium. Cut back on frozen dinners, mixed dishes such as pizza, packaged mixes, canned soup or broths, and salad dressings that have high amounts of sodium.
Use reduced sodium or no-salt-added products.
Use fresh, plain frozen, or canned vegetables with no salt added.
Use fresh or frozen poultry, fish, and lean meat instead of canned, smoked, or processed types.
Limit cured foods (such as bacon and ham) and foods packed in brine (such as pickles, pickled vegetables, olives, and sauerkraut).
Limit condiments (such as MSG, mustard, horseradish, catsup, and barbecue sauce). Limit even the lower-sodium versions of soy sauce and teriyaki sauce. Treat these condiments as you do table salt.
Cook rice, pasta, and hot cereals without salt. Cut back on instant or seasoned rice, pasta, and grain mixes, which usually have added salt.
Be spicy instead of salty. In cooking and at the table, flavor foods with herbs, spices, and lemon, lime, vinegar, or salt-free seasoning blends.
Rinse canned foods such as tuna to remove the sodium.

www.americanheart.org/heart_and_stroke_A_Z_guide/sodium.html; www.eatright.org/erm/erm/00598.html).

Foods at restaurants and fast food outlets typically are highly salted. Some restaurants will comply with requests to not add salt or soy sauces to foods ordered. To lower overall salt intake, eating out should be limited, or on days when eating out, care should be taken that the balance of foods consumed for the day is very low in salt, or restaurants be selected that are willing to reduce sodium in their menus or food choices. Eating fewer sodium-dense foods and cooking more foods at home can result in approaching the daily value of sodium intake. However, to achieve even greater reductions in sodium intake that may be even more beneficial [24], such as 65 mmol (1500 mg/day), or 40% less than the daily value, avoiding ready-to-serve foods and avoiding eating out will be insufficient. To allow individuals greater choices and ability to lower their salt intake and to allow for even lower than daily value levels of sodium intake, it is imperative that the food industry lower the amount of salt it uses in processed foods across all types of foods, including grain products such as breads and ready-to-eat cereals, and for commercial eating establishments to prepare foods with less salt.

COMMUNITY INTERVENTION STUDIES

To achieve broad public health benefits, efficacious methods to lower BP should be shown to be effective in broadly representative populations. Reducing dietary salt should be one approach that is particularly amenable to a population approach, because upwards of 85% of dietary sodium comes from processed foods, a form of environmental exposure.

Two community-intervention salt-reduction trials have been completed in Europe using "quasi-experimental" designs (one intervention, one control community). In the Portuguese Salt Trial [59], two rural communities were compared, with random samples of residents ages 15 to 69 examined pre-intervention, then annually for 2 years. The health education program in the intervention community was facilitated by the fact that 50% of the very high (360 mmol Na per day) salt consumption came from that added in cooking at home, and another one-third was derived from one food item, salted dried codfish. There was also a focus on reducing salt in commercial bread baking. Results of this trial showed 42% lower sodium excretion in the intervention community at 1 year, and significant net reductions of mean BPs of 4 to 5 mmHg at both 1 and 2 years. In contrast, the Belgian salt trial [60] was much less successful in its intervention; there were no net changes in sodium excretion or BP for men, sodium changes for women were modest (about 20% reduction), and net reductions in mean BP (2.9 mmHg SBP and 1.6 mmHg DBP) were not significant. In contrast to the Portuguese trial, the same individuals were not examined at baseline and follow-up, leading to less precise estimation of BP change. A more recent 3-year community trial in urban north China [61] reported significant reductions of SBP (5 mmHg in men and 5 mmHg in women, ages 15 to 64) associated with net reductions in sodium intake of only 14% in men and 6% in women. Communitywide interventions aimed at salt reduction thus appear to be promising, at least in relatively uniform cultures. The success of such efforts in multicultural, highly commercialized settings has not been established.

Another community intervention experiment studied adolescents at two boarding schools [62]. In a crossover design with each phase lasting 1 academic year, sodium intake was reduced 15–20% merely by changes in food purchasing and preparation, with a significant effect on SBP and DBP of about 2 mmhg. This study is encouraging because of the simplicity of the intervention and because prevention is theoretically most attractive when begun in childhood.

CONCLUSIONS

Reducing dietary salt is effective in lowering BP levels (especially systolic pressure, which is more prognostically important than DBP) as well as hypertension incidence. While older persons, African Americans, and possibly women are more responsive to sodium reduction, other predictors of salt sensitivity have little practical application at present. There is no credible, coherent, reproducible evidence for harm from long-term moderate sodium reduction, and more recent evidence suggests benefit for reducing CVD. In addition there is some evidence for benefits from sodium reduction due to effects other than those on BP levels.

Abundant evidence supports the conclusion that there is great potential for reduced dietary sodium to contribute importantly to addressing the populationwide BP problem, which includes the primary prevention of hypertension. To reduce populationwide salt intake several approaches are necessary. Individuals need to be made more aware that reducing salt intake is beneficial, and physicians and health care providers need to advise patients to reduce salt intake as they check blood pressure. Relying solely on individuals to change their behavior regarding salt intake is insufficient, however, and the food industry should gradually lower the amount of salt added to foods during processing and substantially increase the availability of foods lower in sodium. The food service industry likewise should reduce salt use in food preparation practices and increase the availability of meals lower in salt. A combination of increased consumer demand and greater availability of foods and meals lower in salt would help reduce the salt intake of the population.

Modest, gradual, and persistent reductions in sodium intake is one of the most important public health interventions to reduce BP levels and the diseases related to above-optimal BP.

REFERENCES

1. Osborn JL, Greenberg SG. Renal nerves and extracellular volume regulation. In: Izzo JL, Jr, Black HR, eds. Hypertension Primer: The Essentials of High Blood Pressure. Baltimore: Williams and Wilkins, 1999: 89–91.
2. Weinberger MH. Salt sensitivity. In: Izzo JL Jr, Black HR, eds. Hypertension Primer: The Essentials of High Blood Pressure. Baltimore: Williams and Wilkins, 1999: 123–124.
3. Resnick LM. Divalent cations in essential hypertension. In: Izzo JL, Jr, Black HR, eds. Hypertension Primer: The Essentials of High Blood Pressure. Baltimore: Williams and Wilkins, 1999: 125–127.
4. DiPette DJ. Experimental models of hypertension. In: Izzo JL Jr, Black HR, ed. Hypertension Primer: The Essentials of High Blood Pressure. Baltimore: Williams and Wilkins, 1999: 128–130.
5. Denton D, Weisinger R, Mundy NI, Wickings EJ, Dixson A, Moisson P, et al. The effect of increased salt intake on blood pressure of chimpanzees. Nat Med. 1995; 1:1009–1016.
6. Elliott P. Observational studies of salt and blood pressure. Hypertension. 1991; 17(suppl. I):I-3–I-8.
7. Intersalt Cooperative Research Group. Intersalt: an international study of electrolyte excretion and blood pressure. Results for 24 hour urinary sodium and potassium excretion. BMJ. 1988; 297:319–328.
8. Elliott P, Stamler J, Nichols R, Dyer AR, Stamler R, Kesteloot H, et al. Intersalt revisited: further analyses of 24 hour sodium excretion and blood pressure within and across populations. BMJ 1996; 312:1249–1253.
9. Hofman A, Hazebroek A, Valkenburg HA. A randomized trial of sodium intake and blood pressure in newborn infants. JAMA. 1983; 250(3):370–373.
10. Geleijnse JM, Hofman A, Witteman JCM, Valkenburg HA, Grobbee DE. Long-term effects of neonatal sodium restriction on blood pressure. Hypertension 1997; 10(4):913–917.
11. Whelton PK, Appel LJ, Espeland MA, Applegate WB, Ettinger WH Jr, Kostis JB, et al. Sodium reduction and weight loss in the treatment of hypertension in older persons: a randomized controlled Trial of Nonpharmacologic Interventions in the Elderly (TONE). JAMA 1998; 279(11): 839–846.
12. The Trials of Hypertension Prevention Collaborative Research Group. Effects of weight loss and sodium reduction intervention on blood pressure and hypertension incidence in overweight people with high-normal blood pressure: the Trials of Hypertension Prevention, phase II. Arch Int Med 1997; 157:657–667.
13. Midgley JP, Matthew AG, Greenwood CMT, Logan AG. Effect of reduced

dietary sodium on blood pressure: a meta-analysis of randomized controlled trials. JAMA 1996; 275(20):1590–1597.
14. Cutler JA, Follmann D, Allender PS. Randomized trials of sodium reduction: an overview. Am J Clin Nutr 1997; 65(suppl.):643S–651S.
15. Graudal NA, Galloe AM, Garred P. Effects of sodium restriction on blood pressure, renin, aldosterone, catecholamines, cholesterols, and triglyceride: a meta-analysis. JAMA 1998; 279(17):1383–1391.
16. Bompiani GD, Cerasola G, Morici ML, Condorelli M, Trimarco B, De Luca N, et al. Effects of moderate low sodium/high potassium diet on essential hypertension: results of a comparative study. Int J Clin Pharmacol Ther Toxicol 1988; 26:129–132.
17. Geleijnse JM, Witteman JCM, Bak AAA, den Breeijen JH, Grobbee DE. Reduction in blood pressure with a low sodium, high potassium, high magnesium salt in older subjects with mild to moderate hypertension. BMJ 1994; 309:436–440.
18. Whelton PK, He J, Cutler JA, Brancati FL, Appel LJ, Follmann D, et al. Effect of oral potassium on blood pressure: meta-analysis of randomized controlled clinical trials. JAMA 1997; 277(20):1624–1632.
19. Appel LJ, Moore TJ, Obarzanek E, Vollmer WM, Svetkey LP, Sacks FM et al. A clinical trial of the effects of dietary patterns on blood pressure. N Engl J Med 1997; 336:1117–1124.
20. Svetkey LP, Sacks FM, Obarzanek E, Vollmer WM, Appel LJ, Lin P-H, et al. The DASH diet, sodium intake and blood pressure trial (DASH-Sodium): rationale and design. J Am Diet Assoc. 1999; 99(8):S96–S104.
21. Hatch FT, Wertheim AR, Eurman GH, Watkin DM, Froeb HF, Epstein HA. Effects of diet in essential hypertension. III. Alterations in sodium chloride, protein and fat intake. Am J Med 1954; 17:499–513.
22. Kawasaki T, Delea CS, Bartter FC, Smith H. The effect of high-sodium and low-sodium intakes on blood pressure and other related variables inhuman subjects with idiopathic hypertension. Am J Med 1978; 64:193–198.
23. MacGregor GA, Sagnella GA, Markandu ND, Singer DRJ, Cappuccio FP. Double-blind study of three sodium intakes and long-term effects of sodium restriction in essential hypertension. Lancet 1989; ii:1244–1247.
24. Sacks FM, Svetkey LP, Vollmer WM, Appel LJ, Bray GA, Harsha D, et al. Effects on blood pressure of reduced dietary sodium and the Dietary Approaches to Stop Hypertension (DASH) diet. N Engl J Med 2001; 344(1): 3–10.
25. Vollmer WM, Sacks FM, Ard J, Appel LJ, Bray GA, Simons-Morton DG, et al. Effects of dietary patterns and sodium intake on blood pressure: subgroup results of the DASH-Sodium Trial. Ann Int Med 2001; 135(12):1019–1028.
26. Weinberger MH. Salt sensitivity of blood pressure in humans. Hypertension 1996; 27(3):481–490.
27. Luft FC, Weinberger MH. Heterogeneous responses to changes in dietary salt intake: the salt-sensitivity paradigm. Am J Clin Nutr 1997; 65(suppl.): 612S–617S.

28. Weinberger MH, Fineberg NS. Sodium and volume sensitivity of blood pressure: age and pressure change over time. Hypertension 1991; 18(1): 67–71.
29. Overlack A, Ruppert M, Kolloch R, Gobel B, Kraft K, Diehl J, et al. Divergent hemodynamic and hormonal responses to varying salt intake in normotensive subjects. Hypertension 1993; 22(3):331–338.
30. Sharma AM, Schattenfroh S, Kribben A, Distler A. Reliability of salt-sensitivity testing in normotensive subjects. Klin Wochenschr 1989; 67:632–623.
31. Zoccali C, Mallamaci F, Cuzzola F, Leonardis D. Reproducibility of the response to short-term low salt intake in essential hypertension. J Hypertens 1996; 14(12):1455–1459.
32. Mattes RD, Falkner B. Salt-sensitivity classification in normotensive adults. Clin Sci 1999; 96:449–459.
33. Gerdts E, Lund-Johansen P, Omvik P. Reproducibility of salt sensitivity testing using a dietary approach in essential hypertension. J Human Hypertens 1999; 13:375–384.
34. Hunt SC, Cook NR, Oberman A, Cutler JA, Hennekens CH, Allender PS, et al. Angiotensinogen genotype, sodium reduction, weight loss, and prevention of hypertension: Trials of Hypertension Prevention, phase II. Hypertension 1998; 32:393–401.
35. Tobian L. Dietary sodium chloride and potassium have effects on the pathophysiology of hypertension in humans and animals. Am J Clin Nutr 1997; 65:606S–611S.
36. Perry IJ, Beevers DG. Salt intake and stroke: a possible direct effect. J Human Hypertens 1992; 6:23–25.
37. Ferrara LA, de Simone G, Pasanisi F, Mancini M. Left ventricular mass reduction during salt depletion in arterial hypertension. Hypertension 1984; 6:755–759.
38. Liebson PR, Grandits GA, Dianzumba S, Prineas RJ, Grimm RH Jr, Neaton JD, et al. Comparison of five antihypertensive monotherapies and placebo for change in left ventricular mass in patients receiving nutritional-hygienic therapy in the Treatment of Mild Hypertension Study (TOMHS). Circulation 1995; 91:698–706.
39. Alderman MH, Madhavan S, Ooi WL, Cohen H, Sealey JE, Laragh JH. Association of the renin-sodium profile with the risk of myocardial infarction in patients with hypertension. N Engl J Med 1991; 324:1098–1104.
40. Meade TW, Cooper JA, Peart WS. Plasma renin activity and ischemic heart disease. N Engl J Med 1993; 329:616–619.
41. Alderman MH, Madhavan S, Cohen H, Sealey JE, Laragh JH. Low urinary sodium is associated with greater risk of myocardial infarction among treated hypertensive men. Hypertension 1995; 25:1144–1152.
42. Cohen JD, Grandits G, Cutler JA, Neaton JD, Kuller LH, Stamler J. Dietary sodium intake and mortality: MRFIT Follow-up Study results. Circulation 1999; 100(18), I-524.
43. Alderman MH, Cohen H, Madhavan S. Dietary sodium intake and mortality:

the National Health and Nutrition Examination Survey (NHANES I). Lancet 1998; 351:781–785.

44. He J, Ogden LG, Vupputuri S, Bazzano LA, Loria C, Whelton PK. Dietary sodium intake and subsequent risk of cardiovascular disease in overweight adults. JAMA 1999; 282(21):2027–2034.
45. Tuomilehto J, Jousilahti P, Rastenyte D, Moltchanov V, Tanskanen A, Pietinen P, et al. Urinary sodium excretion and cardiovascular mortality in Finland: a prospective study. Lancet 2001; 357:848–851.
45a. Weinberger MH, Fineberg NS, Fineberg SE, Weinberger M. Salt sensitivity puse pressure and death in normal and hypertensive humans. Hypertension 2001; 37:429–432.
46. Antonios TF, MacGregor GA. Salt–more adverse effects. Lancet 1996; 348: 250–251.
47. Blake AJ, Guthrie HA, Smiciklas-Wright H. Accuracy of food portion estimation by overweight and normal-weight subjects. J Am Diet Assoc 1989; 89(7):962–964.
48. Black AE, Goldberg GR, Jebb SA, Livingstone MBE, Cole TJ, Prentice AM. Critical evaluation of energy intake data using fundamental principles of energy physiology: 2. Evaluating the results of published surveys. Eur J Clin Nutr 1991; 45:583–599.
49. Loria CM, Obarzanek E, Ernst ND. Choose and prepare foods with less salt: dietary advice for all Americans. J Nutr 2001; 131(2S-I):536S–551S.
50. Joint National Committee on Prevention, Detection, Evaluation, and Treatment of High Blood Pressure. The Sixth Report of the Joint National Committee on Prevention, Detection, Evaluation, and Treatment of High Blood Pressure. Arch Int Med 1997; 157:2413–2446.
51. Krauss RM, Eckel RH, Howard B, Daniels SR, Deckelbaum RJ, Erdman JW Jr, et al. AHA Dietary Guidelines. Revision 2000: a statement for healthcare professionals from the Nutrition Committee of the American Heart Association. Circulation 2000; 102:2284–2299.
52. The Trials of Hypertension Prevention Collaborative Research Group. The effects of nonpharmacologic interventions on blood pressure of persons with high normal levels: results of the Trials of Hypertension Prevention, phase 1. JAMA 1992; 267(9):1213–1220.
53. Thaler BI, Paulin JM, Phelan EL, Simpson FO. A pilot study to test the feasibility of salt restriction in a community. NZ Med J 1982; 95(721):839–842.
54. Stamler R, Stamler J, Grimm R, Gosch FC, Elmer P, Dyer A, et al. Nutritional therapy for high blood pressure: final report of a four-year randomized controlled trial—the Hypertension Control Program. JAMA 1987; 257(11): 1484–1491.
55. Stamler R, Stamler J, Gosch FC, Civinelli J, Fishman J, McKeever P, et al. Primary prevention of hypertension by nutritional-hygienic means: final report of a randomized, controlled trial. JAMA 1989; 262(13):1801–1807.
56. Mattes RD. The test for salt in humans. Am J Clin Nutr 1997; 65(suppl.):692S–697S.

57. Mattes RD. Discretionary salt and compliance with reduced sodium diet. Nutr Res 1990; 10:1337–1352.
58. Burt VL, Whelton P, Roccella EJ, Brown C, Cutler JA, Higgins M, et al. Prevalence of hypertension in the US adults population: results from the Third National Health and Nutrition Examination Survey, 1988–1991. Hypertension 1995; 25(3):305–313.
59. Forte JG, Miguel JM, Miguel MJ, de Padua F, Rose G. Salt and blood pressure: a community trial. J Human Hypertens 1989; 3:179–184.
60. Staessen J, Bulpitt CJ, Fagard R, Joossens JV, Lijnen P, Amery A. Salt intake and blood pressure in the general population: a controlled intervention trial in two towns. J Hypertens 1988; 6:965–973.
61. Tian H-G, Guo Z-Y, Hu G, Yu S-J, Sun W, Pietinen P, et al. Changes in sodium intake and blood pressure in a community-based intervention project in China. J Human Hypertens 1995; 9:959–968.
62. Ellison RC, Capper AL, Stephenson WP, Goldberg RJ, Hosmer DW Jr, Humphrey KF, et al. Effects on blood pressure of a decrease in sodium use in institutional food preparation: the Exeter-Andover Project. J Clin Epidemiol 1989; 42(3):201–208.

7

Moderation of Alcohol Consumption

Ian B. Puddey
The University of Western Australia and the West Australian Heart Research Institute, Perth, Australia

William C. Cushman
University of Tennessee Health Science Center, Memphis, Tennessee, U.S.A.

INTRODUCTION

The hemodynamic effects of alcohol have been reported at least since the middle of the nineteenth century. In an anonymous editorial in the *British Medical Journal* [1] in 1861, it was stated that "The influence that alcohol exercises on the circulating system is probably one of its most important actions in a therapeutic point of view." In the same editorial the direct effects of alcohol on blood vessels in vitro were described with the observation that "such a state of capillaries would necessarily result in increased tension of the arterial system and fullness of the pulse, the more especially, when taken in connection with the effects produced on the heart itself by the local action of alcohol." In a further article later that same year [2], Dr. Edward Smith observed that alcohol "increases the force of the heart's action, as proved by the fullness and sharpness of the pulse, and by the pulsation at the temples, and in the small arteries of the hand as they lay on the table, and the height to which the foot is jerked when, after taking a glass of spirit and water, we sit with the legs crossed." He speculated that with respect to alcohol "its essential physiological action seems to be directly or indirectly upon the capillary system." A clinical association between excessive alcohol ingestion and hyper-tension was first suggested in 1877 by the observations of Frederick Akbar Mahomed [3], who using a sphygmograph reported a high-tension pulse in "apparently healthy persons, but who, not uncommonly are subjects of the gouty diathesis, dyspeptics, alcoholists, or who possess one or other of the predisposing causes to chronic Bright's disease." The first population-based study of alcohol use and prevalence of hypertension was reported in 1915 by a French surgeon, Lian. He found a linear relationship between the amount of wine regularly ingested by French troops on the western front and the prevalence of hypertension [4]. There has since been a large number of cross-sectional and prospective population studies that have consistently demonstrated a direct and positive relationship between ingestion of alcoholic beverages and an increase in both the level of blood pressure (BP) and the prevalence of hypertension.

CROSS-SECTIONAL STUDIES

After the effects of body weight, the relationship between the amount of alcohol consumed and BP is one of the strongest positive associations of potentially modifiable risk factors for hypertension [5–9]. This relationship usually persists even when other factors are taken into account, such as age, weight (or body mass index), sodium and potassium intake, cigarette smoking, and education. This association is also independent of ethnicity or race, with scores of cross-sectional studies from many different cultures observing the relationship, and reports of an association between alcohol and an increase in BP in whites, blacks, and Asians [5–7].

When regular drinkers alone have been considered, a dose-response relationship has usually been reported between alcohol intake and an increase in the prevalence of hypertension, with increases in BP in association with the consumption of as few as one to two drinks per day [10]. When lifelong nondrinkers and occasional drinkers have been compared to more regular drinkers often a J-shaped relationship has been observed [7,11,12]. In other studies, although no J shape has been seen, curvilinearity of the alcohol–BP relationship has still been demonstrated, with smaller increases of BP with low consumption and larger increases with higher alcohol exposure [13]. The J shape has led to conjecture by some groups that small doses of alcohol may have a BP lowering effect. There are many factors that could potentially result in curvilinearity of the relationship, however studies have often not accounted for distinctions among nondrinkers, light drinkers, and heavier drinkers in dietary habits (including salt intake), level of physical activities, prevalence of overweight, smoking habit, and socioeconomic background. Other confounders include misclassification bias, with subjects underreporting their alcohol intake and being inappropriately included in a non- or light-drinker category. Past heavy drinkers who have now given up drinking may also mistakenly be categorized as nondrinkers. In some studies in which these confounding influences have been carefully taken into account, the J shape or curvilinearity of the alcohol–BP relationship has been attenuated [14].

GENDER EFFECTS

In several cross-sectional studies, curvilinearity of the alcohol–BP relationship has often been more marked in women compared to men [12,15]. In fact, a meta-analysis of 11 population-based studies carried out up until 1993 [16] suggested that in women with low-level drinking there were lower levels of BP and a decrease in the risk of hypertension compared to nondrinkers. Overall, however, associations between alcohol intake and hypertension have not been as extensively evaluated in women as in men, and generally women have been underrepresented in the heavier drinking categories in many of the cross-sectional studies. A large cross-sectional U.S. survey of over 19,000 subjects [17] found that women who reported a prior diagnosis of hypertension also reported consuming significantly less alcohol than women who did not report hypertension. In contrast, self-reported hypertensive men consumed equal or greater amounts of alcohol than self-reported normotensive men. Such gender differences in drinking behavior despite knowledge of higher BP may well have biased cross-sectional surveys that have suggested an influence of gender on the alcohol–BP relationship. A large U.K. study of over 14,000 female employees (the Marks and Spencer Cardiovascular Risk Study) [18] found a decrease in the prevalence of hypertension with consumption of up to 14 drinks per week, but this decrease was largely explained by confounding by age, body mass index (BMI), physical activity, and family history of premature coronary heart disease. The recent large National Health and Nutrition Examination Survey (NHANES) III study [19], which included over 9000 women, found that associations of alcohol intake with both systolic blood pressure and pulse pressure were considerably smaller in women compared to men. A Brazilian study indicated the opposite, with substantially increased levels of blood pressure in women for the same level of intake compared to men [13]. Resolution of the controversy as to whether or not there are unconfounded gender differences awaits a randomized controlled trial, since there have been no randomized controlled trials to date of the effects of alcohol on BP in women and certainly no randomized controlled trials in either men or women to demonstrate that low-level drinking can lower BP compared with abstention.

TEMPORAL RELATIONSHIPS OF ALCOHOL DRINKING TO BLOOD PRESSURE

Some cross-sectional population-based studies have concluded that the effects of alcohol are predominantly related to recent alcohol intake rather than chronic levels of alcohol use [20,21]. Because studies in alcoholic subjects during detoxification have shown that the magnitude of BP is related to the severity of alcohol withdrawal [22,23], this has resulted in speculation that the relationship of alcohol with BP in population-based studies is also largely due to a withdrawal effect. In such studies, however, measures of recent and usual alcohol intake have often been constructed from the same 7-day retrospective diary, raising the possibility that any results have to some extent been influenced by confounding due to recall bias, with more accurate recall of recent alcohol intake. In a Japanese study [24] usual daily alcohol consumption—but not alcohol abstinence—for 1 day prior to BP measurement predicted the finding of higher BP in regular male drinkers, while in an Australian study [25] the relationship between usual weekly alcohol intake and BP was independent of intake within the preceding 24 hr, but a relationship between recent intake and BP was no longer significant after adjustment for usual intake. A study from Brazil [13], which measured the time elapsed since the last drink, identified a biphasic effect, with BP lower in men who had consumed alcohol less than 3 hr before BP measurement, but a higher prevalence of hypertension in men who consumed alcohol 13 to 23 hr before measurement compared to those for whom 24 hr or more had elapsed.

PATTERN OF DRINKING AND BLOOD PRESSURE

The temporal relationships of alcohol to level of BP have also led to conjecture that there is possibly a greater impact on BP of episodic (binge) drinking than regular daily patterns of lower levels of alcohol intake. This was initially highlighted by a British study of the alcohol–BP relationship by day of the week on which BP measurement was made [26]. That study found higher daily BP in heavy weekend drinkers than in moderate daily drinkers, even though total weekly alcohol intake was similar between the two groups. Diagnosis of hypertension was more prevalent on Mondays than on Fridays in moderate and heavy weekend drinkers, while in heavy daily drinkers the prevalence of hypertension was substantially higher on both Monday and Tuesday. The PRIME study, which compared the population of Belfast with those of three French cities [27], has shown similar results. The Northern Irish subjects consumed two-thirds of their alcohol intake on the weekend and had higher BP on a Monday, falling toward Thursday, while the French subjects consumed their alcohol in a more homogenous pattern and had constant BP throughout the week. In another study, using ambulatory BP monitoring, subjects who predominantly concentrated their drinking at the weekend were shown to have higher BP levels throughout a 24-hr period on Monday compared to Thursday [28] (Fig. 1), and this difference was lost when they substantially reduced their alcohol intake.

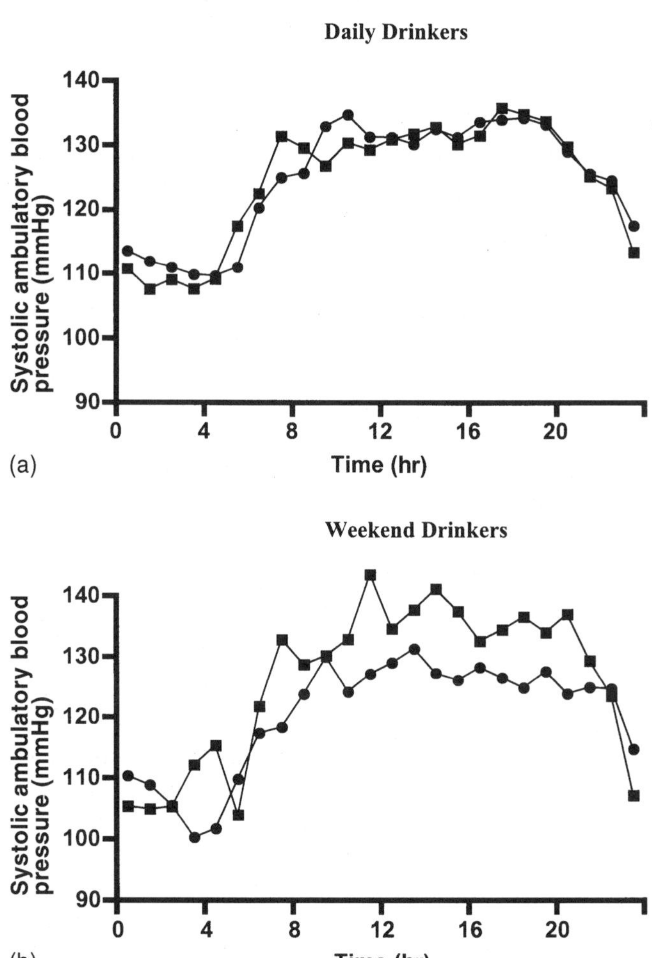

FIGURE 1 The 24-hr ambulatory SBP profile by day of assessment for (a) daily drinkers compared to (b) weekend drinkers; -■- Monday SBP, -●- Thursday SBP. *Source*: Reprinted with permission from Ref. 28.

Other studies have directly compared the effects of heavy daily drinking versus heavy episodic drinking. In the large worldwide Intersalt Study [6], higher BP were seen in heavy drinkers (> 250 g/week) than nondrinkers, irrespective of any alcohol consumed in the previous 24 hr. Compared to nondrinkers, however, those heavy drinkers with a high variability of alcohol intake exhibited even higher BPs than heavy drinkers with low variability in alcohol consumption. A different result was seen in a Finnish study [29], in which daily heavy drinkers (mean alcohol intake of 527 g/week) showed more detrimental BP effects than heavy binge-type weekend drinkers (mean alcohol intake of 289 g/week). Both systolic and diastolic BP were significantly higher (by 8/6 mmHg, respectively) in the daily heavy drinkers, while in heavy weekend drinkers only systolic BP was increased (by 5 mmHg), despite the weekend alcohol consumption being nearly twice as high as in the daily drinkers. In a recent Japanese study of strictly normotensive subjects [30], both episodic alcohol consumption and monthly alcohol consumption showed similar dose-effect relationships with level of BP.

These studies of both the pattern of alcohol consumption and the temporal relationship of alcohol with BP suggest that there is probably both an acute BP elevating effect of the alcohol withdrawal syndrome in episodic and predominantly weekend drinkers and a longer-term but reversible direct pressor effect in regular daily drinkers. Sustained heavy drinking, however, may cause less reversible hypertensive effects, with evidence suggestive of residual chronic pressor effects of alcohol in heavy drinkers and alcoholics, even after subjects have become abstinent [31,32].

ALCOHOL AND AMBULATORY BLOOD PRESSURE

A recent Australian cross-sectional study [33] raised the possibility that the effects of alcohol to elevate BP were only a "white coat" effect, with alcohol consumption related to clinic BP measurement or the difference between clinic and 24-hr mean BP, but not to 24-hr mean BP itself. In two other reports, however, 24-hr BP monitoring in ambulant moderate drinkers confirmed significant changes in BP during either 4 weeks of a substantial decrease in alcohol intake [28] or after a single session of binge drinking (twelve drinks over 6hr) [34]. In the first study [35], 14 drinkers who consumed most part of their alcohol on the weekend were compared with 41 drinkers who drank predominantly on a daily basis. They were studied during either a 4-week period of high alcohol intake or a 4-week period in which there was an approximate 80% reduction in alcohol intake. When switched from high to low alcohol intake, there was a significant decrease in 24-hr ambulatory BP, which was of similar magnitude in both the weekend and daily drinkers. In the second study [34] 24-hr BP was higher during the 6-hr intoxication period but lower over the ensuing 6hr and no different the following day. A similar biphasic pattern has been suggested on ambulatory BP monitoring in several other acute studies [36–40]. In some, acute vasodilatory effects of alcohol have predominated [38,39], with an early fall in BP after drinking, although the metabolic consequences of acetaldehyde dehydrogenase deficiency with tachycardia and acute flushing characteristic of many Japanese subjects may have influenced some of these results. An overall conclusion from these studies is that there is an acute depressor effect of alcohol followed by an increase in BP toward the second half of a 24-hr period. Other cross-sectional studies of alcohol consumption in relation to 24-hr ambulatory BP have identified alcohol–BP relationships independent of any white coat effects [41], while studies in heavy drinkers and alcoholics consistently report falls in 24-hr or daytime BP following abstention [42–44]. Other studies have reported heightened BP variability after alcohol [44,45], even when no overall effect on 24-hr BP has been seen [45].

BEVERAGE PREFERENCE

The alcohol–BP relationship has been observed no matter what type of alcoholic beverage has been ingested, with reports of an increase in BP with alcohol in predominantly wine-drinking French [46] or Italians [47], beer-drinking Australians [10] or Germans [48,49], and sake-drinking Japanese [50]. There are suggestions, however, that wine has a lesser effect on BP, with speculation that this may reflect the high levels of vasodilator and antioxidant flavonoids seen particularly in red wine. The first report was from the Lipid Research Clinics Prevalence Study [21], in which regression analysis was used to assess the relative associations with BP in those who reported consuming only one type of alcoholic beverage. The coefficients for beer and spirits were both positive and statistically significant in men, while the coefficient for wine was positive for systolic BP and negative for diastolic BP, with neither result statistically significant. A recent report from the PRIME study [51] also found a lesser association of wine with BP compared to beer. Although each of these studies adjusted for conventional risk factors such as age, BMI, smoking, and education, they did not consider differences in diet by beverage preference. There is now considerable evidence that this may be a powerful determinant of differences in hypertension incidence and cardiovascular risk between those who prefer wine to beer or spirits, with wine drinkers more likely to have a healthier diet [52].

PROSPECTIVE POPULATION STUDIES

The evidence from prospective population studies that the regular consumption of alcohol results in an increased long-term risk for developing hypertension is persuasive. In 1999 a meta-analysis of three careful prospective studies reported a 40% increase in relative risk of hypertension in those drinking 25 g of alcohol per day and a more than four-fold increase in risk in those drinking 100 g of alcohol per day [53]. In several further recent large-scale prospective studies from Japan [54–56] and the United States [57] up to two-fold increases in the the risk of hypertension with intakes of 30 to 50 g of alcohol per day have been reported. In the Atherosclerosis Risk in Communities (ARIC) study [57] it was estimated that in subjects drinking 30 g/day or more, one in five cases of hypertension could be attributed to the consumption of alcohol alone. A change in drinking status during follow-up has also been associated with changes in BP with increases in those who initiate drinking [58,59] and decreases in those who lessen their intake or become abstinent [56,60]. A further recent Canadian report [61] compared the consequences of drinking eight or more drinks in one sitting to a nonbinge pattern of drinking, and after an 8-year follow-up period the binge pattern of drinking increased the risk of hypertension in men but not women. In the ARIC study, the relative long-term risks for developing hypertension with intakes of alcohol $\geq$ 210g/week appeared similar for both men and women.

INTERVENTION STUDIES

Short-term controlled intervention studies to reduce alcohol intake in moderate to heavy drinkers provide strong support for the suggestion from cross-sectional and prospective population studies of a direct causal link between chronic alcohol consumption and raised BP. Such studies have consistently demonstrated a decline in BP within 1 to 2 weeks of alcohol restriction [62,63], with further gradual declines in BP after 4 to 6 weeks. In longer-term randomized controlled interventions the results have not been as consistent. In an 18-week study in which alcohol restriction (by four to five standard drinks per day) was combined with caloric restriction (reducing weight by 7.5 kg), the two interventions had an additive effect to reduce BP by approximately 10 mmHg [64] (Fig. 2). In contrast, the largest and longest randomized, controlled trial to date, the Prevention and Treatment of Hypertension Study (PATHS) [65], observed smaller and insignificant falls in BP during a 6-month intervention (0.9/0.6 mmHg decrease for systolic and diastolic BP, respectively). This U.S. National Institutes of Health and Veterans Affairs Cooperative Studies Program trial included 641 moderate to heavy drinkers with diastolic BP of 80 to 99 mmHg. Anyone with evidence of alcoholism, complications of excess alcohol intake, or significant cardiovascular or psychiatric diseases was excluded. Although the difference in alcohol intake was highly significant, it averaged only 1.3 drinks per day, the shortfall resulting in part because the control group lowered alcohol intake more than anticipated. In most other controlled trials of alcohol reduction and BP,

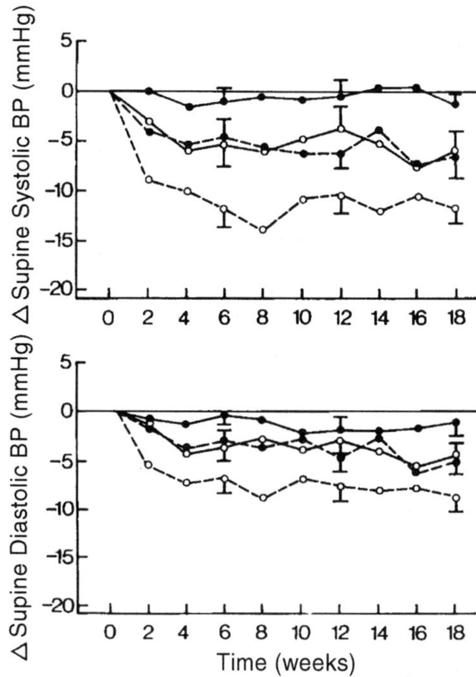

FIGURE 2 Line graph shows change in mean ± standard error of the mean (SEM) systolic (top) and diastolic (bottom) blood pressure in four study groups: ●—●, normal alcohol intake/normal caloric intake (n = 20); ●—●, normal alcohol intake/low caloric intake (n = 22); ○—○, low alcohol intake/normal caloric intake (n = 21); ○—○, low alcohol intake/low caloric intake (n = 23). *Source*: Reprinted with permission from Ref. 64.

baseline levels of alcohol intake have been higher and changes in alcohol intake larger than in PATHS.

The first meta-analysis of randomized controlled trials of the effects of alcohol reduction on BP was recently published [66], with 15 trials meeting the inclusion criteria [28,62–65,67–75]. Men were the sole participants in 12 of these trials, and by far the majority in the remaining three trials. In seven studies subjects were hypertensive and in six studies they were normotensive, while in two studies they were either normotensive or hypertensive. In six trials subjects were taking antihypertensive medication. The median duration of the trials was 8 weeks, during which subjects reduced their alcohol consumption by a median 76% from a base intake of three to six standard drinks per day. This resulted in a pooled effect estimate of the effects of alcohol reduction on BP of 3.31/2.04 mmHg (Fig. 3). The magnitude of this

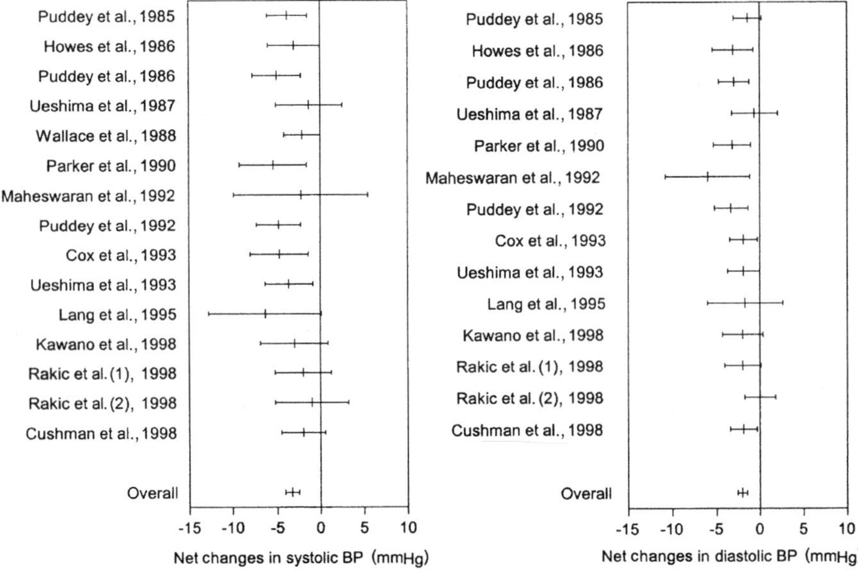

FIGURE 3 Average net change in systolic BP (left) and diastolic BP (right) and corresponding 95% confidence intervals (CIs) related to alcohol reduction intervention in 15 randomized controlled trials. Net change was calculated as the difference of the baseline minus follow-up levels of BP for the intervention and control groups (parallel trials) or the difference in BP levels at the end of the intervention and control treatment periods (crossover trials). The overall effect represents a pooled estimate obtained by summing the average net change for each trial, weighted by the inverse of its variance. *Source*: Reprinted with permission from Ref. 66.

effect was similar in hypertensive and normotensive subjects and of similar magnitude in treated vs. untreated hypertensive subjects, with evidence of a dose-response relationship between the falls in BP and the reduction in alcohol intake. The fall in BP in these intervention studies corresponds well within the predicted estimates from large cross-sectional population studies such as Intersalt [6], in which subjects consuming 2.8 to 4.8 drinks per day exhibited BP 2.7/1.6 mmHg higher than nondrinkers.

ALCOHOL-NUTRIENT-LIFESTYLE INTERVENTIONS

Population-based studies suggest that the relationship between alcohol and increasing levels of BP is additive to the effects of obesity [7,10] and the oral contraceptive pill [76]. Such studies have also suggested that a BP increase with alcohol is additive to the effects of a sedentary lifestyle [77,78], although in an intervention study a simultaneous increase in fitness using exercise training, together with alcohol restriction, did not lead to lower BP than that achieved with alcohol restriction alone [68]. In another study a past history of alcoholism sensitized subjects to the BP-raising effect of salt [79], but in a group of men who were moderate regular drinkers, a short-term and moderate reduction in sodium intake in addition to a substantial decrease in alcohol did not lead to a greater fall in BP than that seen with alcohol restriction alone [67].

Smoking and alcohol interactions to influence the level of BP remain controversial. In an Australian study, in a population of working men, both nondrinkers and heavy drinkers who smoked had lower BP than those who did not smoke [10]. In contrast, a series of cross-sectional German studies have suggested that cigarette smoking may sensitize both male and female drinkers to the BP-raising effects of alcohol [48,49,80]. The psychological construct, job strain, in which subjects have high work demands but little decision latitude, has also been reported to sensitize subjects to an increase in BP with regular alcohol use [81], and psychometric factors may well need consideration in attempts to understand the interrelationships of alcohol and smoking with BP. In this regard, Arkwright et al. [82] reported that introverted drinkers who were nonsmokers had the highest levels of BP, but that this was not seen in drinkers who also smoked cigarettes.

Interactions between dietary calcium intake and alcohol consumption also remain controversial. In an analysis from the Honolulu Heart Program, Criqui et al. [83] found that calcium intake was associated with BP only in subjects with absent to light levels of alcohol intake. In contrast, the alcohol–BP association was independent of calcium intake. The findings of Hamet et al. [84] in a Canadian population differed, with the observation of a striking alcohol–calcium interaction with the impact of alcohol consumption on BP significantly attenuated in those subjects with intakes of calcium >800 mg/1000 kcal/day. Such an interaction received further credence from a prospective analysis of incident hypertension in the NHANES I Epidemiologic Follow-up Study [85], in which a protective effect of dietary calcium on hypertension ($OR=0.84$) was only seen in subjects who were not daily drinkers. Multivariate modeling suggested that this inhibitory effect of daily alcohol use on the protective relation between calcium intake and the risk of hypertension was seen even among younger and leaner subjects, with a 1 g/day increase in calcium intake associated with a 41% reduction in risk of hypertension in such subjects if they were not daily drinkers.

ALCOHOL AND HYPERTENSIVE TARGET-ORGAN DISEASE

The regular consumption of alcohol has been consistently associated with a decrease in risk for coronary artery disease. In a recent meta-analysis the peak protective effect was observed at an intake of 20 g per day [86], with a continued protective effect up to 72 g per day but an increase in coronary risk at intakes greater than 89 g per day. Large prospective studies have also reported antiatherosclerotic effects of light regular alcohol consumption in the peripheral [87,88] and renal vasculature [89]. These antiatherosclerotic effects may be related to increases in high-density lipoprotein (HDL-C) and its major apolipoproteins A-I and A-II [90], decreases in fibrinogen [91], and reduced platelet aggregability [92]. At higher levels of intake, however, any epidemiologically observed benefits of alcohol are reversed. The extent to which this may be due to alcohol-related hypertension is speculative, but statistical modeling of data from the Honolulu Heart Program [93] suggests that while 50% of the decrease in coronary risk with alcohol can be accounted for by an increase in HDL-C, this is counterbalanced in part by a 17% increase in risk due to higher systolic BP.

Similarly, with respect to cerebrovascular disease, light to moderate consumption confers protection against ischemic strokes [94]. Heavier consumption, on the other hand (especially binge drinking), increases the risk of both ischemic strokes and hemorrhagic events [95–97], an effect that to some extent may be due to alcohol-related hypertension. In a Japanese study [98] heavy drinking acted synergistically with hypertension to increase the risk of cerebral hemorrhage and infarction two- and three-fold, respectively. In contrast, in a British study of patients attending a hypertension clinic [99] there was a 40% decrease in relative risk of stroke seen in drinkers, with the lowest risk of stroke mortality at intakes of 1 to 10 units per week. Overall, however, that population sample included few heavy drinkers, and any beneficial effects of alcohol were offset at intakes >21 units/week by an increasing incidence of noncirculatory causes of death.

Alcohol-related hypertension may also contribute to the association of increasing alcohol intake with either increased left ventricular mass [41,100] or electrocardiographic evidence of left ventricular hypertrophy [101], although in these studies such associations were still present after controlling for level of BP. With respect to hypertensive nephrosclerosis, results from the Honolulu Heart Program [89] suggest that alcohol intake is negatively associated with the degree of renal arteriolar hyalinization. Similar to the scenario for coronary heart disease, effects of alcohol to reduce the risk of intrarenal atherosclerotic vascular changes may therefore mitigate against any detrimental effects on the kidney of alcohol-related increases in BP. There are several reports, however, that heavy alcohol use can increase the risk of microalbuminuria [41,102], an effect that in one of these studies appeared to be mediated by alcohol-related increases in BP [41]. In contrast, in a case control study in Maryland the finding of an increase in risk of end-stage renal disease with increasing alcohol intake [35] was independent of any effects of alcohol on hypertension.

GENE–ENVIRONMENT INTERACTIONS

Apolipoprotein E polymorphisms have been reported as determinants of the alcohol–BP relationship [103], with the E2/E3 and E3/E3 genotypes in Finnish subjects identified with stronger alcohol–BP relationships than E4/E3 subjects. In an intervention study, however, no relationship between decreases in BP with alcohol restriction and apolipoprotein E genotype were found [104]. Diminished aldehyde dehydrogenase activity due to the presence of the ADH2 polymorphism results in a high prevalence of a flushing response with tachycardia after alcohol ingestion in Japanese subjects. As a consequence this polymorphism has also been investigated in relation to alcohol-related hypertension [105,106]. Results to date have been mixed primarily because of the confounding caused by a substantially reduced alcohol intake in subjects who have the polymorphism. In a predominantly white North American population slow metabolism of alcohol due to the presence of the alcohol dehydrogenase type 3 polymorphism was associated with a decrease in risk of myocardial infarction, probably because of higher HDL-Cholesterol levels [107], but the implications of this polymorphism for alcohol-related hypertension have not been reported. Further insights into potential genetic determinants of the alcohol–BP relationship in both Asian and European populations may be anticipated from the combined approach of assessing genetic variation in both aldehyde dehydrogenase and alcohol dehydrogenase, the two major enzymes responsible for alcohol metabolism.

ANIMAL STUDIES AND POTENTIAL MECHANISMS

The predominant animal model utilized to explore possible mechanisms of alcohol-related hypertension has been the rat. This model has provided useful insights into potentially relevant etiological factors, but has proved controversial because of inconsistencies in BP outcomes between studies. In fact, in one of the inaugural studies carried out to ascertain effects of chronic ethanol feeding, in both normotensive Wistar Kyoto rats (WKY) and spontaneously hypertensive rats (SHR) [108], no significant effects on BP were seen after 80 days of ad libitum feeding of alcohol 10% v/v in the drinking water. In contrast, Chan and Sutter [109] have identified a pressor response in Wistar rats after 12 weeks of alcohol feeding. In that study alcohol was incrementally increased to 20% v/v in the drinking water over an initial 3 weeks and maintained at this level during a final 9 weeks.

This group [110,111] and others [112,113] have been able to reproduce this finding in Wistar rats in several subsequent studies that have focused on possible mechanisms of alcohol-related hypertension. In one study the BP increase was associated with slight increases in calcium pump activity, together with decreased membrane cholesterol content [110]. These were thought to be compensatory changes in response to the known acute fluidizing effects of alcohol on cell membranes, with altered lipid composition ultimately resulting in increased Ca^{2+}/Mg^{2+}-ATPase activity. Changes in membrane lipid composition with alterations in the polyunsaturated to saturated fatty acid ratio were directly related to the BP changes with alcohol in another study [112], suggesting altered membrane function or diminished availability of arachidonic acid precursors as potential mechanisms for alcohol-induced hypertension. Alcohol-induced increases in vascular smooth muscle calcium uptake, together with an increase in BP, have since been seen in WKY rats fed lower doses of alcohol [114], namely 5–10% v/v ad libitum in the drinking water, over a period of 7 to 14 weeks. These studies also identified renal arteriolar vascular smooth muscle hyperplasia in alcohol-fed rats that could be reversed by the administration of a calcium entry blocker, verapamil, but not by discontinuation of the alcohol intake [115]. The increase in BP, renal vascular changes, and the increase in intracellular calcium could also be reversed by coadministration of n-acetyl cysteine [116], suggesting an important role for the metabolism of alcohol to acetaldehyde for alcohol-induced hypertension in this model. Of interest, this group of investigators has also been able to identify a pressor response to alcohol in WKY rats, even with the administration of as little as 1% alcohol v/v over a period of 14 weeks [117]. In that study coadministration of dietary vitamin B6 (which augments methionine metabolism to cysteine) also decreased tissue acetaldehyde conjugates, prevented an increase in intracellular calcium levels, and counteracted both the increase in blood pressure and renal arteriolar changes. Other investigators have reported that magnesium supplementation can prevent the development of alcohol-induced hypertension in Wistar rats, possibly by counteracting an alcohol-induced increase in intracellular calcium and suppression of sodium pump activity [113]. Using the Wistar rat model, a synergy has also been demonstrated with chronic heat stress to induce more severe hypertension, with evidence that both the stress and chronic alcohol feeding simultaneously increase BP through chronic activation of the sympathetic nervous system [118].

Chronic alcohol administration (33% calories in a liquid diet over 30 days) to male Sprague Dawley rats had no effect on basal BP but impaired arterial baroreceptor responses [119], with the suggestion that such an effect may be an important prelude to subsequent BP elevation. After 12 weeks of alcohol administration this mechanism was clearly identified in Wistar rats, but was less evident in Sprague Dawley rats [120], although in both strains chronic alcohol feeding led to modest increases in BP.

Increases in BP in the Wistar rat have not been confirmed when each animal has been pair-fed with a control animal, with each study group identical for both isocaloric and fluid intake diets [121]. With this approach a relative decrease in BP has been seen within 3 weeks. A hypotensive effect of high-dose alcohol has also been evident in a number of other studies in the SHR with stroke-prone SHR and WKY rats [122–124]. Sanderson et al. [122] fed both SHR and WKY animals either no alcohol or alcohol as a 5% or 20% v/v solution for 8 or 16 weeks. In the SHR there was no difference in BP after 8 weeks, but by 16 weeks the 20% alcohol significantly lowered BP. Howe et al. [123,124] have similarly reported a retardation of the rise in BP normally seen in SHR or stroke-prone SHRs. They fed alcohol ad libitum in the drinking water at concentrations of 5% v/v at 4 to 5 weeks of age, 10% at 6 weeks, and 15% from 7 to 22 weeks. Lower BP relative to controls was evident from 12 weeks. These lower BPs may have been due to a myocardial depressant effect of alcohol, a phenomenon known to be augmented in the setting of hypertension [125,126]. They may also have resulted from lower weight gain when rats are fed alcohol ad libitum [127], and appear to have developed despite heightened heart rate responses to stress [127] or enhanced vascular contractility [121] after alcohol feeding in these strains.

The hypotensive response in SHRs contrasted with a rise in BP lasting several days after a sudden withdrawal of alcohol [123]. Similarly, although no increase in BP was seen in Sprague-Dawley rats fed a 30% alcohol solution twice daily by gavage, a hypertensive response was reported 24 hr after cessation of alcohol feeding [128]. Some of the differences between rat models may therefore relate not only to the dose of alcohol used and its means of administration but also to the timing of BP measurement in relation to the last intake of alcohol—a withdrawal pressor response also characteristic of the alcohol withdrawal syndrome in man. A further confounding factor in animal studies may relate to gender. Often this has been unspecified or studies were confined to males. Acute administration of ethanol intragastrically has resulted in hypotensive responses in female Sprague-Dawley rats, together with evidence of myocardial depression, but not in males, despite identical blood alcohol concentrations [129]. These differences have since been shown to be estrogen-dependent, but the etiology is yet to be characterized [130].

HUMAN STUDIES OF POTENTIAL MECHANISMS

Given the rapid onset and offset of alcohol-related hypertension evident in both animal and human studies, it is likely that any effects of alcohol on BP are not mediated by long-term structural alterations but by neural, hormonal, or other reversible physiologic changes affecting vascular tone and/or heart rate and cardiac output. The precise nature of these mechanisms needs further elucidation, but the studies in humans to date lend credence to some of the mechanisms suggested by animal studies and concur with a multifactorial basis for the pathogenesis of alcohol-related hypertension.

One of the more widely appreciated physiological changes relates to cutaneous vasodilatation, with a ruddy face and flushed peripheries often observed soon after acute alcohol ingestion. Graf and Strom [131] studied the influence of alcohol on skin and muscle blood flow in the human forearm and found an increase in hand blood flow but no significant influence on resting forearm blood flow. If alcohol is injected directly into the brachial artery rather than given orally, however, vasoconstriction is observed in both the forearm muscles and in the hand [131,132]. Cutaneous vasodilatory effects may therefore depend on alcohol metabolism to acetaldehyde, and need to be considered against alternative findings (mainly confined to animals) of vasoconstrictor effects of alcohol when other vascular sites (hepatic, pancreatic, and renal) have been studied.

Other studies in man have assessed the acute and subacute effects of alcohol on the pressor responses to α and β receptor agonists. Eisenhofer et al. [133] measured the acute effects of ethanol on the circulatory responses to isoprenaline. Alcohol (1 ml/kg) increased forearm blood flow measured by forearm venous occlusion plethysmography, but had no influence on the increase in forearm blood flow caused by isoprenaline. Howes and Reid [134] studied the effects of 4 days of alcohol ingestion (80 g/day) and reported an increase in the dose of noradrenaline necessary to raise blood pressure by 20 mmHg. It was inferred from these studies that alcohol acutely depressed α adrenoreceptor-mediated vasoconstriction but had no effect on β receptor mediated vasodilation. A report by Arkwright et al. [135], however, suggests any longer-term effects of alcohol on vascular reactivity are unlikely. In a case-control study of drinking and nondrinking males matched for age and weight, they compared BP responses to a series of standardized physiologic stressors and demonstrated very similar results despite significantly higher resting BP in the drinkers. More recently there has been a focus on the potential effects of alcohol and alcoholic beverages to modulate endothelial function rather than just vascular smooth muscle reactivity [136]. Whether endothelial dysfunction is a cause or consequence of hypertension needs further resolution, but a potential direct influence of alcohol to either improve or impair endothelial function may be more relevant to ultimate effects of alcohol on atherogenesis rather than BP.

Increased sympathetic nervous system activity has been implicated in the hypertension typical of acute alcoholic withdrawal [137], but attempts to demonstrate sympathetic nervous system activation as the basis for chronic pressor effects of regular alcohol use have not produced consistent results. Resting and stimulated catecholamine levels were similar in drinkers and nondrinkers in the previously cited study of Arkwright et al. [135], and plasma catecholamine levels did not change during 7 days of regular alcohol consumption in an intervention study in normotensive males [69]. After the acute ingestion of alcohol increases in plasma adrenaline or noradrenaline have been reported by some groups [138–140] but not by others [141,142]. In one study, the acute ingestion of alcohol increased heart rate and sympathetic nerve activity as measured by skeletal muscle microneurography but did not increase BP, probably because of the acute vasodilator effects of alcohol [143]. Acute intravenous infusion of alcohol, however, caused both a pressor response and an increase in sympathetic nerve activation, measured again by using intraneural electrodes [144]. Interestingly, the increase in BP in that study occurred as the plasma alcohol concentration was falling and could be blocked by prior administration of dexamethasone, causing the investigators to postulate that it may have been mediated by the release of corticotropin-releasing hormone, resulting in a centrally mediated sympathoexcitatory effect.

Either acute or chronic stimulation by alcohol of the renin-angiotensin axis has also been explored as a possible contributory mechanism. An increase in plasma renin activity after acute ingestion, however, appears secondary to changes in fluid and electrolyte balance rather than a consequence of direct stimulation by alcohol of renin release [139], and no differences in plasma renin activity have been seen in controlled comparisons of drinkers and nondrinkers [135]. Stimulation of adrenal cortisol secretion by alcohol has also been invoked, but again in the acute setting this appears more likely a nonspecific stress response, and chronically, plasma cortisol levels have been similar in heavy drinkers compared to nondrinking controls [135]. The phenomenon of alcohol-related pseudo-Cushing's syndrome suggests a role for chronic stimulation of adrenal cortisol release in alcohol-related hypertension, but appears more likely a result of the effects of coexistent alcoholic liver disease on cortisol metabolism.

Magnesium depletion with hypomagnesemia and magnesuria are well described with chronic alcohol consumption [145,146], with evidence of reduced intracellular levels of magnesium as a consequence [147]. In an uncontrolled intervention in hypertensive Japanese drinkers [148], a fall in decrease during 4 weeks of alcohol restriction correlated with an increase in intraerythrocyte magnesium and a decrease in intraerythrocyte sodium. The authors proposed that alcohol-related hypertension may result from cellular magnesium deficiency in drinkers with inactivation of the sodium pump, an increase in intracellular sodium, and an increase in vascular tone. Altura and Altura [149] argue that by competing with Ca^{2+} for membrane-binding sites and by modulating Ca binding and release from the sarcoplasmic reticular membranes, intracellular free Mg^{2+} can act to maintain low resting levels of intracellular free Ca^{2+} and trigger muscle contraction or relaxation. This suggests another mechanism whereby alcohol—by decreasing Mg^{2+} levels—may increase resting vascular tone and level of BP. This mechanism may also be relevant to alcohol-induced cerebrovascular spasm and the relationship between binge drinking and stroke [150]. Alternative membrane effects of alcohol to increase intracellular sodium concentration and heighten vascular tone include reported associations of alcohol intake and reduced sodium–lithium counter transport activity [151] and effects of both acute and chronic alcohol intake on membrane Na^+-K^+-ATP-ase activity [152]. The latter may also cause changes in both vascular tone and renal sodium handling by the kidney, and further contribute to any increase in BP.

In a population-based study in healthy volunteers alcohol intake was an independent predictor of lower baroreflex activity [153], and a decrease in baroreflex sensitivity has been reported in acute studies in man in association with an increase in pressor responsiveness [154]. These results support the previously discussed animal studies [120] and suggest a decrease in baroreflex sensitivity as another potential mechanism for the development of raised BP with alcohol in humans.

PRACTICAL RECOMMENDATIONS FOR INTERVENTION

The size of the fall in BP with alcohol restriction compares favorably to that seen in meta-analytic overviews of the effects on BP of sodium restriction [155], potassium supplementation [156], weight reduction [157], or increased physical activity [158]. The magnitude of the anticipated BP reduction should also be interpreted in the light of estimates that populationwide falls of BP of 2 to 3 mmHg are likely to result in a 17% decrease in the prevalence of hypertension, a 6% reduction in the risk of coronary heart disease, and a 15% reduction in the risk of a transient ischemic attack or stroke [159]. Reduction in alcohol intake at a population level with a corresponding improvement in community control of hypertension over a 6-year period has been reported in an uncontrolled Italian study [160]. In a controlled study in France, hypertensive excessive drinkers in a working population were given specific advice to decrease their alcohol intake [74], and over a 2-year period a reduction in alcohol intake of just over one unit per day (relative to the controls) was found to be an effective means for reducing systolic BP over the long term. Community-based approaches to hypertension prevention and control that have a reduction in alcohol intake as a major focus are therefore feasible and achievable.

At the level of the individual hypertensive patient, all primary care physicians should routinely discuss alcohol consumption and recommend limitation of excessive intake whenever it occurs. If doubt exists with respect to patient's self-reports of alcohol intake, biomarkers such as γ-glutamyl transpeptidase, carbohydrate-deficient transferrin, and erythrocyte mean corpuscular volume may be clinically helpful. Furthermore, if excessive alcohol intake is suspected as an important contributory factor to any patient's hypertension, he or she should be reassessed after a period of a substantial reduction in alcohol intake before any diagnosis of sustained essential hypertension is confirmed and before opting for any pharmacological therapy.

When weighing the balance of risks and benefits of alcohol for cardiovascular disease the current World Health Organization–International Society of Hypertension guidelines suggest that hypertensive patients who drink should limit their alcohol intake to 20 to 30g/day for men and 10 to 20 g/day for women, which is a maximum of approximately two standard drinks/day for men and 1.5 drinks/day for women [161]. These recommendations represent a reasonable balance between the potential efficacy of this intervention for BP reduction versus the apparent protection against atherosclerosis associated with consumption within this range. These guidelines have also been framed for hypertensive patients in the knowledge that such a reduction in alcohol intake can be achieved with relative ease by nondependent drinkers and that there will be a simultaneous reduction in risk from the many other detrimental health and psychosocial consequences of heavier drinking. Those who are not hypertensive and who follow the suggested guidelines should also anticipate a reduction in their risk of developing hypertension as well as other alcohol-related problems, and within these limits beneficial cardiovascular effects of alcohol should outweigh any adverse effects on BP.

REFERENCES

1. Alcohol: its actions and uses. Br Med J 1861;1:364–366.
2. Smith E. On the detection and use of alcohol. Br Med J 1861;2:472–473, 537–538.
3. Mahomed FA. The sphygmographic evidence of arterio-capillary fibrosis. Trans Path Soc 1877;28:394.
4. Lian C. L'alcoolisme, cause d'hypertension arterielle. Bull Acad Med 1915;74:525–528.
5. MacMahon S. Alcohol consumption and hypertension. Hypertension 1987;9:111–121.
6. Marmot MG, Elliott P, Shipley MJ, Dyer AR, Ueshima H, Beevers DG, et al. Alcohol and blood pressure: the INTERSALT study. Br Med J 1994; 308:1263–1267.

7. Klatsky AL, Friedman GD, Siegelaub AB, Gerard MJ. Alcohol consumption and blood pressure. N Engl J Med 1977;296:1194–1200.
8. Arkwright PD, Beilin LJ, Rouse I, Armstrong B, Vandongen R. Alcohol and blood pressure in a working population. Clin Exp Pharmacol Physiol 1981;8:451–454.
9. Friedman GD, Klatsky AL, Siegelaub AB. Alcohol, tobacco, and hypertension. Hypertension 1982;4:III143–III150
10. Arkwright PD, Beilin LJ, Rouse I, Armstrong BK, Vandongen R. Effects of alcohol use and other aspects of lifestyle on blood pressure levels and prevalence of hypertension in a working population. Circulation 1982; 66:60–66.
11. Fortmann S, Haskell W, Vranizan K, Brown B, Farquhar J. The association of blood pressure and dietary alcohol: differences by age, sex, and estrogen use. Am J Epidemiol 1983;118:497–507.
12. Harburg E, Ozgoren F, Hawthorne V, Schork A. Community norms of alcohol usage and blood pressure: Tecumseh, Michigan. Am J Pub Health 1980;70:813–820.
13. Moreira LB, Fuchs FD, Moraes RS, Bredemeier M, Duncan BB. Alcohol intake and blood pressure—the importance of time elapsed since last drink. J Hypertens 1998;16:175–180.
14. Cooke KM, Frost GW, Stokes GS. Blood pressure and its relationship to low levels of alcohol consumption. Clin Exp Pharmacol Physiol 1983;10: 229–233.
15. Klatsky A, Friedman G, Siegelaub A, Gerard M. Alcohol consumption and blood pressure—Kaiser-Permanente multiphasic health examination data. N Engl J Med 1977;296(21):1194–1200.
16. Holman CDJ, English DR, Milne E, Winter MG. Meta-analysis of alcohol and all-cause mortality—a validation of NHMRC recommendations. Med J Aust 1996;164:141–145.
17. Laforge R, Williams GD, Dufour MC. Alcohol consumption, gender and self-reported hypertension. Drug Alcohol Depend 1990;26:235–249.
18. Nanchahal K, Ashton WD, Wood DAE. Alcohol consumption, metabolic cardiovascular risk factors and hypertension in women. Internat J Epidemiol 2000;29:57–64.
19. Hajjar IM, Grim CE, George V, Kotchen TA. Impact of diet on blood pressure and age-related changes in blood pressure in the US population: analysis of NHANES III. Arch Intern Med 2001;161:589–593.
20. Maheswaran R, Gill JS, Davies P, Beevers DG. High blood pressure due to alcohol. A rapidly reversible effect. Hypertension 1991;17:787–792.
21. Criqui MH, Wallace RB, Mishkel M, Barrett-Connor E, Heiss G. Alcohol consumption and blood pressure. the Lipid Research Clinics Prevalence Study. Hypertension 1981;3:557–565.
22. Saunders JB, Beevers DG, Paton A. Factors influencing blood pressure in chronic alcoholics. Clin Sci 1979;57 suppl. 5:295s–298s.
23. Potter JF, Bannan LT, Beevers DG. The effect of a non-selective lipophilic

beta-blocker on the blood pressure and noradrenaline, vasopressin, cortisol and renin release during alcohol withdrawal. Clin Exp Hypertens 1984;6: 1147–1160.

24. Choudhury SR, Ueshima H, Okayama A, Kita Y, Miyoshi Y. Relationship between blood pressure and alcohol consumption on the previous day in Japanese men. Hypertens 1998;21:175–178.
25. Puddey IB, Jenner DA, Beilin LJ, Vandongen R. An appraisal of the effects of usual vs recent alcohol intake on blood pressure. Clin Exp Pharmacol Physiol 1988;15:261–264.
26. Wannamethee G, Shaper AG. Alcohol intake and variations in blood pressure by day of examination. J Human Hypertens 1991;5:59–67.
27. Marques-Vidal P, Arveiler D, Evans A, Amouyel P, Ferrieres J, Ducimetiere P. Different alcohol drinking and blood pressure relationships in France and Northern Ireland: the PRIME Study. Hypertension 2001;38: 1361–1366.
28. Rakic V, Puddey IB, Burke V, Dimmitt SB, Beilin LJ. Influence of pattern of alcohol intake on blood pressure in regular drinkers—a controlled trial. J Hypertens 1998;16:165–174.
29. Seppa K, Laippala P, Sillanaukee P. Drinking pattern and blood pressure. Am J Hypertens 1994;7:249–254.
30. Okubo Y, Miyamoto T, Suwazono Y, Kobayashi E, Nogawa K. Alcohol consumption and blood pressure in Japanese men. Alcohol 2001;23: 149–156.
31. King AC, Parsons OA, Bernardy NC, Lovallo WR. Drinking history is related to persistent blood pressure dysregulation in postwithdrawal alcoholics. Alc Clin Exp Res 1994;18:1172–1176.
32. York JL, Hirsch JA. Residual pressor effects of chronic alcohol in detoxified alcoholics. Hypertension 1996;28:133–138.
33. Ryan JM, Howes LG. White coat effect of alcohol. Am J Hypertens 2000;13:1135–1138.
34. Seppa K, Sillanaukee P. Binge drinking and ambulatory blood pressure. Hypertension 1999;33:79–82.
35. Perneger TV, Whelton PK, Puddey IB, Klag MJ. Risk of end-stage renal disease associated with alcohol consumption. Am J Epidemiol 1999;150: 1275–1281.
36. Abe H, Kawano Y, Kojima S, Ashida T, Kuramochi M, Matsuoka H, et al. Biphasic effects of repeated alcohol intake on 24-hr blood pressure in hypertensive patients. Circulation 1994;89:2626–2633.
37. Rosito GA, Fuchs FD, Duncan BB. Dose-dependent biphasic effect of ethanol on 24-h blood pressure in normotensive subjects. Am J Hypertens 1999;12:236–240.
38. O'Callaghan CJ, Phillips PA, Krum H, Howes LG. The effects of short-term alcohol intake on clinic and ambulatory blood pressure in normotensive "social" drinkers. Am J Hypertens 1995;8:572–577.
39. Kawano Y, Abe H, Kojima S, Ashida T, Yoshida K, Imanishi M, et al. Acute

depressor effect of alcohol in patients with essential hypertension. Hypertension 1992;20:219–226.
40. Kawano Y, Abe H, Kojima S, Yoshimi H, Sanai T, Kimura G, et al. Different effects of alcohol and salt on 24-hour blood pressure and heart rate in hypertensive patients. Hypertens Res 1996;19:255–261.
41. Vriz O, Piccolo D, Cozzutti E, Milani L, Gelisio R, Pegoraro F, et al. The effects of alcohol consumption on ambulatory blood pressure and target organs in subjects with borderline to mild hypertension. Am J Hypertens 1998;11:230–234.
42. Aguilera MT, De la Sierra A, Coca A, Estruch R, Fernández-Solá J, Urbano-Márquez A. Effect of alcohol abstinence on blood pressure: assessment by 24-hour ambulatory blood pressure monitoring. Hypertension 1999;33:653–657.
43. Rajzer M, Kaweckajaszcz K, Czarnecka D, Dragan J, Betkowska B. Blood pressure, insulin resistance and left ventricular function in alcoholics. J Hypertens 1997;15:1219–1226.
44. Maiorano G, Bartolomucci F, Contursi V, Saracino E, Agostinacchio E. Effect of alcohol consumption versus abstinence on 24-h blood pressure profile in normotensive alcoholic patients. Am J Hypertens 1995;8:80–81.
45. Howes LG, Krum H, Phillips PA. Effects of regular alcohol consumption on 24 hour ambulatory blood pressure recordings. Clin Exp Pharmacol Physiol 1990;17:247–250.
46. Lang T, Degoulet P, Aime F, Devries C, Jacquinet-Salord M-C, Fouriaud C. Relationship between alcohol consumption and hypertension prevalence and control in a French population. J Chron Dis 1987;40:713–720.
47. Trevisan M, Krogh V, Farinaro E, Panico S, Mancini M. Alcohol consumption, drinking pattern and blood pressure: analysis of data from the Italian National Research Council Study. Int J Epidemiol 1987;16:520–527.
48. Cairns V, Keil U, Kleinbaum D, Doering A, Stieber J. Alcohol consumption as a risk factor for high blood pressure: Munich Blood Pressure Study. Hypertension 1984;6:124–131.
49. Keil U, Chambless L, Remmers A. Alcohol and blood pressure: results from the Luebeck blood pressure study. Prev Med 1989;18:1–10.
50. Ueshima H, Shimamoto T, Iida M, Konishi M, Tanigaki M, Doi MTK, et al. Alcohol intake and hypertension among urban and rural Japanese populations. J Chron Dis 1984;37:585–592.
51. Marques-Vidal P, Montaye M, Haas B, Bingham A, Evans A, Juhan-Vague I, et al. Relationships between alcoholic beverages and cardiovascular risk factor levels in middle-aged men, the PRIME study. Atherosclerosis 2001;157: 431–440.
52. Tjonneland A, Gronbaek M, Stripp C, Overvad K. Wine intake and diet in a random sample of 48763 Danish men and women. Am J Clin Nutr 1999;69:49–54.
53. Corrao G, Bagnardi V, Zambon A, Arico S. Exploring the dose-response

relationship between alcohol consumption and the risk of several alcohol-related conditions: a meta-analysis. Addiction 1999;94:1551–1573.
54. Nakanishi N, Yoshida H, Nakamura K, Suzuki K, Tatara K. Alcohol consumption and risk for hypertension in middle-aged Japanese men. J Hypertens 2001;19:851–855.
55. Tsuruta M, Adachi H, Hirai Y, Fujiura Y, Imaizumi T. Association between alcohol intake and development of hypertension in Japanese normotensive men: 12-year follow-up study. Am J Hypertens 2000;13:482–487.
56. Okubo Y, Suwazono Y, Kobayashi E, Nogawa K. Alcohol consumption and blood pressure change: 5-year follow-up study of the association in normotensive workers. J Hum Hypertens 2001;15:367–372.
57. Fuchs FD, Chambless LE, Whelton PK, Nieto FJ, Heiss G. Alcohol consumption and the incidence of hypertension: the Atherosclerosis Risk in Communities Study. Hypertension 2001;37:1242–1250.
58. Gordon T, Kannel W. Drinking and its relation to smoking, BP, blood lipids, and uric acid—the Framingham Study. Arch Int Med 1983;143: 1366–1374.
59. Gordon T, Doyle JT. Alcohol consumption and its relationship to smoking, weight, blood pressure, and blood lipids: the Albany Study. Arch Int Med 1986;146 :262–265.
60. Curtis AB, James SA, Strogatz DS, Raghunathan TE, Harlow S. Alcohol consumption and changes in blood pressure among African Americans—the Pitt County Study. Am J Epidemiol 1997;146:727–733.
61. Murray RP, Connett JE, Tyas SL, Bond R, Ekuma O, Silversides CK, et al. Alcohol volume, drinking pattern, and cardiovascular disease morbidity and mortality: is there a U-shaped function? Am J Epidemiol 2002;155: 242–248.
62. Puddey IB, Beilin LJ, Vandongen R, Rouse IL, Rogers P. Evidence for a direct effect of alcohol consumption on blood pressure in normotensive men: a randomized controlled trial. Hypertension 1985;7:707–713.
63. Puddey IB, Beilin LJ, Vandongen R. Regular alcohol use raises blood pressure in treated hypertensive subjects: a randomised controlled trial. Lancet 1987;1:647–651.
64. Puddey IB, Parker M, Beilin LJ, Vandongen R, Masarei JR. Effects of alcohol and caloric restrictions on blood pressure and serum lipids in overweight men. Hypertension 1992;20:533–541.
65. Cushman WC, Cutler JA, Hanna E, Bingham SF, Follmann D, Harford T, et al. Prevention and Treatment of Hypertension Study (PATHS): effects of an alcohol treatment program on blood pressure. Arch Int Med 1998; 158:1197–1207.
66. Xin X, He J, Frontini MG, Ogden LG, Motsamai OI, Whelton PK. Effects of alcohol reduction on blood pressure: a meta-analysis of randomized controlled trials. Hypertension 2001;38:1112–1117.
67. Parker M, Puddey IB, Beilin LJ, Vandongen R. Two-way factorial study of alcohol and salt restriction in treated hypertensive men. Hypertension 1990;16:398–406.
68. Cox KL, Puddey IB, Morton AR, Beilin LJ, Vandongen R, Masarei JR. The

combined effects of aerobic exercise and alcohol restriction on blood pressure and serum lipids: a two-way factorial study in sedentary men. J Hypertens 1993;11:191–201.
69. Howes LG, Reid JL. Changes in blood pressure and autonomic reflexes following regular, moderate alcohol consumption. J Hypertens 1985;4: 421–425.
70. Ueshima H, Ogihara T, Baba S, Tabuchi Y, Mikawa K, Hashizume K, et al. The effect of reduced alcohol consumption on blood pressure: a randomised, controlled, single blind study. J Human Hypertens 1987;1:113–119.
71. Wallace P, Cutler S, Haines A. Randomised controlled trial of general practitioner intervention in patients with excessive alcohol consumption. Br Med J 1988;297:663–668.
72. Maheswaran R, Beevers M, Beevers DG. Effectiveness of advice to reduce alcohol consumption in hypertensive patients. Hypertension 1992;19:79–84.
73. Ueshima H, Mikawa K, Baba S, Sasaki S, Ozawa H, Tsushima MKA, et al. Effect of reduced alcohol consumption on blood pressure in untreated hypertensive men. Hypertension 1993;21:248–252.
74. Lang T, Nicaud V, Darne B, Rueff B. Improving hypertension control among excessive alcohol drinkers: a randomised controlled trial in France. J of Epidemiol & Comm Health 1995;49:610–616.
75. Kawano Y, Abe H, Takishita S, Omae T. Effects of alcohol restriction on 24-hour ambulatory blood pressure in Japanese men with hypertension. Am J Med 1998;105:307–311.
76. Wallace RB, Barrett-Connor E, Criqui M, Wahl P, Hoover J, Hunninghake D, et al. Alteration in blood pressures associated with combined alcohol and oral contraceptive use—the Lipid Research Clinics Prevalence Study. J Chron Dis 1982;35:251–257.
77. Hartung GH, Kohl HW, Blair SN, Lawrence SJ, Harrist RB. Exercise tolerance and alcohol intake. Blood pressure relation. Hypertension 1990;16: 501–507.
78. Sobocinski K, Gruchow H, Anderson A, Barboriak J. Associations of aerobic exercise and alcohol consumption with systolic blood pressure in employed males. J Hypertens 1986;4(suppl. 5):S358–S360
79. Di Gennaro C, Barilli A, Giuffredi C, Gatti C, Montanari A, Vescovi PP. Sodium sensitivity of blood pressure in long-term detoxified alcoholics. Hypertension 2000;35:869–874.
80. Keil U, Chambless L, Filipiak B, Hartel U. Alcohol and blood pressure and its interaction with smoking and other behavioural variables: results from the MONICA Augsburg Survey 1984–1985. J Hypertens 1991;9:491–498.
81. Schnall PL, Schwartz JE, Landsbergis PA, Warren K, Pickering TG. Relation between job strain, alcohol and ambulatory blood pressure. Hypertension 1992;19:488–494.
82. Arkwright PD, Beilin LJ, Rouse IL, Vandongen R. Alcohol, personality and predisposition to essential hypertension. J Hypertens 1983;1:365–371.
83. Criqui MH, Langer RD, Reed DM. Dietary alcohol, calcium and potassium:

independent and combined effects on blood pressure. Circulation 1989;80: 609–614.
84. Hamet P, Mongeau E, Lambert J, Bellavance F, Daignault-Gelinas M, Ledoux M, et al. Interactions among calcium, sodium, and alcohol intake as determinants of blood pressure. Hypertension 1991;17:I150–I154.
85. Dwyer JH, Li L, Dwyer KM, Curtin LR, Feinleib M. Dietary calcium, alcohol, and incidence of treated hypertension in the NHANES I epidemiologic follow-up study. Am J Epidemiol 1996;144:828–838.
86. Corrao G, Rubbiati L, Bagnardi V, Zambon A, Poikolainen K. Alcohol and coronary heart disease: a meta-analysis. Addiction 2000;95:1505–1523.
87. Djousse L, Levy D, Murabito JM, Cupples LA, Ellison RC. Alcohol consumption and risk of intermittent claudication in the Framingham Heart Study. Circulation 2000;102:3092–3097.
88. Mingardi R, Avogaro A, Noventa F, Strazzabosco M, Stocchiero CTA, Erle G. Alcohol intake is associated with a lower prevalence of peripheral vascular disease in non-insulin dependent diabetic women. Nutr Metab Cardiovasc Dis 1997;7:301–308.
89. Burchfiel CM, Tracy RE, Chyou PH, Strong JP. Cardivascular risk factors and hyalinization of renal arterioles at autopsy—the Honolulu Heart Program. Arterioscler Thromb Vasc Biol 1997;17:760–768.
90. Masarei JR, Puddey IB, Rouse IL, Lynch WJ, Vandongen R, Beilin LJ. Effects of alcohol consumption on serum lipoprotein-lipid and apolipoprotein concentrations: results from an intervention study in healthy subjects. Atherosclerosis 1986;60:79–87.
91. Dimmitt SB, Rakic V, Puddey IB, Baker R, Oostryck R, Adams MJ, et al. The effects of alcohol on coagulation and fibrinolytic factors—a controlled trial. Blood Coag Fibrinol 1998;9:39–45.
92. Renaud SC, Beswick AD, Fehily AM, Sharp DS, Elwood PC. Alcohol and platelet aggregation: the Caerphilly Prospective Heart Disease Study. Am J Clin Nutr 1992;55:1012–1017.
93. Langer RD, Criqui MH, Reed DM. Lipoproteins and blood pressure as biological pathways for effect of moderate alcohol consumption on coronary heart disease. Circulation 1992;85:910–915.
94. Berger K, Ajani UA, Kase CS, Gaziano JM, Buring JE, Glynn RJ, et al. Light-to-moderate alcohol consumption and risk of stroke among U.S. male physicians. N Engl J Med 1999;341:1557–1564.
95. Gill JS, Shipley MJ, Tsementzis SA, Hornby RS, Gill SK, Hitchcock ER, et al. Alcohol consumption—a risk factor for hemorrhagic and non-hemorrhagic stroke. Am J Med 1991;90:489–497.
96. Hansagi H, Romelsjo A, Gerhardsson de Verdier M, Andreasson S, Leifman A. Alcohol consumption and stroke mortality: 20-year follow-up of 15,077 men and women. Stroke 1995;26:1768–1773.
97. Palomaki H, Kaste M. Regular light-to-moderate intake of alcohol and the risk of ischemic stroke: is there a beneficial effect? Stroke 1993;24: 1828–1832.

98. Kiyohara Y, Kato I, Iwamoto H, Nakayama K, Fujishima M. The impact of alcohol and hypertension on stroke incidence in a general Japanese population: the Hisayama Study. Stroke 1995;26:368–372.
99. Palmer AJ, Fletcher AE, Bulpitt CJ, Beevers DG, Coles EC, Ledingham JGPJ, et al. Alcohol intake and cardiovascular mortality in hypertensive patients: report from the Department of Health Hypertension Care Computing Project. J Hypertens 1995;13:957–964.
100. Manolio TA, Levy D, Garrison RJ, Castelli WP, Kannel WB. Relation of alcohol intake to left ventricular mass: the Framingham Study. J Am Coll Cardiol 1991;17:717–721.
101. Ishimitsu T, Yoshida K, Nakamura M, Tsukada K, Yagi S, Ohrui M, et al. Effects of alcohol intake on organ injuries in normotensive and hypertensive human subjects. Clin Sci 1997;93:541–547.
102. Klein R, Klein BE, Moss SE. Prevalence of microalbuminuria in older-onset diabetes. Diab Care 1993;16:1325–1330.
103. Kauma H, Savolainen MJ, Rantala AO, Kervinen K, Reunanen A, Kesaniemi YA. Apolipoprotein E phenotype determines the effect of alcohol on blood pressure in middle-aged men. Am J Hypertens 1998;11: 1334–1343.
104. Puddey IB, Rakic V, Dimmitt SB, Burke V, Beilin LJ, Van Bockxmeer F. Apolipoprotein E genotype and the blood pressure raising effect of alcohol. Am J Hypertens 1999;12:946–947.
105. Tsuritani I, Ikai E, Date T, Suzuki Y, Ishizaki M, Yamada Y. Polymorphism in ALDH2-genotype in Japanese men and the alcohol–blood pressure relationship. Am J Hypertens 1995;8:1053–1059.
106. Okayama A, Ueshima H, Yamakawa M, Kita Y. Low-km aldehyde dehydrogenase deficiency does not influence the elevation of blood pressure by alcohol. J Hum Hypertens 1994;8:205–208.
107. Hines LM, Stampfer MJ, Ma J, Gaziano JM, Ridker PM, Hankinson SE, et al. Genetic variation in alcohol dehydrogenase and the beneficial effect of moderate alcohol consumption on myocardial infarction. N Engl J Med 2001;344:549–555.
108. Khetarpal V, Volicer L. Effects of ethanol on blood pressure of normal and hypertensive rats. J Stud Alc 1979;40(7):732–736.
109. Chan TC, Sutter MC. The effects of chronic ethanol consumption on cardiac function. Can J Physiol Pharmacol 1982;60:777–782.
110. Chan TC, Sutter MC. Ethanol consumption and blood pressure. Life Sci 1983;33:1965–1973.
111. Chan TC, Godin DV, Sutter MC. Erythrocyte membrane properties of the chronic alcoholic rat. Drug Alcohol Depend 1983;12:249–257.
112. Puddey IB, Burke V, Croft K, Beilin LJ. Increased blood pressure and changes in membrane lipids associated with chronic ethanol treatment of rats. Clin Exp Pharmacol Physiol 1995;22:655–657.
113. Hsieh ST, Sano H, Saito K, Kubota Y, Yokoyama M. Magnesium supplementation prevents the development of alcohol-induced hypertension. Hypertension 1992;19:175–182.

114. Vasdev S, Sampson CA, Prabhakaran VM. Platelet-free calcium and vascular calcium uptake in ehtanol-induced hypertensive rats. Hypertension 1991;18: 116–122.
115. Vasdev S, Gupta IP, Sampson CA, Longerich L, Parai S. Ethanol induced hypertension in rats: reversibility and role of intracellular cytosolic calcium. Artery 1993;20:19–43.
116. Vasdev S, Mian T, Longerich L, Prabhakaran V, Parai S. N-acetyl cysteine attenuates ethanol induced hypertension in rats. Artery 1995;21:312–336.
117. Vasdev S, Wadhawan S, Ford CA, Parai S, Longerich L, Gadag V. Dietary vitamin B6 supplementation prevents ethanol-induced hypertension in rats. Nutr Metab Cardiovasc Dus 1999;9:55–63.
118. Chan TC, Wall RA, Sutter MC. Chronic ethanol consumption, stress, and hypertension. Hypertension 1985;7:519–524.
119. Abdel-Rahman A-RA, Dar MS, Wooles WR. Effect of chronic ethanol administration on arterial baroreceptor function and pressor and depressor responsiveness in rats. J Pharmacol Exper Ther 1984;232:194–201.
120. Abdel-Rahman AA, Wooles WR. Ethanol-induced hypertension involves impairment of baroreceptors. Hypertension 1987;10:67–73.
121. Hatton DC, Bukoski RD, Edgar S, McCarron DA. Chronic alcohol consumption lowers blood pressure but enhances vascular contractility in Wistar rats. J Hypertens 1992;10:529–537.
122. Sanderson JE, Jones JV, Graham DI. Effect of chronic alcohol ingestion on the heart and blood pressure of spontaneously hypertensive rats. Clin Exp Hypertens 1983;5:673–689.
123. Howe PRC, Rogers PF, Smith RM. Effects of chronic alcohol consumption and alcohol withdrawal on blood pressure in stroke-prone spontaneously hypertensive rats. J Hypertens 1989;7:387–393.
124. Howe PR, Rogers PF, Smith RM. Antihypertensive effect of alcohol in spontaneously hypertensive rats. Hypertension 1989;13:607–611.
125. Jones JV, Raine AEG, Sanderson JE, Carretta R, Graham DI. Adverse effect of chronic alcohol ingestion on cardiac performance in spontaneously hypertensive rats. J Hypertens 1988;6:419–422.
126. Ren J, Brown RA. Hypertension augments ethanol-induced depression of cell shortening and intracellular Ca(2+) transients in adult rat ventricular myocytes. Biochem Biophys Res Commun 1999;261:202–208.
127. Beilin LJ, Hoffmann P, Nilsson H, Skarphedinsson J, Folkow B. Effect of chronic ethanol consumption upon cardiovascular reactivity, heart rate and blood pressure in spontaneously hypertensive and Wistar-Kyoto rats. J Hypertens 1992;10:645–650.
128. Crandall DL, Ferraro GD, Lozito RJ, Cervoni P, Clark LT. Cardiovascular effects of intermittent drinking: assessment of a novel animal model of human alcoholism. J Hypertens 1989;7:683–687.
129. el-Mas MM, Abdel-Rahman A-RA. Sexually dimorphic hemodynamic effects of intragastric ethanol in conscious rats. Clin Exp Hypertens 1999; 21:1429–1445.

130. El Mas MM, Abdel-Rahman AA. Estrogen-dependent hypotensive effects of ethanol in conscious female rats. Alcohol Clin Exp Res 1999;23:624–632.
131. Graf K, Strom G. Effect of ethanol ingestion on arm blood flow in healthy young men at rest and during leg work. Acta Pharmacol et Toxicol 1960;17:115–120.
132. Gillespie JA. Vasodilator properties of alcohol. Br Med J 1967;2:274–277.
133. Eisenhofer G, Lambie DG, Johnson RH. No effect of ethanol ingestion on β-adrenoceptor-mediated circulatory responses to isoprenaline in man. Brit J Clin Pharmacol 1985;20:684–687.
134. Howes LG, Reid JL. Decreased vascular responsiveness to noradrenaline following regular ethanol consumption. Brit J Clin Pharmacol 1985;20:669–674.
135. Arkwright PD, Beilin LJ, Vandongen R, Rouse IL, Lalor C. The pressor effect of moderate alcohol consumption in man: a search for mechanisms. Circulation 1982;66:515–519.
136. Puddey IB, Zilkens RR, Burke V, Beilin LJ. Alcohol intake and endothelial function: A brief review. Clin Exp Pharmacol Physiol 2001;28:1020–1024.
137. Bannan LT, Potter JF, Beevers DG, Saunders JB, Walters JRF, Ingram MC. Effect of alcohol withdrawal on blood pressure, plasma renin activity, aldosterone, cortisol and dopamine α-hydroxylase. Clin Sci 1984;66:659–63.
138. Ireland MA, Vandongen R, Davidson L, Beilin LJ, Rouse IL. Acute effects of moderate alcohol consumption on blood pressure and plasma catecholamines. Clin Sci 1984;66:643–648.
139. Puddey IB, Vandongen R, Beilin LJ, Rouse IL. Alcohol stimulation of renin release in man: its relation to the hemodynamic, electrolyte, and sympatho-adrenal responses to drinking. J Clin Endocrinol Metab 1985;61:37–42.
140. Howes LG, Reid JL. Changes in plasma free 3,4-dihydroxyphenylethylene glycol and noradrenaline levels after acute alcohol administration. Clin Sci 1985;69:423–428.
141. Potter JF, Macdonald IA, Beevers DG. Alcohol raises blood pressure in hypertensive patients. J Hypertens 1986;4:435–441.
142. Stott DJ, Ball SG, Inglis GC, Davies DL, Fraser R, Murray GD, et al. Effects of a single moderate dose of alcohol on blood pressure, heart rate and associated metabolic and endocrine changes. Clin Sci 1987;73:411–416.
143. van de Borne P, Mark AL, Montano N, Mion D, Somers VK. Effects of alcohol on sympathetic activity, hemodynamics, and chemoreflex sensitivity. Hypertension 1997;29:1278–1283.
144. Randin D, Vollenweider P, Tappy L, Jequier E, Nicod P, Scherrer U. Suppression of alcohol-induced hypertension by dexamethasone. N Engl J Med 1995;332:1733–1737.
145. Kalbfleisch JM, Lindeman RD, Ginn HE, Smith WO. Effects of ethanol administration on urinary excretion of magnesium and other electrolytes in alcoholic and normal subjects. J Clin Invest 1963;42:1471–1475.
146. Flink EB. Magnesium deficiency in alcoholism. Alcohol Clin Exp Res 1986;10:590–594.

147. Shane SR, Flink EB. Magnesium deficiency in alcohol addiction and withdrawal. Magnes Trace Elem 1991;10:263–268.
148. Hsieh ST, Saito K, Miyajima T, Lin CM, Yhokoyama M. Effects of alcohol moderation on blood pressure and intracellular cations in mild essential hypertension. Am J Hypertens 1995;8:696–703.
149. Altura BM, Altura BT. Mechanisms of alcohol-induced-hypertension: importance of intracellular cations and magnesium. National Institute on Alcohol Abuse and Alcoholism RM31, Alcohol and the Cardiovascular System, Zahkari and Wassef eds. Bethesda, MD: NIH, 1996;27:591–614.
150. Ema M, Gebrewold A, Altura BT, Zhang A, Altura BM. Alcohol-induced vascular damage of brain is ameliorated by administration of magnesium. Alcohol 1998;15:95–103.
151. Trevisan M, Laurenzi M. Correlates of sodium-lithium countertransport. Findings from the Gubbio Epidemiological Study. The Gubbio Collaborative Study Group. Circulation 1991;84:2011–2019.
152. Rodrigo R, Thielemann L, Olea M, Munoz P, Cereceda M, Orellana M. Effects of ethanol ingestion on renal regulation of water and electrolytes. Archives of Medical Research 1998;29:209–218.
153. Kardos A, Watterich G, de Menezes R, Csanady M, Casadei B, Rudas L. Determinants of spontaneous baroreflex sensitivity in a healthy working population. Hypertension 2001;37:911–916.
154. Abdel-Rahman AR, Merrill RH, Wooles WR. Effect of acute ethanol administration on the baroreceptor reflex control of heart rate in normotensive human volunteers. Clin Sci 1987;72:113–122.
155. Graudal NA, Galloe AM, Garred P. Effects of sodium restriction on blood pressure, renin, aldosterone, catecholamines, cholesterols, and triglyceride: a meta-analysis. JAMA 1998;279:1383–1391.
156. Whelton PK, He J, Cutler JA, Brancati FL, Appel LJ, Follmann D, et al. Effects of oral potassium on blood pressure—meta-analysis of randomized controlled clinical trials. JAMA 1997;277:1624–1632.
157. Mulrow CD, Chiquette E, Angel L, Cornell J, Summerbell C, Grimm R, et al. Dieting to reduce body weight for controlling hypertension in adults. Cochrane Database System Rev 2000;CD000484
158. Whelton SP, Chin A, He J. Effect of aerobic exercise on blood pressure: a meta-analysis of randomized controlled trials. Circulation 2001;103: 1369-c
159. Cook NR, Cohen J, Herbert PR, Taylor JO, Hennekens CH. Implications of small reductions in diastolic blood pressure for primary prevention. Arch Int Med 1995;155:701–709.
160. Menotti A, Lanti M, Zanchetti A, Puddu PE, Cirillo M, Mancini M, et al. Impact of the Gubbio population study on community control of blood pressure and hypertension. Gubbio Study Research Group. J Hypertens 2001;19:843–850.
161. Guidelines Subcommittee. 1999 World Health Organization–International Society of Hypertension guidelines for the management of hypertension. J Hypertens 1999;17:151–183.

8

Physical Activity

Kazuko Ishikawa-Takata and Toshiki Ohta
National Institute of Health and Nutrition, Shinjyuku, Tokyo, Japan

PHYSICAL ACTIVITY

Mechanism of the Depressor Effect of Physical Activity

Not much is known about the various underlying mechanisms for the hypotensive effects of physical activity. Many studies are underway to elucidate these mechanisms, however.

Blood pressure is determined by cardiac output and peripheral vascular resistance. In essential hypertension, there is an increase in pressor substances and a decrease in depressor substances. Blood pressure is thought to decrease if a decrease in cardiac output, a decrease in peripheral resistance, a reduction in pressor substances, or an increase in depressor substances occurs.

Hagberg et al. [1] considered a decrease in cardiac output to be the main mechanism for reduced blood pressure, while Nelson et al. [2] took a decrease in peripheral resistance to be the main mechanism. Arakawa [3] found no decrease in peripheral resistance from exercise. These differences are thought to be due to individual differences in salt intake and the condition of hypertension, as well as in the intensity of the exercise [4]. O'Sullivan and Bell suggested that the regulation of peripheral resistance by reductions in sympathetic drive and by neural and nonneural effects is the mechanism for the hypotensive effect of exercise [5].

Exercise can be expected to produce a decrease in pressor substances, an increase in depressor substances, and a decrease in body fluids. Typical pressor substances are norepinephrine and an ouabainlike substance, and typical depressor substances are taurine, prostaglandin E, dopamine, and kallicrein. Arakawa [3] summarizes the dynamics of each of these substances during exercise. A decrease in plasma norepinephrine that probably reflects changes in sympathetic nerve activity was seen in 20 controlled studies. Exercise caused increases in plasma prostaglandin E and serum taurine, and decreases in plasma endogenous ouabainlike substance. Arakawa concluded that norepinephrine decreased in response to these changes. All three of these substances are known to sedate sympathetic nerve activity. Ouabainlike substance is a natriuretic hormone that is released in response to excessive intake of sodium or water. In another study by Arakawa et al., the plasma level of ouabainlike substance was twice as great in hypertension patients than in normotensive people, but this decreased significantly after 7 weeks of exercise [6].

Taurine is one type of amino acid. Arakawa concluded in his review [3] that taurine lowers blood pressure by modulating sympathetic activity, and actions of central angiotensin II, and by increasing urinary sodium excretion. Tanabe et al. showed a 26% increase in serum taurine concentration from 10 weeks of mild exercise [7]. In his review, Arakawa concluded that exercise increased prostaglandin E, that the release of norepinephrine at sympathetic nerve endings was possible, and that there was an increase in urinary dopamine excretion after 4 weeks of exercise. This increase in dopamine preceded a decrease in the atrial natriuretic peptide level, after which sodium excretion increased. There was insufficient data for kallikrein.

Physical activity causes a decrease in the amount of body fluids, and as a result there is decreased cardiac output and lower blood pressure. The decreased body fluids are thought to be due to increased dopamine and kallikrein in the urine in addition to the above-mentioned ouabainlike substance and increased taurine [3]. As discussed above, physical activity is thought to help correct the unbalanced blood pressure regulation in the body.

Moreover, in recent years Brett et al. demonstrated a strong correlation between changes in blood pressure during exercise and the reduction in total cholesterol and insulin resistance in the plasma [8], and clinical trials have shown that aerobic exercise by people with hypertension improves insulin resistance and insulin levels. There is therefore a strong possibility that physical exercise contributes to lowering blood pressure.

Intervention Studies on the Depressor Effect of Physical Activity

There have been many intervention studies to investigate the effect of increased physical activity, but some of these studies have been poorly designed. Since 1994, there have been numerous meta-analyses of intervention studies of physical activity. Here we will review the effect of physical activity in people with hypertension based on the main studies among them.

The results of intervention studies on physical activity are greatly affected by the experimental design. Kelley and Tran [9] and Fagard [10] compared randomized control studies (RCTs), in which the exercise and control groups were properly randomized, and studies that were not randomized, and showed that there tended to be less hypotensive effect in properly conducted RCTs than in studies in which there are numerous methodological deficiencies.

Fagard [11] conducted a meta-analysis of randomized control studies in 1999. This analysis covered 44 studies with subjects aged 21 to 79 years, exercise intervention periods of 4 to 52 weeks, and exercise sessions lasting 15 to 70 min (mainly walking, jogging, running, and cycling). Exercise intensity was 30–85%, with a mean of 65%. Among these subjects, the depressor effect of exercise in people with hypertension was –7.4 mmHg (95% confidence interval (CI): –10.5, –4.3) and –5.8 mmHg (–8.0, –3.5) for systolic and diastolic pressure, respectively.

Whelton et al. conducted a meta-analysis of randomized controlled trials investigating the effect of aerobic exercise on blood pressure that were published before September 2001 [12]. This analysis covered 54 studies, with patients 21 to 79 years of age and intervention periods of 3 weeks to 2 years. Of these 54 studies, 47 included hypertensive subjects and 28 included normotensive subjects. Antihypertensive medication was administered in four trials. Overall, the change in blood pressure was −3.84 mmHg (95% CI: −4.97, −2.72) in systolic pressure and −2.58 mmHg (95% CI: −3.35, −1.81) in diastolic pressure (Figs. 1, 2).

The results of other meta-analyses of high-quality studies on people with hypertension are summarized in Fig. 3. In these studies, the decrease in systolic pressure ranged from −0.8 to −13.0 mmHg, and in diastolic pressure from −3.7 to −8.0 mmHg.

It has similarly been reported from meta-analyses of progressive resistance trials that exercise reduces systolic and diastolic blood pressure by –3 mmHg (95% bootstrap CI: −4, −1) and −3 mmHg (95% bootstrap CI: −4, −1), respectively [16].

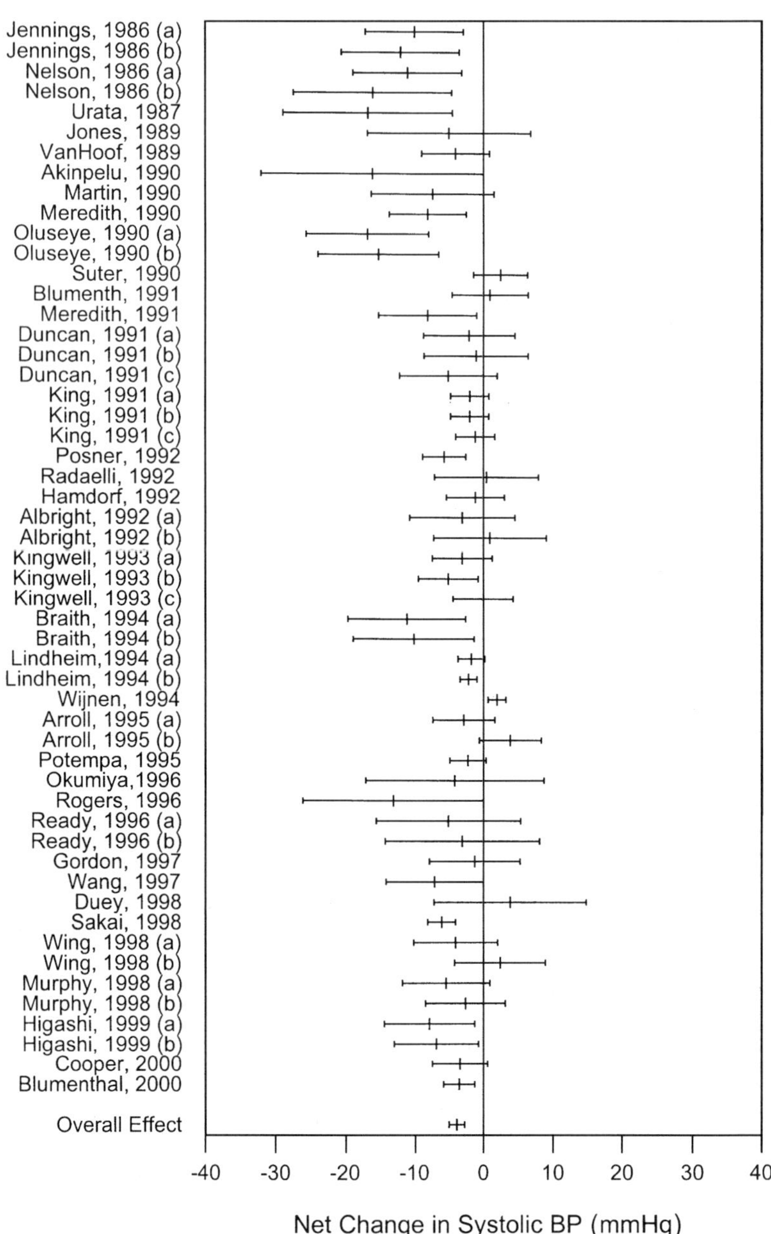

FIGURE 1 Average net change in systolic blood pressure and corresponding 95% CIs related to aerobic exercise intervention in 53 randomized, controlled trials. *Source*: Ref. 12.

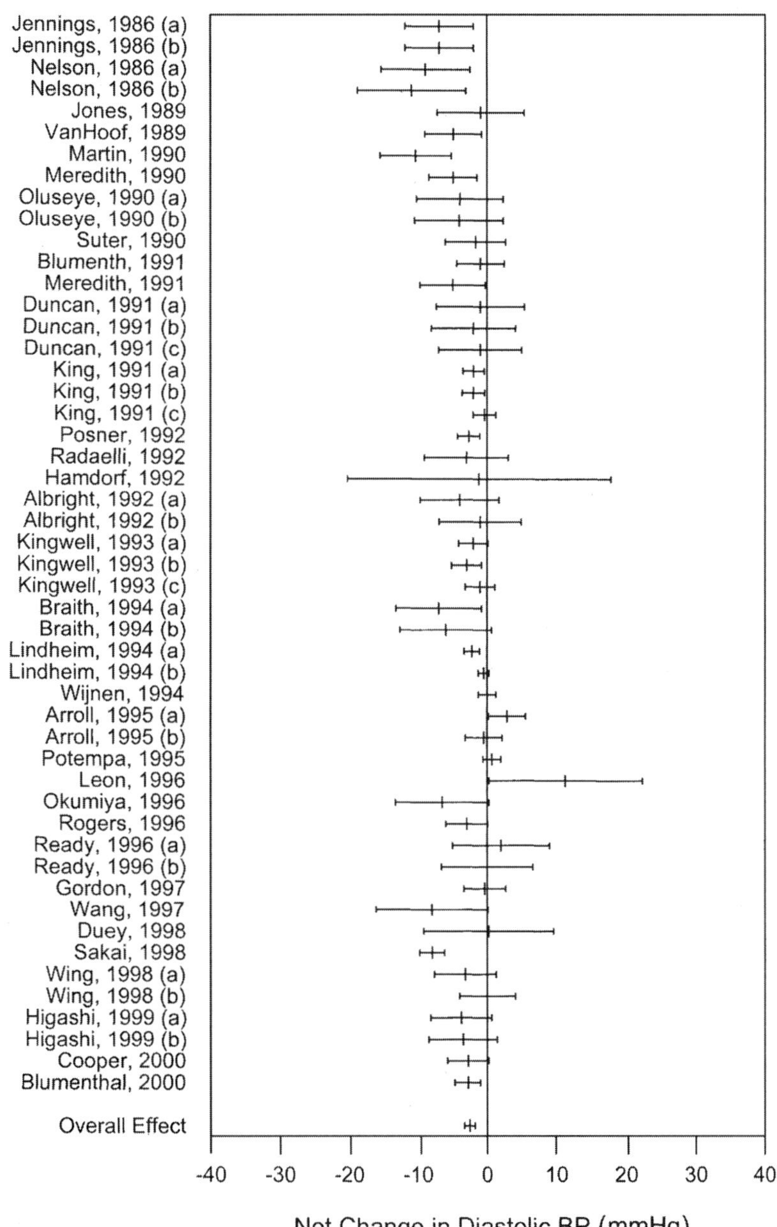

FIGURE 2 Average net change in diastolic blood pressure and corresponding 95% CIs related to aerobic exercise intervention in 50 randomized, controlled trials. *Source*: Ref. 12.

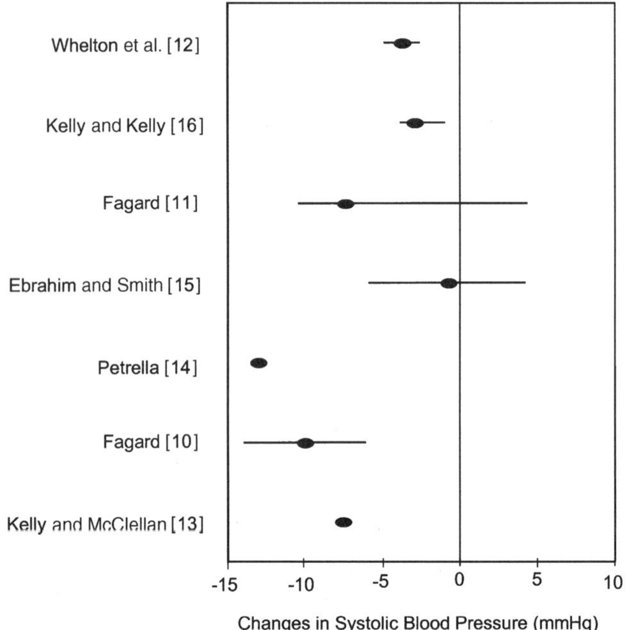

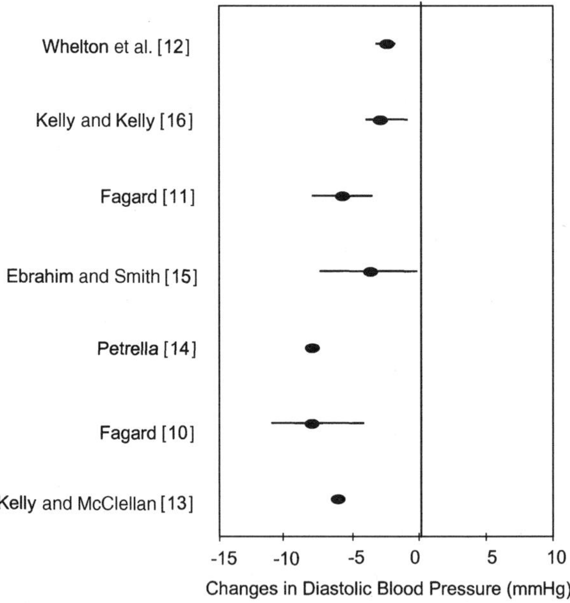

FIGURE 3 Summary of meta-analyses of the depressor effect of exercise in hypertensive subjects. *Source*: Refs. 10–16.

Factors Affecting the Magnitude of the Depressor Effect

According to Fagard and Tipton [17], determinants of the training-induced change in blood pressure are the level of blood pressure, demographic and anthropometric characteristics, and characteristics of the training program.

Fagard and Tipton [17] reported that the depressor effect of aerobic training in systolic/diastolic pressure was –3.2/–3.1 mmHg in normotensive people, compared with –6.2/–6.9 mmHg in those with borderline hypertension and –9.9/–7.6 mmHg in those with hypertension. Similar results were reported from meta-analyses by Fagard [10] and Petrella [14]. Moreover, Fagard [18] found in his review a correlation ($r = 0.74$, $p = 0.001$) between systolic pressure before training and the amount of decrease in blood pressure (Fig. 4). These findings indicate that the higher the blood pressure before the intervention with physical activity, the greater the hypotensive effect due to that exercise.

Among the demographic characteristics, for the effect of age, data from a meta-analysis indicate that the magnitude of blood pressure reduction is greater in middle-aged hypertensive subjects than in both younger and older subjects [19,20]. There were few data for the young and aged, however. In contrast, other meta-analyses by different investigators

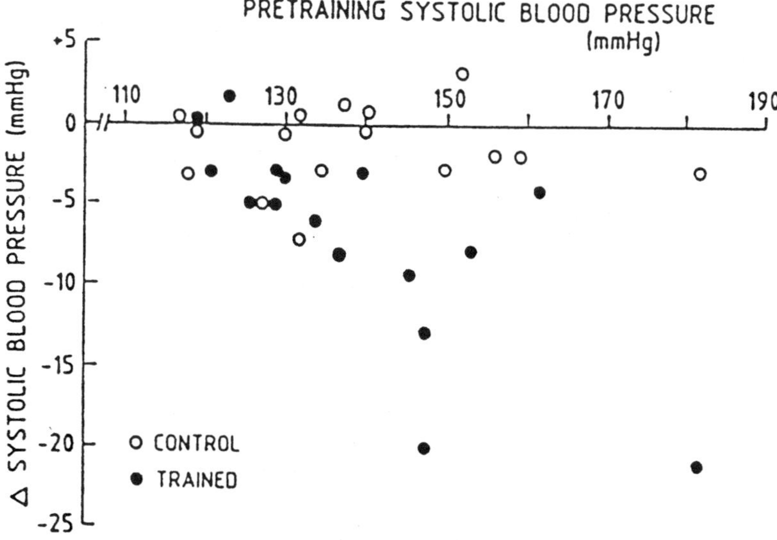

FIGURE 4 Changes of systolic blood pressure versus pretraining systolic blood pressure; open circles represent control observations, closed circles are data for subjects who underwent training. *Source*: Ref. 18.

revealed that exercise-induced changes in blood pressure did not seem to be age-dependent [14,17]. In any case, there has been no study aimed at investigating the age difference. With regard to gender, Petrella [14] found in a meta-analysis that the reduction in blood pressure after training was similar among men and women. In hypertensive adolescents, females did not have as great a reduction in diastolic blood pressure as their male counterparts [21]. Hagberg wrote in a review [20], however, that because estrogen is known to modulate blood pressure, it is possible that the effects of exercise training on blood pressure will differ between men and women. In this review by Hagberg as well as in another meta-analysis [17], the data generally support the conclusion that blood pressure is reduced with exercise training somewhat more and somewhat more consistently in women with hypertension than in men. We conducted a physical activity program in which hypertensive subjects, corresponding to stages 1 or 2 based on the criteria of the sixth report of the Joint National Committee on Prevention, Detection, Evaluation, and Treatment of High Blood Pressure (JNC VI) [22], exercised at an intensity of 50% of maximal oxygen consumption. In this study, exercise and control groups were each divided according to sex and age (30 to 49 and 50 to 69 years), and the sex and age differences in the effects of physical activity were investigated [23]. The level of change in blood pressure was adjusted by the baseline blood pressure, exercise time, and level of change in body weight and salt intake, and a comparison was made by sex and age (Fig. 5). There was no significant change in blood pressure in the control group. In the exercise groups, no sex difference was seen in either systolic or diastolic pressure, but the decreases were larger in subjects aged 30 to 49 years than in those aged 50 to 69 years in both the fourth and eighth weeks. In the group 50 to 69 years of age, the depressor effect of exercise was smaller or appeared later than in the younger group.

Fagard and Tipton [17] concluded that the initial body weight and amount of change in body weight affected the change in blood pressure, whereas Whelton et al. [12] found that the hypotensive effect of exercise was independent of changes in body weight (the details of which will be left for another section).

The characteristics of the training programs used in studies are summarized in the meta-analyses of Fagard [24], Petrella [14], Whelton et al. [12], and Halbert et al. [25], and the review of Hagberg [20]. Fagard [24] concluded that the interstudy differences among most studies were not related to the number of weeks, time for each session, or intensity of the exercise. If one looks at investigations comparing the number of weeks in individual studies, however, blood pressure decreased by the same amount with exercise of 30 to 60 min three to five times per week, regardless of the number of weeks. When exercise was done seven times per week, there was

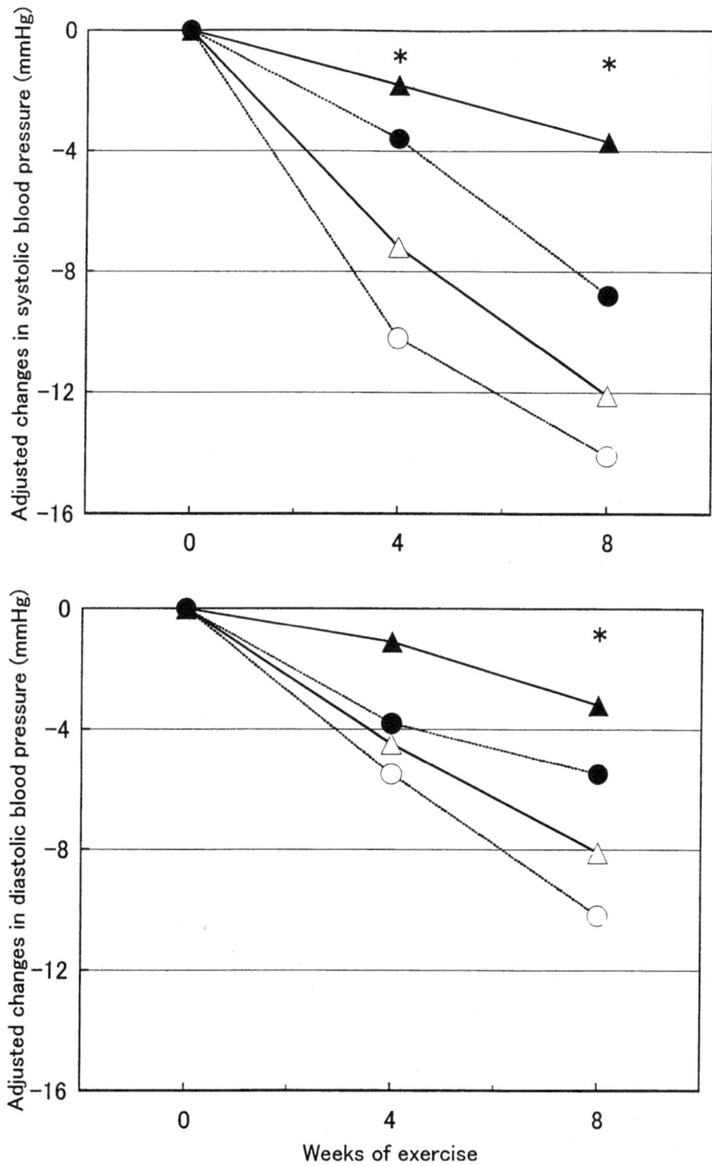

FIGURE 5 Time courses of systolic and diastolic blood pressure reduction with exercise training. Changes were adjusted for baseline blood pressure, exercise duration, and changes in body mass and salt intake. Open triangles, 30- to 49-year-old men; closed triangles, 50- to 69-year-old men; open circles, 30- to 49-year-old women; closed circles, 50- to 69-year-old women. Note: Age difference was significant (p <0.01). *Source*: Ref. 23.

a slight but real reduction in blood pressure compared with exercise done three times per week. Petrella [14] and Halbert et al. [25] showed a sufficient effect with an exercise frequency of three times per week. With greater frequencies of exercise, the effect increased only slightly.

When investigating the effect of the period of training, Petrella [14] found that the effect of exercise seen in studies with intervention for more than 20 weeks was already present after 10 weeks. Similarly, Hagberg et al. [20] stated that for both systolic and diastolic blood pressure, significant and substantial reductions were already evident after only 1 to 10 weeks of exercise training. It would thus appear that the effects of exercise are seen at about the tenth week (Table 1). In the meta-analysis of Whelton et al., a smaller effect was seen in trials with a follow-up of more than 24 weeks than in those with short (< 10 weeks) or medium (10 to 24 weeks) follow-up times [12]. One reason for this may be that in the shorter trials the exercise sessions were supervised, whereas in the longer trials exercise was done independently.

Fagard [24] reported that in several studies there was a greater depressor effect with light exercise of 40% than with intense exercise of 70%. There is disagreement among these results, however, and he concluded that there are insufficient research data. Petrella [14] and Hagberg

TABLE 1 Summary of Effects of Exercise Training Length on Systolic and Diastolic Blood Pressure in Patients with Hypertension

	Training length (weeks)		
	1 to 10	11 to 20	20+
Systolic BP			
Average weighted reduction (mmHg)[a]	9.8	10.9	11.1
Groups reducing (%)[b]	67	78	75
Total sample size[c]	299	773	212
Diastolic BP			
Average weighted reduction (mmHg)[a]	8.4	7.9	9.1
Group reducing (%)[b]	90	78	86
Total sample size[c]	229	818	214

[a] The average weighted reduction is the average reduction in BP with exercise training weighting the average for the sample size of each study and assigning a value of zero to the change for studies with insignificant reduction.
[b] The percentage of groups reducing is the percentage of the total number of groups that reduced BP significantly with exercise training.
[c] The total sample size is the number of hypertensive individuals (systolic BP > 140; diastolic BP >90 mmHg) in the studies.
Source: Ref. 20

et al. [20] reported the possibility that light exercise is more effective than moderate exercise in people with hypertension (Table 2).

Most intervention studies on the hypotensive effect of physical exercise consider mainly aerobic exercise, and because of this studies using aerobic exercise are selected for nearly all meta-analyses. Commonly used types of aerobic exercise are walking, jogging, and cycling. Jennings [26] has pointed out that despite the many recommendations for swimming, the effect of swimming is based only on studies using other types of exercise. Swimming is recommended because it is inexpensive, uses many muscles, and does not put a great load on the joints because of the small load from body weight. At the same time, characteristics of swimming are that the face is put in the water, a horizontal body position is adopted, the body must absorb pressure from the water, the conductivity of water is high, and the amount of exercise done by the arms is considerable. Jennings therefore concluded that the research on swimming was needed.

Tanaka et al. [27] studied 18 middle-aged people with mild hypertension who swam for exercise for 10 weeks, and observed decreases in systolic pressure of 6.6 mmHg and diastolic pressure of 2.5 mmHg. This

TABLE 2 Summary of Effects of Exercise Training Intensity on Systolic and Diastolic Blood Pressure in Patients with Hypertension

	Training intensity	
	<70% Vo_{2max}	>70% VO_{2max}
Systolic BP		
Average weighted reduction (mmHg)[a]	11.1	7.6
Groups reducing (%)[b]	79	75
Total sample size[c]	684	386
Diastolic BP		
Average weighted reduction (mmHg)[a]	7.6	6.7
Groups reducing (%)[b]	81	81
Total sample size[c]	764	317

Note: Vo_{2max} = maximal oxygen uptake.

[a] The average weighted reduction is the average reduction in BP, with exercise training weighting the average for the sample size of each study and assigning a value of zero to the change for studies with insignificant reduction.

[b] The percentage of groups reducing is the percentage of the total number of groups that reduced BP significantly with exercise training.

[c] The total sample size is the number of hypertensive individuals (systolic BP >140; diastolic BP >90 mmHg) in the studies.

Source: Ref. 20

improvement in blood pressure was somewhat smaller than that in studies employing exercise on land.

Similarly, we conducted a study with female subjects corresponding to JNC VI stage 1 or 2 hypertension in which the subjects performed exercise of a similar level of intensity on land (walking, cycling, calisthenics, etc.) and in water (swimming, water walking, etc.) for 2 months [28]. The results showed a significant decrease in both systolic and diastolic blood pressure compared with the nonexercise control group from both exercise on land and in water. The amount of the decrease was significantly greater in the group that exercised on land than in the group that exercised in water, however. The intensity of the water exercise in this study was based on the study of Holmer et al. [29], with a value 10 beats lower than the target heart rate on land, but it is possible that a setting of this intensity was not appropriate. On the other hand, the compliance of the participants in the water exercise was very good, and water exercise has the advantage of a light load for people who are obese or are not used to exercise.

There have also been several studies investigating the depressor effect of exercise other than aerobic exercise, such as resistance training and circuit weight training, and there are reports of a depressor effect from resistance training as well. Kelly and Kelly [16] conducted a meta-analysis of 11 randomized control studies with resistance exercise only for more than 4 weeks. The intervention period was 6 to 30 weeks. The exercise frequency was two to five times per week, and the exercise time per session was 20 to 60 min. The exercise intensity was 30–90% of the one-repetition maximum. Exercises of six to 11 types were done for one to four sets. As a result, there was a slight decrease in blood pressure, with systolic blood pressure declining by 3 mmHg (bootstrap CI; −4, −1), and diastolic pressure also declining by 3 mmHg (bootstrap CI; −4, −1). Kelly and Kelly emphasized that no elevation was seen in blood pressure with resistance exercise, but in this analysis the number of hypertensive subjects was small, and they concluded that more studies with hypertensive subjects should be done.

Harris and Holly [30] had 10 male subjects with borderline hypertension conduct circuit weight training for 9 weeks, and reported no change in systolic pressure but a significant decrease of 7% in diastolic pressure. Hagberg et al. [31] had six adolescents with persistent essential hypertension conduct endurance training for about 5 months, followed by weight training for about 5 months. They found that systolic pressure decreased by 17 ± 4 mmHg from the pretraining level, and by 4 ± 4 mmHg compared with the level after endurance training, but that blood pressure rose again after the exercise was stopped. Hagberg et al. [31] stated that the decrease in blood pressure from weight training was due to the decrease in systemic vascular resistance.

In an article outlining resistance training safety and assessment guidelines for cardiac and coronary prone patients, Kelemen [32] wrote that aerobic exercise was a mild method for the control of blood pressure in hypertension patients, and that resistance training had been avoided to that point because of the elevation in blood pressure that occurs when heavy weights are lifted. Blood pressure during exercise was higher during circuit weight training than endurance training, but was within the clinically allowable range. Moreover, there was an increasing amount of research showing a significant depressor effect from resistance training. The form of resistance exercise recommended was circuit weight training. He also said that exercise using moderate weights set at 30–50% of the one-repetition maximum was safe and effective and that machine weights were preferable to free weights. In addition, he urged that all people should undergo screening before starting this training.

In recent years, there has been research comparing the effects of physical exercise in individuals with different genotypes. Hagberg et al. [33] had 18 obese people with hypertension exercise three times a week over 9 months. They then compared the hypotensive effect of exercise by angiotensin-converting enzyme, apolipoprotein E, and lipoprotein lipase genotype. They reported that for any of the genes investigated the hypo-

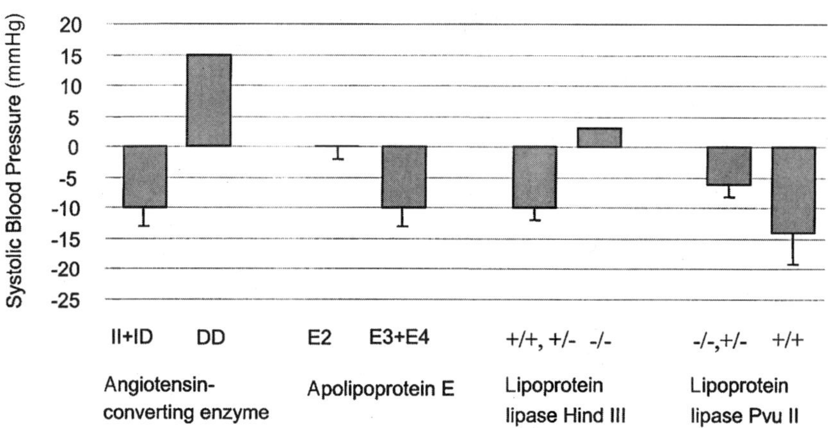

FIGURE 6 Changes in systolic blood pressure with exercise among different genotype groups. Changes with exercise training between genotype groups ($p<0.05$). *Note*: ID, insertion/deletion; DD, deletion/deletion; II, insertion/insertion; E2, apolipoprotein E2; E3, apolipoprotein E3; E4, apolipoprotein E4. *Source*: Ref. 33.

tensive effect of exercise differed according to genotype, with the most marked difference seen with the lipoprotein lipase Hind III type (Fig. 6). It is said that blood pressure decreases with exercise in 75% of hypertensives, and in the remaining 25% does not change [34]. By considering genotype it thus may be possible in the future to develop individualized physical activity programs.

Recommendations for Physical Activity as a Treatment for Hypertension

The report of JNC VI [22] recommends lifestyle modification as the first treatment step for people with high normal and stage I hypertension who have no or one other risk factor (Table 3). Lifestyle modification includes the following five considerations: alcohol intake, tobacco intake, diet related to sodium and potassium, relaxation, and physical activity. Recommendations for physical activity are intermediate exercise (40–60% of maximal oxygen consumption), such as walking fast for 30 to 45 min almost daily.

The 1999 World Health Organization–International Society of Hypertension guidelines for the management of hypertension [35] recommend a modest level of regular aerobic exercise, such as fast walking or swimming for 30 to 45 min three to four times per week for sedentary persons. This mild exercise can more effectively reduce blood pressure than such strenuous exercise as running or jogging, and lower systolic blood pressure 4 to 8 mmHg. It also states that isometric exercise such as heavy weightlifting can have a pressor effect and should be avoided.

The position stand of the American College of Sports Medicine (ASCM) [34] states that endurance training is effective not only for mild essential hypertension but for secondary hypertension due to renal dysfunction, and recommends large muscle activities three to five times per week for 20 to 60 min per session at an intensity of 50–85% of maximal oxygen consumption. They also state that exercise training at somewhat lower intensities (40–70% of maximal oxygen consumption) appears to lower blood pressure as much—or more—than exercise at higher intensities, which may be especially important in such specific hypertensive populations as the elderly.

In Japan, national health insurance began covering exercise therapy for hypertension in April 1996, and guidelines were subsequently published [36]. These include walking as a main aerobic exercise conducted at a 50% heart rate reserve with a target of a total of at least 120 min per week, or more than 8000 steps per day. It is also desirable that physical activity, including daily life activities, be increased by 200 kcal/day, especially for people who have little physical activity.

TABLE 3 Risk Stratification and Treatment

Blood pressure stages (mmHg)	Risk group A (no risk factors: no TOD/CCD)[a]	Risk group B (at least one risk factor, not including diabetes; no TOD/CCD)	Risk group C (TOD/CCD and/or diabetes, with or without other risk factors)
High-normal (130–139/85–89)	Lifestyle modification	Lifestyle modification	Drug therapy[c]
Stage 1 (140–159/90–99)	Lifestyle modification (up to 12 months)	Lifestyle modification[b] (up to 6 months)	Drug therapy
Stage 2 and 3 (≥160/≥100)	Drug therapy	Drug therapy	Drug therapy

Note: For example, a patient with diabetes and a blood pressure of 124/94 mmHg plus left ventricular hypertrophy should be classified as having stage 1 hypertension with target organ disease (left ventricular hypertophy) and with another major risk.
[a] TOD/CCD indicates target organ disease/clinical cardiovascular disease.
[b] For patients with multiple risk factors, clinicians should consider drug as initial therapy plus lifestyle modifications.
[c] For those with heart failure, renal insufficiency, or diabetes.
Source: Ref. 22

PHYSICAL ACTIVITY FOR THE PREVENTION OF HYPERTENSION

Mechanism of the Preventive Effect from Physical Activity

To the authors' knowledge there have been no studies investigating the mechanism of the preventive effect on hypertension of physical activity. In the people with hypertension indicated above, however, the physical changes that occur as a result of physical activity are thought to prevent persistently occurring hypertension.

Cohort Studies on Preventing the Development of Hypertension

Cohort studies with a sufficiently large number of people and observation periods are needed to investigate the preventive effect of physical activity on the development of hypertension. Moreover, hypertension is not only influenced by physical activity; adjustments must also be made for various confounding factors, including body weight, smoking and alcohol habits, and family history. It is thus very difficult to investigate the intensity and duration of the physical activity required for a preventive effect. Here we will introduce cohort studies examining differences in the onset of hypertension according to level of physical activity (Fig. 7).

Paffenbarger et al. [37] observed 14,998 male alumni of Harvard University for 6 to 10 years, and found no relation between the development of hypertension and exercise history (stair climbing, walking, or light

FIGURE 7 Incidence of hypertension according to the level of physical activity. Open circles are reference, closed circles are incidence rate, and horizontal bars indicate the 95% confidence interval: (a) adjusted for age; (b) physical activity index includes stairs ascended, blocks walked daily, hr per week of light and vigorous sports activity, yard work, and the like; (c) adjusted for age. Total leisure time physical activity was assessed from the questions concerning conditioning exercise, sports, physical recreation, different leisure time and household chores, and commuting to and from work. Only the risk among men is shown; (d) leisure time included frequency of television watching, walking, bicycling, and walking or bicycling to and from work or shopping. Incidence rate was adjusted for age, education, baseline systolic and diastolic blood pressure, and study field; (e) adjusted for age, body mass index, alcohol consumption, leisure-time physical activity, smoking status, fasting glucose level, and systolic and diastolic blood pressure; (f) adjusted for age, body mass index, smoking status, alcohol consumption, family history, and baseline blood pressure. *Source*: Refs. 36–42.

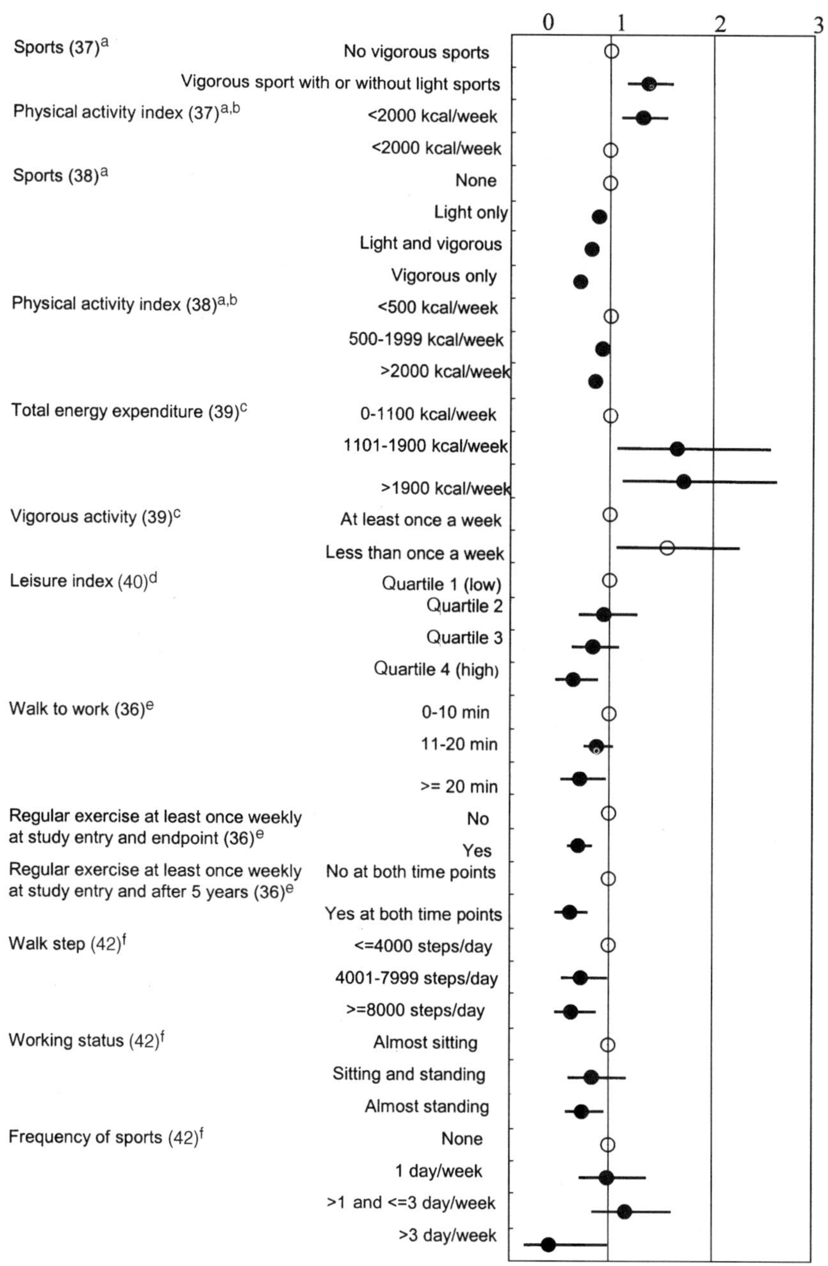
0
1
2
3
Sports (37)a
No vigorous sports
Vigorous sport with or without light sports
Physical activity index (37)a,b
<2000 kcal/week
<2000 kcal/week
Sports (38)a
None
Light only
Light and vigorous
Vigorous only
Physical activity index (38)a,b
<500 kcal/week
500-1999 kcal/week
>2000 kcal/week
Total energy expenditure (39)c
0-1100 kcal/week
1101-1900 kcal/week
>1900 kcal/week
Vigorous activity (39)c
At least once a week
Less than once a week
Leisure index (40)d
Quartile 1 (low)
Quartile 2
Quartile 3
Quartile 4 (high)
Walk to work (36)e
0-10 min
11-20 min
>= 20 min
Regular exercise at least once weekly at study entry and endpoint (36)e
No
Yes
Regular exercise at least once weekly at study entry and after 5 years (36)e
No at both time points
Yes at both time points
Walk step (42)f
<=4000 steps/day
4001-7999 steps/day
>=8000 steps/day
Working status (42)f
Almost sitting
Sitting and standing
Almost standing
Frequency of sports (42)f
None
1 day/week
>1 and <=3 day/week
>3 day/week

sports) while at college. They also reported that subjects who did no vigorous exercise during the observational period had a 35% higher risk of onset of hypertension than did those who exercised. In addition, they calculated the energy consumed per week from the amount of stair climbing and walking, sports activities, and housework, and compared the development of hypertension. Those who consumed less than 2000 kcal of energy per week had a 30% higher risk of developing hypertension than those who consumed 2000 kcal or more did. Paffenbargar et al. [38] observed 5463 alumni of the University of Pennsylvania over 15 years from 1962 to 1976 in a study of physical activity and the onset of hypertension. They found no relationship between the development of hypertension and walking distance or number of steps climbed. People who did vigorous sports had a 30% lower risk, however, and those who did vigorous and light sports a 19% lower risk. When adjustments were made for age and body mass index (BMI), people who did vigorous sports for 1 to 2 hr per week had a lower risk of hypertension than those who did not; however, those who exercised more than that amount showed no additional beneficial effect of exercise. Walking, stair climbing, and sports activities were converted to energy consumption, and the weekly energy consumption and risk of developing hypertension were compared. This revealed that the greater the weekly energy consumption, the lower the risk of developing hypertension. People with a weekly consumption of 2000 kcal or more had a 15% lower risk of hypertension, but this value was not statistically significant.

In a study of 2500 middle-aged Finnish men and women, Haapanen et al. detected a higher risk of developing hypertension in men in groups with the least weekly amounts of leisure time activity or no vigorous activity. No similar trend was seen, however, in the women in these groups [39].

Later, Pereira et al. [40] divided activity into leisure activities (watching television, walking, cycling, etc.), sports activities, and work activities, and investigated the relationship of each of them with the development of hypertension. Among white men, the results suggested that with leisure activities only, the development of hypertension was 36% lower in the group that was most active than in the group with the least activity. This tendency was not seen, however, in women or African Americans.

In research in Japan, Hayashi et al. [41] followed 6017 male employees age 35 to 63 years of one company for 6 to 16 years, and investigated the relationship between physical activity and the development of hypertension. Hypertension was 29% lower in men who walked more than 20 min to work than in those who walked less than 10 min to work. Moreover, there was 30% less hypertension in men who exercised once per week at the start of the observation period than in those who did not exercise. Those who exercised at least once per week both at the start of the observation period and 5 years later had a 39% lower rate of hypertension than men who were not exercising at either of these times.

We followed 3106 male employees of one company for 4 years in an investigation of the relationship between physical activity and hypertension [42]. A comparison by number of steps walked per day showed that, compared with men who walked fewer than 4000 steps per day, those who walked 4000 to 8000 steps per day had a 27% lower risk of developing hypertension and those who walked more than 8000 steps per day a 37% lower risk. Looking at the amount of physical activity during work, the risk was 26% lower in men who worked "mostly standing" than in those who worked "mostly sitting." Among leisure activities, the risk of hypertension was decreased by 59% in men who exercised three or more times per week compared with those who did no exercise at all, but no difference was seen according to the intensity of the exercise.

Data from various countries thus show a lower incidence of hypertension among people who perform relatively intense exercise. In addition, data from Japan show that even light exercise, such as walking a great amount, reduces the risk of developing hypertension. These differences are thought to be affected by race, living habits, and degree of obesity, and further study is necessary for a proper investigation of the amount of exercise needed to prevent the development of hypertension.

Recommendations for the Prevention of Hypertension

The report of JNC VI [22] does not clearly recommend an amount of physical activity, but states that sedentary normotensive individuals have a 20–50% increased risk of suffering from hypertension than more active and fit people.

The ACSM position stand [43] recommends the following quantity and quality of exercise for developing and maintaining cardiorespiratory and muscular fitness in healthy people:

1. Frequency of three to five times a week.
2. Intensity of 60–90% of maximum heart rate or 50–85% of maximal oxygen consumption or maximum heart rate reserve.
3. Continuous aerobic activity for 60 to 90 min. The duration of exercise is also influenced by the exercise intensity, and for adults who are not athletes a lower- to moderate-intensity activity is recommended over high-intensity exercise.
4. Exercises that use large muscle groups are easier to continue.
5. Moderate-intensity strength training to increase or maintain fat-free mass is necessary in exercise programs for adults. For the major muscle groups, eight to 10 sets of eight to 12 repetitions done twice weekly are recommended.

The surgeon general's report [44] states with regard to the effect of physical activity on blood pressure that physical activity prevents or delays the development of high blood pressure. It also recommends a moderate amount of physical activity, such as 30 min of brisk walking or raking leaves, 15 min of running, or 45 min of playing volleyball on most, if not all, days of the week. Furthermore, among healthier people additional health benefits can be gained through greater amounts of physical activity. People who can maintain a regular regimen of activity of longer duration or of more vigorous intensity are likely to derive greater benefit.

REFERENCES

1. Hagberg JM, Montain SJ, Martin WH, Ehsani AA. Effect of exercise training in 60- to 69-year-old persons with essential hypertension. Am J Cardiol 1989; 64: 348–353.
2. Nelson L, Jennings GL, Esler MD, Korner PI. Effect of changing levels of physical activity on blood pressure and hemodynamics in essential hypertension. Lancet 1986; ii: 473–476.
3. Arakawa K. Antihypertensive mechanism of exercise. J Hypertens 1993; 11: 223–329.
4. Arakawa K. Effect of exercise on hypertension and associated complications. Hypertens Res 1996; 19 (suppl. I): S87–S91.
5. O'Sullivan SE, Bell C. The effects of exercise and training on human cardiovascular reflex control. J Auton Nerv Syst 2000; 81: 16–24.
6. Koga M, Ideishi M, Matsusaki M, Tashiro E, Kinoshita A, Ikeda M, Tanaka H, Shindo M, Arakawa K. Mild exercise decreases plasma endogenous digitalislike substance in hypertensive individuals. Hypertension 1992; 19 (suppl. II): II231–II236.
7. Tanabe Y, Urata H, Kiyonag A, Ikeda M, Tanaka H, Shindo M, Arakawa K. Changes in serum concentrations of taurine and other amino acids in clinical antihypertensive exercise therapy. Clin Exp Hypertens A 1989; 11: 149–165.
8. Brett SE, Ritter JM, Chowienczyk PJ. Diastolic blood pressure changes during exercise positively correlate with serum cholesterol and insulin resistance. Circulation 2000; 101: 1462–1467.
9. Kelley G, Tran ZV. Aerobic exercise and normotensive adults: a meta-analysis. Med Sci Sports Exerc 1995; 27: 1371–1377.
10. Fagard RH. Prescription and results of physical activity. J Cardiovasc Pharmacol 1995; 25: S20–S27.
11. Fagard RH. Physical activity in the prevention and treatment of hypertension in the obese. Med Sci Sports Exerc 1999; 31: S624–S630.
12. Whelton SP, Chin A, Xin X, He J. Effect of aerobic exercise on blood pressure: a meta-analysis of randomized, controlled trials. Ann Int Med 2002; 136: 493–503.

13. Kelly G, McClellan P. Antihypertensive effects of aerobic exercise: a brief meta-analytic review of randomized controlled trials. AJH 1994; 7: 115–119.
14. Petrella RJ. How effective is exercise training for the treatment of hypertension? Clin J Sport Med 1998; 8: 224–231.
15. Ebrahim S, Smith GD. Lowering blood pressure: a systematic review of sustained effects of non-pharmacological interventions. J Publ Health Med 1998; 20: 441–448.
16. Kelly GA, Kelly KS. Progressive resistance exercise and resting blood pressure: a meta-analysis of randomized controlled trials. Hypertension 2000; 35: 838–843.
17. Fagard RH, Tipton CM. Physical activity, fitness, and hypertension. In: Brouchard C, Shephard RJ, Stephens T, eds. Physical Activity, Fitness, and Health. Champaign, IL: Human Kinetics, 1994: 633–655.
18. Fagard R. Habitual physical activity, training, and blood pressure in normo- and hypertension. Int J Sports Med 1985; 6: 57–67.
19. Hagberg JM, Brown MD. Does exercise training play a role in the treatment of essential hypertension? Cardiovasc Risk 1995; 2: 296–302.
20. Hagberg JM, Park J, Brown MD. The role of exercise training in the treatment of hypertension: an update. Sports Med 2000; 30: 193–206.
21. Hagberg JM, Goldring D, Ehsani AA, Heath GW, Hernandez A, Schechtman K, Holloszy JO. Effects of exercise training on the blood pressure and hemodynamic features of hypertensive adolescents. Am J Cardiol 1983; 52: 763–768.
22. The Joint National Committee on Prevention, Detection, Evaluation, and Treatment of High Blood Pressure. The Sixth Report of the Joint National Committee on Prevention, Detection, Evaluation, and Treatment of High Blood Pressure. Arch Int Med 1997; 157: 2413–2446.
23. Ishikawa K, Ohta T, Zhang J, Hashimoto S, Tanaka H. Influence of age and gender on exercise training-induced blood pressure reduction in systemic hypertension. Am J Cardiol 1999; 84: 192–196.
24. Fagard RH. Exercise characteristics and the blood pressure response to dynamic physical training. Med Sci Sports Exerc 2001; 6 (suppl.): S484–S492.
25. Halbert JA, Silagy CA, Finucane P, Withers RT, Hamdorf PA, Andrews GR. The effectiveness of exercise training in lowering blood pressure: a meta–analysis of randomized controlled trials of 4 weeks or longer. J Hum Hypertens 1997; 11: 641–649.
26. Jennings GL. Exercise and blood pressure: walk, run or swim? J Hypertens 1997; 15: 567–569.
27. Tanaka H, Bassett DR, Howley ET, Thompson DL, Ashraf M, Rawson FL. Swimming training lowers the resting blood pressure in individuals with hypertension. J Hypertens 1997; 15: 651–657.
28. Ishikawa K, Ohta T, Kato M. Comparison of training-induced blood pressure reduction between land-based and aqua exercises in hypertensive women. Nippon Rinsyo Sport Igaku Kaishi 1999; 7: 76–80.
29. Holmer I, Stein EM, Saltin B, Ekblom B, Astrand PO. Hemodynamic and

respiratory responses compared in swimming and running. J Appl Physiol 1974; 37: 49–54.
30. Harris KA, Holly RG. Physiological response to circuit weight training in borderline hypertensive subjects. Med Sci Sports Exerc 1987; 19: 246–252.
31. Hagberg JM, Ehsani AA, Goldring D, Hernandez A, Sinacore DR, Holloszy JO. Effect of weight training on blood pressure and hemodynamics in hypertensive adolescents. J Pediatr 1984; 104: 147–151.
32. Kelemen MH. Resistive training safety and assessment guidelines for cardiac and coronary prone patients. Med Sci Sports Exerc 1989; 21: 675–677.
33. Hagberg JM, Ferrell RE, Dengel DR, Wilund KR. Exercise training-induced blood pressure and plasma lipid improvements in hypertensives may be genotype dependent. Hypertension 1999; 34: 18–23.
34. American College of Sports Medicine. Position stand. Physical activity, physical fitness, and hypertension. Med Sci Sorts Exerc 1993; 25: i–x.
35. 1999 World Health Organization–International Society of Hypertension. Guidelines for the management of hypertension. J Hypertens 1999: 17: 151–183.
36. Japan Medical Association. Guidelines for exercise therapy. Tokyo: Nippon Iji Shinposha, 1996.
37. Paffenbarger RS, Wing AL, Hyde RT, Jung DL. Physical activity and incidence of hypertension in college alumni. Am J Epidemiol 1983; 117: 245–257.
38. Paffenbarger RS, Jung DL, Leung RW, Hyde RT. Physical activity and hypertension: an epidemiological view. Ann Med 1991; 23: 319–327.
39. Haapanen N, Milunpalo S, Vuori I, Oja P, Pasanen M. Association of leisure time physical activity with the risk of coronary heart disease, hypertension and diabetes in middle-aged men and women. Int J Epidemiol 1997; 739–747.
40. Pereira MA, Folsom AR, McGovern PG, Carpenter M, Arnett DK, Liao D, Szklo M, Hutchinson RG. Physical activity and incident hypertension in black and white adults: the atherosclerosis risk in communities' study. Prev Med 1999; 28: 304–312.
41. Hayashi T, Tsumura K, Suematsu C, Okada K, Fujii S, Endo G. Walking to work and the risk for hypertension in men: the Osaka Health Survey. Ann Int Med 1999; 130: 21–26.
42. Ishikawa K, Ohta T. Physical activity and blood pressure. Nippon Rinsho 2000; 58 (suppl.): 353–359.
43. American College of Sports Medicine Position Stand. The recommended quantity and quality of exercise for developing and maintaining cardiorespiratory and muscular fitness in healthy adults. Med Sci Sports Exerc 1990; 22: 265–274.
44. U.S. Department of Health and Human Service, Centers for Disease Control and Prevention, National Center for Chronic Disease Prevention and Health Promotion, the President's Council on Physical Fitness and Sports. Physical activity and health: a report of the surgeon general. Pittsburgh: Superintendent of Documents, 1996.

9

Potassium Supplementation

Paul K. Whelton and Jiang He
Tulane University School of Public Health and Tropical Medicine,
New Orleans, Louisiana, U.S.A.

INTRODUCTION

Hypertension is an important worldwide public health problem because of its high prevalence and the concomitant increase in the risk of cardiovascular–renal disease [1–4]. Nutritional factors have been identified as the most important environmental determinant of blood pressure and the risk of hypertension [5–7]. The relationship of overweight, high salt intake, and alcohol consumption to elevated blood pressure has been established in both observational studies and clinical trials. A reduction in exposure to these risk factors has been recommended as an important approach to preventing hypertension [7]. The relationship of other dietary nutrients to blood pressure, however, including potassium, calcium, magnesium, and macronutrients, has not been well established [5–7].

Over 70 years ago Addison first reported that a high potassium intake could exert an antihypertensive effect [8]. Since then, numerous observational epidemiologic studies, randomized controlled trials, and animal experiments have been conducted to investigate this issue. This review will examine the available evidence for a relationship between potassium intake and blood pressure from studies conducted in human populations. In addition, the effect of potassium intake on the risk of cardiovascular disease will be discussed.

OBSERVATIONAL EPIDEMIOLOGICAL STUDIES

Observational epidemiologic studies have examined the relationship between dietary potassium intake and blood pressure in many populations. Most of these studies found an inverse association between dietary potassium intake (or urinary potassium excretion) and blood pressure within and across populations. The epidemiologic evidence linking potassium intake to blood pressure initially came from studies in low-blood-pressure populations.

Studies in Low-Blood-Pressure Populations

More than 20 populations with low average blood pressures and little or no rise in blood pressure with age throughout adulthood have been reported from isolated areas around the world. Hypertension is virtually absent in these populations. Typically, they consist of individuals who consume a diet that is low in sodium and high in potassium [9–16]. In general, urinary sodium excretion has been low and potassium excretion high among those populations. Oliver and colleagues studied blood pressure in a group of 506 Yanomamo Indians living in the tropical equatorial rain forest of northern Brazil [9]. They found that mean blood pressure was low (systolic blood pressure varied from 93 to 108 mmHg and diastolic blood pressure from 59 to 69 mmHg among different age groups) and did not increase with age. Indeed, both systolic and diastolic blood pressure declined with age in both men and women, although the change was not statistically significant except for systolic blood pressure in women ($p < 0.01$). In a subgroup of 26 study participants, 24-hr urinary sodium excretion was 1.02 mmol, and potassium excretion was 152.2 mmol [9]. Truswell and co-authors reported a low-blood-pressure population in southwest African Kung bushmen [11]. Mean 24-hr urinary sodium excretion was 29 to 31 mmol, and the corresponding potassium excretion was 70 to 103 mmol, based on data from 10 subjects [11].

The INTERSALT study, which used standardized methods to measure blood pressure and urinary electrolytes, provided an opportunity to compare these variables in four isolated populations (Yanomamo and Xingu Indians of Brazil and rural populations in Kenya and Papua New Guinea) with corresponding data from acculturated populations [13]. Compared to the other 48 INTERSALT populations, the four remote populations had a lower mean systolic blood pressure of 103 versus 120 mmHg and a lower mean diastolic blood pressure of 63 versus 74 mmHg, respectively [13]. Mean urinary sodium excretion varied from 1 to 60 mmol/24 hr in the four remote populations, which was substantially lower than the average level for the remaining INTERSALT populations (mean of 166 mmol/24 hr). Urinary potassium excretion in three of the four low-blood-pressure populations (60 to 69 mmol/24 hr) was higher than the mean potassium value of 54 mmol observed in the other 48 INTERSALT populations. The level in Kenya, 32 mmol in men and 35 mmol in women, was below that of the other remote population samples and of the average INTERSALT value for urinary potassium excretion.

The authors have conducted several large population-based studies in an isolated population of Yi farmers in southwestern China [14–16]. In one such study, data on blood pressure and 24-hr urinary electrolytes were collected over three consecutive days [14]. Mean systolic and diastolic blood pressure was 99.4 and 63.2 mmHg, respectively, in the Yi farmers living in high mountain areas compared to a mean systolic and diastolic blood pressure of 108.6 and 71.3 mmHg among their counterparts living in urban settings. Mean urinary excretion of sodium and potassium was 73.9 mmol/24 hr and 58.6 mmol/24 hr, respectively, in Yi farmers compared to 159.4 mmol/24 hr and 28.3 mmol/24 hr in the Yi urban residents [14].

Studies in Other Populations

Studies that have compared potassium intake and blood pressure within a given population provide strong evidence for a causal relationship between potassium intake and blood pressure. One of the earliest such studies was conducted by Walker and his colleagues [17]. In this study, blood pressure and urinary potassium were measured among 574 ambulatory subjects. An inverse relationship was identified between urinary potassium and diastolic blood pressure ($r = -0.23$, $p < 0.001$). In addition, urinary potassium was significantly lower in hypertensives compared to normotensives [17]. Watson et al. studied 662 adolescent females in Hinds County, Mississippi, and noted an inverse correlation between 24-hr urinary potassium excretion and systolic blood pressure and a positive correlation between the urinary sodium/potassium ratio and systolic blood pressure [18]. As has been demonstrated in subsequent studies, the associations were stronger for the sodium/potassium ratio than for potassium alone [15,19–23]. These observations suggest that both dietary potassium intake as well as the ratio of sodium to potassium are important in the pathogenesis of high blood pressure.

The INTERSALT study has provided the most precise and accurate estimates of the effect of potassium on blood pressure [21,22]. Blood pressure and a single measurement of 24-hr urinary potassium excretion were obtained in 10,079 men and women aged 20 to 59 years sampled from 52 populations around the world using a standardized protocol with central training of observers, a central laboratory, and extensive quality control. In addition, a random sample of 807 participants completed second visits, at which blood pressure was remeasured and a repeat 24-hr urine specimen was collected. This subsample provided reliability data to correct for regression dilution bias. The relationship between potassium excretion and blood pressure was estimated using regression analysis techniques in individual subjects within each population, and the results of these regression analyses in all 52 populations were pooled. After adjustment for age, sex, body mass index, alcohol consumption, and urinary sodium excretion and correction for regression dilution bias, a 50 mmol per day difference in urinary potassium excretion was associated with a 3.36 mmHg lower systolic blood pressure and 1.87 mmHg lower diastolic blood pressure.

Lower potassium intake has been implicated in the higher prevalence of hypertension in African Americans [23–25]. Grim and colleagues studied blood pressure and electrolyte intake in a random sample of the African-American and white populations of Evans County, Georgia [24]. The prevalence of hypertension was higher in African Americans compared to their counterparts who were white. Sodium intake, assessed by collecting duplicate diets and 24-hr urine specimens, was similar in African Americans and whites. Potassium, however, was significantly lower in African Americans compared to whites: 24 versus 40 mmol/24 hr for men, and 27 versus 36 mmol/24 hr for women, respectively [24]. Likewise, in the Veterans Administration Cooperative Study on Antihypertensive Agents urinary 24-hr sodium excretion was similar in 407 African-American and 216 white untreated hypertensives, but the African Americans excreted 62% less potassium than their counterparts who were white: 45 versus 73 mmol/24 hr [25].

Most of the previously mentioned studies utilized a cross-sectional design and could not provide information on the temporal relationship between potassium intake and blood pressure. Two prospective studies provide important additional data that address this question, however [26,27]. The effect of baseline dietary potassium intake, as assessed by dietary questionnaire, on subsequent incidence of hypertension during 4 years of follow-up was examined in 58,218 predominantly white women, aged 34 to 59 years, who were participants in the Nurses' Health Study [26]. Compared to those with a potassium intake of $<2{,}000$ mg/day, the relative risk of hypertension was 0.77 ($p < 0.001$) in women whose potassium intake was $\geq 3{,}200$ mg/day, after adjustment for age, body mass index, and alcohol consumption. The relative risk increased to 1.05, however, and was no longer statistically significant after further adjustment for dietary intake of calcium, magnesium, and fiber [26]. In the Health Professionals Study, the relationship between dietary potassium intake and 4-year incidence of hypertension was investigated in 30,681 predominantly white men, aged 40 to 75 years old [27]. After adjustment for age, body mass index, and alcohol intake, men with a potassium intake ≥3,600 mg/day had a significantly lower risk of hypertension (relative risk = 0.65) compared to those with an intake of <2,400 mg/day ($p < 0.01$). Following further adjustment for dietary intake of calcium, magnesium, and fiber, the relative risk was 0.83 and was no longer significant [27]. Because of the high correlation between dietary nutrients, the adjusted relative risk of hypertension on dietary potassium intake might have been overadjusted in the Nurses' Health Study and the Health Professionals Study [28].

RANDOMIZED CONTROLLED TRIALS

Randomized controlled trials provide an opportunity to study the effect of potassium on blood pressure without the potentially confounding influence of concurrent changes in other dietary nutrients. Trials evaluating both the effects of potassium depletion and potassium supplementation have been conducted in humans.

Potassium Depletion

Krishna et al. investigated the effects of potassium depletion on blood pressure in normotensives and hypertensives who were maintained on their usual level of sodium intake [29,30]. In a randomized crossover trial, 10 normotensive men were randomly assigned to isocaloric diets that provided either 10 mmol or 90 mmol of potassium per day. Sodium consumption was maintained at the subjects' usual level of intake (120 to 200 mmol per day). Mean arterial blood pressure did not change significantly during normal potassium intake, but it increased over the 9 days of low potassium intake from 91 to 95 mmHg ($P < 0.05$). Both mean arterial ($P < 0.01$) and diastolic ($P < 0.005$) blood pressure were significantly higher following the low potassium diet compared to the normal potassium diet. This study suggests that short-term potassium depletion increases blood pressure in normotensive men [29]. In another double-blind, randomized crossover study [30], 12 hypertensive patients were placed on a 10-day isocaloric diet that provided a daily potassium intake of either 16 mmol or 96 mmol. Intake of sodium (120 mmol/day) and other minerals was kept constant. During the period of low potassium intake, systolic blood pressure increased ($P = 0.01$) by 7 mmHg (95% CI: 3 to 11 mmHg) and diastolic pressure increased ($P = 0.04$) by 6 mmHg (95% CI: 1 to 11 mmHg). This study indicates that dietary potassium restriction increases blood pressure in patients with essential hypertension.

Potassium Supplementation

The first randomized controlled trial to evaluate the effect of potassium supplementation in lowering blood pressure was conducted in 1980 [31]. Since then, results from at least 33 such trials have been reported [32]. Most of these trials have found that potassium supplementation reduced systolic and diastolic blood pressure in both normotensives and hypertensives, although the reduction in many of them did not reach a conventional level of statistical significance because their sample size was too small to provide sufficient statistical power. Pooling of results from individual trials allows for more precise and accurate estimation of intervention effect and exploration of the basis for heterogeneity in the outcome.

The authors conducted a meta-analysis of 33 randomized controlled trials (2565 participants) published between 1981 and 1995 [32]. Twenty-one trials were conducted in hypertensives (1560 participants) and 12 in normotensives (1005 participants) (Fig. 1). The dose of potassium prescribed in the intervention arm was ∃60 mmol/day in all but two trials. The weighted mean net change in urinary potassium excretion for intervention versus control, however, was 53 mmol/24 hr in the 31 trials with available urinary electrolyte excretion information. Overall, potassium supplementation was associated with a significant reduction in mean (95% CI) systolic and diastolic blood pressure of −4.4 (−2.5 to −6.4) and −2.4 (−0.7 to −4.2) mmHg, respectively (Table 1). An extreme effect of potassium in lowering systolic (−41 mmHg) and diastolic (−17 mmHg) blood pressure was observed in one trial [33]. After exclusion of the results from this outlier trial, potassium supplementation was associated with a mean systolic blood pressure reduction of −3.11 (95% CI: −1.91 to −4.31) mmHg and diastolic blood pressure reduction of −1.97 (95% CI: −0.52 to −3.42) mmHg [32]. Subgroup analysis suggested the treatment effects were enhanced in hypertensives, blacks, and participants consuming a high intake of sodium (Fig. 2). A dose-response relationship between change in 24-hr urinary potassium and effect size was found in trials in which the participants were consuming a diet high in sodium ($p < 0.001$). This meta-analysis provides strong evidence in support of the hypothesis that potassium supplementation reduces blood pressure.

Potassium and Risk of Cardiovascular Disease

Khaw and Barrett-Connor examined the relationship between the 24-hr dietary potassium intake at baseline and subsequent stroke-associated mortality in a population-based cohort of 859 men and women (aged 50 to 79 years) in a retirement community in southern California [34]. After

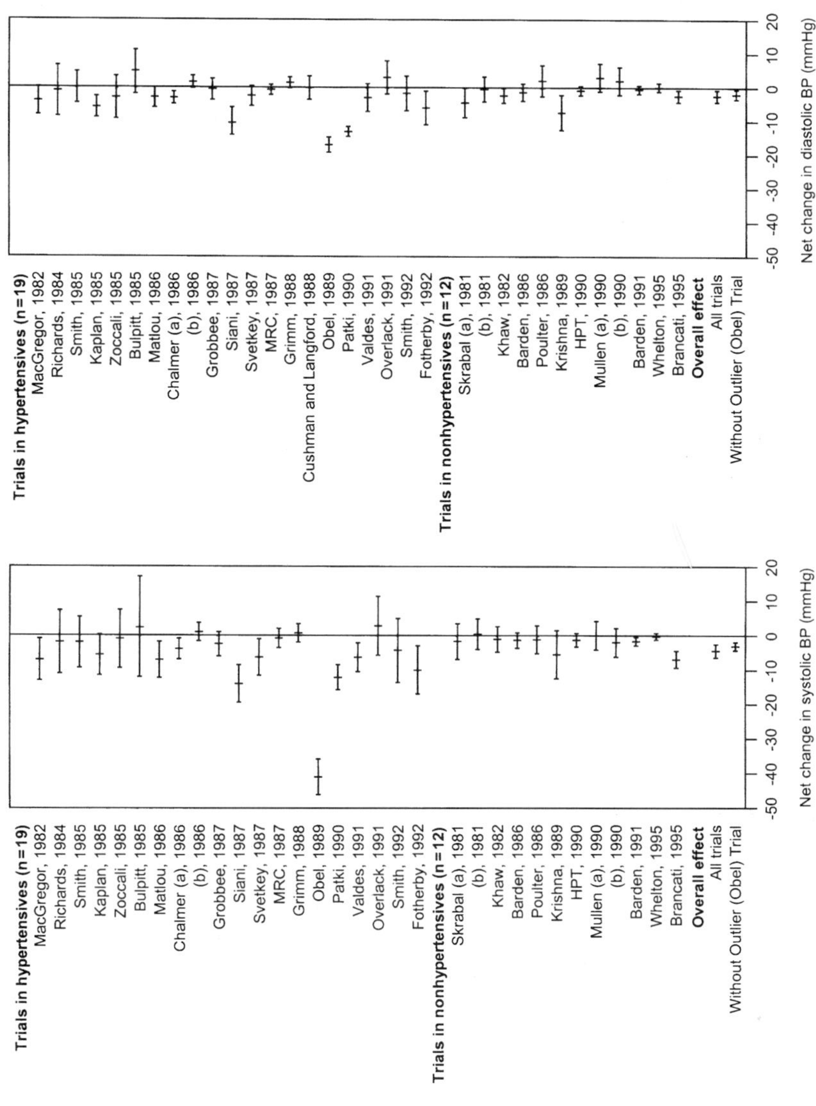

FIGURE 1 Average net change and corresponding 95% confidence interval in systolic blood pressure (left panel) and diastolic blood pressure (right panel) after treatment with oral potassium supplementation in 33 randomized controlled trials.

TABLE 1 Mean Net Systolic and Diastolic Blood Pressure Changes in Trials Using Different Exclusion Criteria

	Systolic BP (mmHg)			Diastolic BP (mmHg)		
	Number	Net change (95% CI)	p Value	Number	Net change (95% CI)	p Value
All trials	32	−4.44 (−2.53 to −6.36)	<0.001	33	−2.45 (−0.74 to −4.16)	<0.01
All trials without outlier[a]	31	−3.11 (−1.91 to −4.31)	<0.001	32	−1.97 (−0.52 to −3.42)	<0.01
Trials with net change in urinary K≥20 mmol/24 hr[a]	28	−4.91 (−2.69 to −7.12)	<0.001	29	−2.71 (−0.71 to −4.71)	<0.01
Trials in which no antihypertensive medications were administered	28	−4.85 (−2.74 to −6.95)	<0.001	29	−2.71 (−0.80 to −4.61)	<0.01

[a] Trial of Obel [33] excluded.

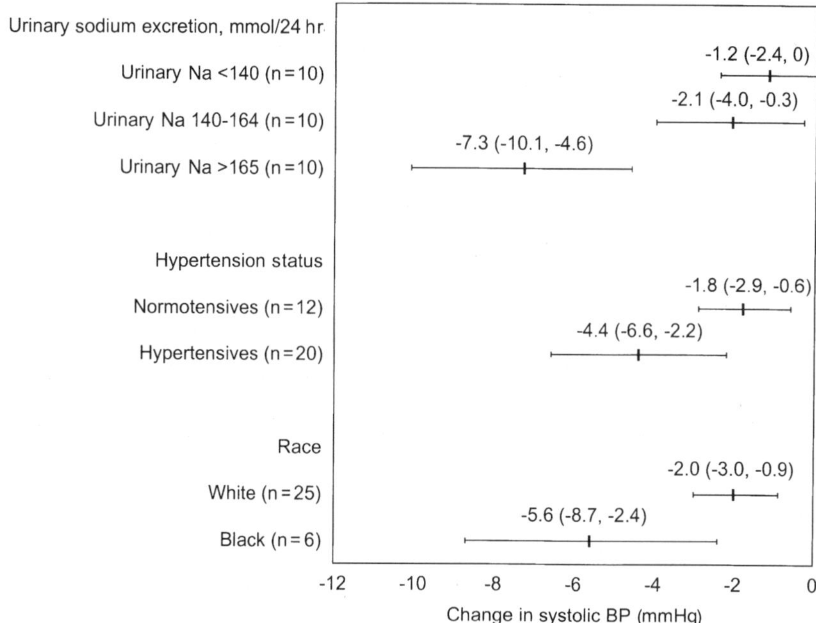

FIGURE 2 Mean net systolic blood pressure changes in subgroups of trials defined by participant and study design characteristics.

12 years, 24 stroke-associated deaths had occurred. The relative risks of stroke-associated mortality in the lowest compared to the top two tertiles of potassium intake at baseline were 2.6 ($P=0.16$) for men and 4.8 ($P=0.01$) for women. In multivariate analyses, a 10-mmol increase in daily potassium intake was associated with a 40% reduction in the risk of stroke-associated mortality ($P<0.001$). This effect was independent of known cardiovascular risk factors, including age, sex, blood pressure, blood cholesterol level, obesity, fasting blood glucose level, cigarette smoking, and a number of dietary variables, including intake of calories, fat, protein, fiber, calcium, magnesium, and alcohol. These findings suggest that a high intake of potassium from food sources may protect against stroke-associated death [34].

Several ecological analyses have also identified an inverse relation between potassium intake and stroke mortality, or a positive relation between the sodium/potassium ratio and stroke mortality [35,36]. Xie et al. conducted an ecological study using mean 24-hr urinary potassium and sodium excretion from the INTERSALT study and age-standardized stroke mortality for 45 to 74-year-old men and women from 25 countries. A significant and inverse correlation was identified between mean 24-hr urinary potassium excretion and stroke mortality in women, while a positive correlation was found between the sodium/potassium ratio and stroke mortality in women [35]. In the WHO Cardiovascular Diseases and Alimentary Comparison Study, age-adjusted stroke mortality rates were significantly and positively related to mean sodium/potassium ratio in both sexes ($p < 0.05$) across 19 centers in 14 countries [36].

In the first National Health and Nutrition Examination Survey Epidemiologic Follow-Up Study, Bazzano and colleagues examined the relationship between dietary potassium intake and the risk of stroke in a representative sample of 9805 U.S. men and women [37]. Dietary potassium and total energy intake were estimated at baseline by using a 24-hr dietary recall. Incidence data for stroke and coronary heart disease were obtained from medical records and death certificates. Over an average of 19 years of follow-up, 927 stroke events and 1847 coronary heart disease events were documented. Overall, stroke hazard was significantly different among quartiles of potassium intake (likelihood ratio $P = 0.03$); however, a test of linear trend across quartiles did not reach a customary level of statistical significance ($P = 0.14$). Participants consuming a low potassium diet at baseline (< 34.6 mmol potassium per day) experienced a 28% higher hazard of stroke (hazard ratio 1.28, 95% CI 1.11 to 1.47; $P < 0.001$) than other participants, after adjustment for established cardiovascular disease risk factors. These findings suggest that low dietary potassium intake is associated with an increased risk of stroke.

CONCLUSION

Data from numerous observational epidemiological studies and randomized controlled clinical trials suggest that low potassium intake may play a role in the genesis of hypertension. Low potassium intake also has been associated with an increased risk of stroke mortality in a prospective study and in several ecological analyses. While recognizing the need for additional information, the existing body of evidence favors the notion that potassium supplementation should be included as part of the recommendations for treatment and prevention of hypertension. Potassium supplementation may be especially useful in lowering blood pressure in blacks and those with difficulty reducing their dietary intake of sodium. Increased dietary potassium may also have a direct or indirect, blood pressure-related, beneficial effect in reducing the risk of stroke in the general population.

REFERENCES

1. Whelton PK, He J, Klag MJ. Blood pressure in Westernized populations. In: Swales JD, ed. Textbook of Hypertension. Oxford: Blackwell Scientific Publications, 1994:11–21.
2. MacMahon S, Peto R, Cutler J, et al. Blood pressure, stroke, and coronary heart disease. Part 1. prolonged differences in blood pressure: prospective observational studies corrected for the regression dilution bias. Lancet 1990; 335:765–774.
3. Whelton PK, He J. Blood pressure reduction treatment trials. In: Hennekens C, Buring J, Furberg C, Manson J, eds. Clinical Trials in Cardiovascular Disease. Philadelphia: Saunders, 1999:341–159.
4. Klag MJ, Whelton PK, Randall BL, et al. A prospective study of blood pressure and incidence of end-stage renal disease in 332,544 men. N Engl J Med 1996;334:13–18.
5. Beilin L. Diet and hypertension: critical concepts and controversies. J Hyperten 1987;5:S447–S457.
6. Kotchen TA, Kotchen JM, Boegehold MA. Nutrition and hypertension prevention. Hypertension 1991;18 (suppl. I):I-115–I-120.
7. Whelton PK, He J, Appel LJ, Cutler JA, Havas S, Kotchen TA, Roccella EJ, Stout R, Vallbona C, Winston MC, Karimbakas J. Primary prevention of hypertension. clinical and public health advisory from the National High Blood Pressure Education Program. JAMA 2002;288:1882–1888.
8. Addison WLT. The use of sodium chloride, potassium chloride, sodium bromide and potassium bromide in cases of arterial hypertension which are amenable to potassium chloride. Can Med Assoc J 1928;18:281–285.
9. Oliver WJ, Cohen EL, Neel JV. Blood pressure, sodium intake, and sodium related hormones in the Yanomamo Indians, a "no-salt" culture. Circulation 1975;52:146–151.
10. Prior IA, Evans JG, Harvey HPB, et al. Sodium intake and blood pressure in two Polynesian populations. New Engl J Med 1968;279:515–529.
11. Truswell AS, Kennelly BM, Hansen JD, et al. Blood pressure of Kung bushmen in northern Botswana. Am Heart J 1972;84:5–12.
12. Poulter N, Khaw KT, Hopwood BEC, et al. Blood pressure and associated factors in a rural Kenyan community. Hypertension 1984;6:810–813.
13. Carvalho JJM, Baruzzi RG, Howard PF, et al. Blood pressure in four remote populations in the INTERSALT study. Hypertension 1989; 14:283–246.
14. He J, Tell GS, Tang YC, et al. Relation of electrolytes to blood pressure in men: the Yi People study. Hypertension 1991;17:378–385.
15. He J, Tell GS, Tang YC, et al. Effect of migration on blood pressure: the Yi People Study. Epidemiology 1991;2:88–97.
16. He J, Klag MJ, Whelton PK, et al. Migration, blood pressure pattern and hypertension: the Yi Migrant Study. Am J Epidemiol 1991;134:1085–1101.
17. Walker WG, Whelton PK, Saito H, et al. Relation between blood pressure and renin, renin substrate, angiotensin II, aldosterone and urinary sodium and potassium in 574 ambulatory subjects. Hypertension 1979; 1:287–291.

18. Watson RL, Langford HG, Abernethy J, et al. Urinary electrolytes, body weight, and blood pressure: pooled cross-sectional results among four groups of adolescent females. Hypertension 1980;2:93–98.
19. Kesteloot H, Huang DX, Li YL, et al. The relationship between cations and blood pressure in the People's Republic of China. Hypertension 1987;9:654–659.
20. Smith WCS, Crombie IK, Tavendale RT, et al. Urinary electrolyte excretion, alcohol consumption, and blood pressure in the Scottish heart health study. BMJ 1988;297:329–330.
21. Intersalt Cooperative Research Group. Intersalt: an international study of electrolyte excretion and blood pressure. Results for 24 hour urinary sodium and potassium excretion. BMJ 1988;297:319–328.
22. Dyer AR, Elliott P, Shipley M, et al. Body mass index and associations of sodium and potassium with blood pressure in INTERSALT. Hypertension 1994;23:729–736.
23. Langford HG. Dietary potassium and hypertension: epidemiologic data. Ann Int Med 1983; 98 (part 2):770–772.
24. Grim CE, Luft FC, Miller JZ, et al. Racial differences in blood pressure in Evans County, Georgia: relationship to sodium and potassium intake and plasma renin activity. J Chronic Dis 1980;33:87.
25. Veterans Administration Cooperative Study Group on Antihypertensive Agents. Urinary and serum electrolytes in untreated black and white hypertensives. J Chronic Dis 1987;40:839–847.
26. Witteman JCM, Willett WC, Stampfer MJ, et al. A prospective study of nutritional factors and hypertension among US women. Circulation 1989;80: 1320–1327.
27. Ascherio A, Rimm EB, Giovannucci EL, et al. A prospective study of nutritional factors and hypertension among US men. Circulation 1992;86: 1475–1484.
28. Reed D, McGee D, Yano K, et al. Diet, blood pressure, and multicollinearity. Hypertension 1985;7:405–410.
29. Krishna GG, Miller E, Kapoor SC. Potassium depletion elevates blood pressure in normotensives. N Engl J Med 1989;320:1177–1182.
30. Krishna GG, Kapoor SC: Potassium depletion exacerbates essential hypertension. Ann Int Med 1991;115:77–83.
31. Burstyn P, Hornall D, Watchorn C. Sodium and potassium intake and blood pressure. BMJ 1980;2:537–539.
32. Whelton PK, He J, Cutler JA, Brancati FL, Appel LJ, Follmann D, Klag MJ. Effects of oral potassium on blood pressure: meta-analysis of randomized, controlled clinical trials. JAMA 1997;277:1624–1632.
33. Obel AO. Placebo-controlled trial of potassium supplements in black patients with mild essential hypertension. J Cardiovasc Pharmacol 1989;14:294–296.
34. Khaw KT, Barrett-Connor E. Dietary potassium and stroke-associated mortality: a 12-year prospective population study. N Engl J Med 1987;316: 235–240.

35. Xie JX, Sasaki S, Joossens JV, et al. The relationship between urinary cations obtained from the INTERSALT study and cerebrovascular mortality. J Hum Hypertens 1992;6:17–21.
36. Yamori Y, Nara Y, Mizushima S, et al. Nutritional factors for stroke and major cardiovascular diseases: international epidemiological comparison of dietary prevention. Health Rep 1994;6:22–27.
37. Bazzano LA, He J, Ogden LG, Loria C, Vupputuri S, Myers L, Whelton PK. Dietary potassium intake and risk of stroke in US men and women: National Health and Nutrition Examination Survey I epidemiologic follow-up study. Stroke 2001; 32:1473–1480.

10

Calcium and Magnesium Supplementation

Francesco P. Cappuccio
St. George's Hospital Medical School, London, England

INTRODUCTION

Among lifestyle and environmental factors that may have important roles in the cause of hypertension, calcium and magnesium intake have received considerable attention. Early and more recent reports relating harder drinking water to lower mortality from cardiovascular causes generated interest in the association between calcium, as well as magnesium, and blood pressure [1–4]. Potential antihypertensive effects of dietary calcium and/or magnesium are of interest because the intake of both calcium and magnesium can be increased with simple dietary means.

Observational epidemiological studies have been carried out in the past 30 years to explore the association among calcium, magnesium, and blood pressure, its consistency across populations, its size of effect, and its specificity [5]. Furthermore, randomized controlled clinical trials of calcium or magnesium supplementation have investigated both the cause and effect relationship and the size of the effect [5]. The present chapter briefly reviews the evidence and explores the implications for the prevention and treatment of hypertension in patients and populations.

CALCIUM

Association Between Calcium Intake and Blood Pressure in Observational Studies

A large number of epidemiological studies have looked at the possible association between dietary calcium intake and blood pressure levels. (See Refs. 5–7 for a review.) Most of the studies have been cross-sectional, examining the association between dietary calcium and blood pressure as an outcome at one particular time. Similarly, some studies have also used a casecontrol design with hypertension as the disease. A limited number of studies have been prospective. In such studies it was possible to determine whether the incidence of hypertension in a given period of time of follow-up was different in groups exposed to different levels of dietary calcium intake assessed at the baseline. Whichever design, these studies established associations rather than cause and effect relationships. To establish causality a set of criteria must be met, including the existence and strength of statistical association between the exposure and its effect, the specificity of the association, the consistency of the association, the presence of a dose-response relationship, a time order (effect follows cause), and the possible biological mechanism. Harder evidence of causality can then be provided by a different study design, such as randomized clinical trials. Furthermore, the observational studies have employed different methods of assessing dietary intake of calcium [5–7]. The different techniques for assessing dietary intake have advantages and disadvantages [8], but all methods are subject to recall and reporting errors, to interviewer and nonresponse bias, to sample error, and to wide intraindividual variability in food intake. Such limitations make these techniques inaccurate in characterizing an individual's intake and may tend to underestimate the true intake of a dietary component [8]. In reviewing observational epidemiological studies it must be considered that confounders may play an important role, and that high intercorrelation of certain nutrients may constitute an additional problem in studying the epidemiology of diet and blood pressure [9]. Considering all these caveats, however, when looking at pooled data from observational studies of the relationship between dietary calcium intake and blood pressure, there is a wide representation of studies carried out in geographically diverse populations from the five continents. The individuals surveyed included males and females who ranged from as young as 6 months of age to as old as 80, and the ethnic groups studied included Caucasians, blacks, Japanese, Chinese, and Hispanics. Also, sample sizes of the different studies vary from 55 to over 58,000 people studied [6,7]. Figure 1 shows the size of the association between calcium intake and blood pressure in a number of population-based observational studies. The data report an average regression coefficient indicating

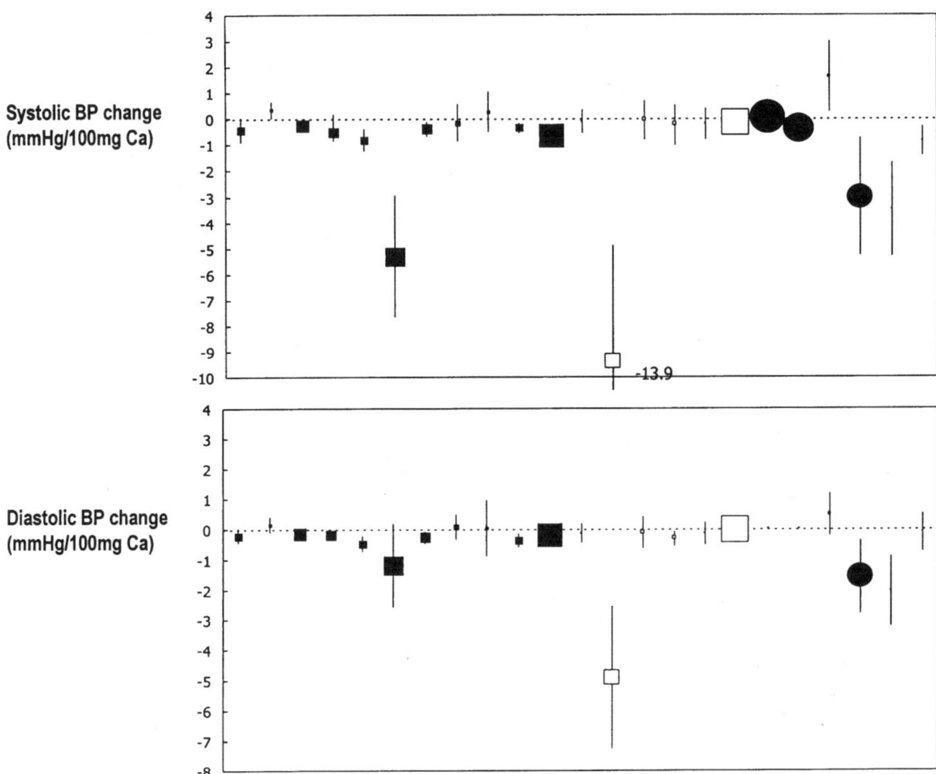

FIGURE 1 Association between calcium intake and blood pressure in observational studies: overview of population-based studies of the associations between dietary calcium intake and blood pressure, and average regression coefficients (mmHg/100 mg calcium) and 95% confidence intervals. The size of the square is proportional to the sample size. *Note*: Closed squares = men; open squares = women; closed circles = men and women combined. *Source*: Redrawn from Ref. 6 with corrections [10,11].

the change in blood pressure for a 100-mg change in dietary calcium intake [6,10,11]. An attempt to summarize the results of these studies is constrained by important methodological differences, as well as by a significant heterogeneity in these studies. Although more studies report inverse associations between dietary calcium intake and either systolic or diastolic blood pressure than either a direct association or no association [7], there are many inconsistencies in these results. For instance, seven independent analyses of the National Health and Nutrition Examination Survey (NHANES) I and II data sets have looked at the association between dietary calcium intake and blood pressure or hypertension. (See Ref. 5 for a review.) A great degree of inconsistency was found when comparing the results of these different analyses of approximately the same data sets. Some reported inverse associations between dietary calcium and blood pressure (some systolic, some diastolic), although not all could hold after adjustment for confounders. One analysis even reported a positive association.

The inconsistencies among studies could also be due to inadequacies in the methods used to assess dietary calcium intake (current versus past or usual intake). The strength of the associations (where found) was variable, and several studies did not control for important potential confounding variables, such as alcohol, age, social class, or body weight, which may produce spurious associations. Some of the studies had a small sample size and may not have had the statistical power to detect a sizeable difference in the association between dietary calcium and blood pressure. The specificity of such associations could be questioned because of the multicolinearity between nutrients in the diet, which could lead to spurious associations and make interpretation of these results difficult. No dose-response data are available, and temporality is difficult to assess, as only a few studies had a prospective design and their results were as inconsistent as those from nonprospective studies. The overall view is that there is a modest inverse association between dietary calcium intake and blood pressure. The estimate of effects in men may lie between −0.01 (95% CI −0.02 to −0.003) mmHg change in systolic blood pressure per 100 mg calcium change [6] and −0.38 (−0.44 to −0.25) mmHg per 100 mg calcium [10] and in women between −0.15 (−0.20 to −0.10) ((6) and −0.16 (−0.19 to −0.12) mmHg per 100 mg calcium [10]. The estimate of effects for diastolic blood pressure are smaller, and may lie between −0.01 (95% CI −0.02 to −0.001) mmHg change in blood pressure per 100 mg calcium change [6] and −0.03 (−0.25 to −0.12) mmHg per 100 mg calcium [10], and in women between −0.06 (−0.10 to −0.01) [6] and −0.02 (−0.11 to −0.03) mmHg per 100 mg calcium [10]. In conclusion, although there might be an indication for an inverse association between dietary calcium and blood pressure, studies of associations cannot establish the cause and effect relationship but can only direct toward the formulation of a clear hypothesis to test in a properly controlled clinical trial.

Effect of Calcium Supplementation on Blood Pressure in Clinical Trials

Randomized controlled clinical trials can overcome some of the problems of interpreting observational data, including time order and various sources of confounding. They can provide more direct evidence for causality in the short term and can demonstrate benefit for the individual. A large number of clinical trials have been performed worldwide looking at the potential effect of a calcium supplement on blood pressure in both normotensive and hypertensive groups. Due to the discrepancy in the overall results some authors have carried out quantitative overviews (meta-analyses) to increase statistical power, to resolve the uncertainty on the overall direction of the effect, and to improve the estimate of the effect size. Unlike observational studies it has been possible to summarize the results of intervention trials in which the main outcome is the blood pressure change following a period of oral calcium supplementation. Since 1989 at least five increasingly larger meta-analyses have been performed [12–16], and one large trial also has been carried out Trial of Hypertension Prevention (TOHP) [17]. Since the original meta-analysis by Cappuccio et al. in 1989 [12], which was based on a small overall sample size (n = 391), the published trials have increased over time, leading to the latest meta-analysis by Griffith et al., published in 1999 [16], with a much larger sample size (n > 4,000). The five meta-analyses differ for important aspects regarding the inclusion criteria. While the first three studies [12–14] limited the pooled analysis to randomized and placebo-controlled trials, the latest [16] was inclusive of *all* trials of calcium supplementation of 2 weeks' duration or longer. They included trials not controlled versus placebo, with the likelihood of a bias toward an overestimate of effect. They estimate a fall in blood pressure of −1.4 mmHg (95% CI −2.2 to −0.7) for systolic and −0.8 mmHg (−1.4 to −0.2) for diastolic for an oral calcium supplement of approximately 1,000 mg per day. A more conservative estimate is reported by Allender et al. in placebo-controlled trials only [−0.89 mmHg (−1.74 to −0.05) for systolic and −0.18 mmHg (−0.75 to +0.40) for diastolic][14]. In spite of these important differences in inclusion criteria, the results of the different meta-analyses are compatible with each other, although the confidence intervals have narrowed with the increase in the sample sizes (Fig. 2). The TOHP study was the sole large intervention trial that could stand alone in the comparison of effect sizes, given its large sample size. The trial failed to confirm a beneficial effect on blood pressure of oral calcium supplementation [−0.5 mmHg (−1.8 to +0.9) systolic and +0.2 mmHg (−0.7 to +1.1) diastolic](Fig. 2).

The complete overlap of confidence intervals between the first and last meta-analyses as well as the TOHP study appear to confirm the very small effect that an oral calcium supplement exerts on blood pressure levels, mainly systolic. It is nevertheless of interest to note the sharp contrast in the conclusions drawn by the different authors. While Cappuccio et al. [12], Cutler and Brittain [13], Allender et al. [14], and the TOHP Collaborative Research Group [17] agree in considering the evidence insufficient to support the use of calcium supplementation for the prevention and treatment of hypertension, Bucher et al. [15], using similar data and similar results, feel that

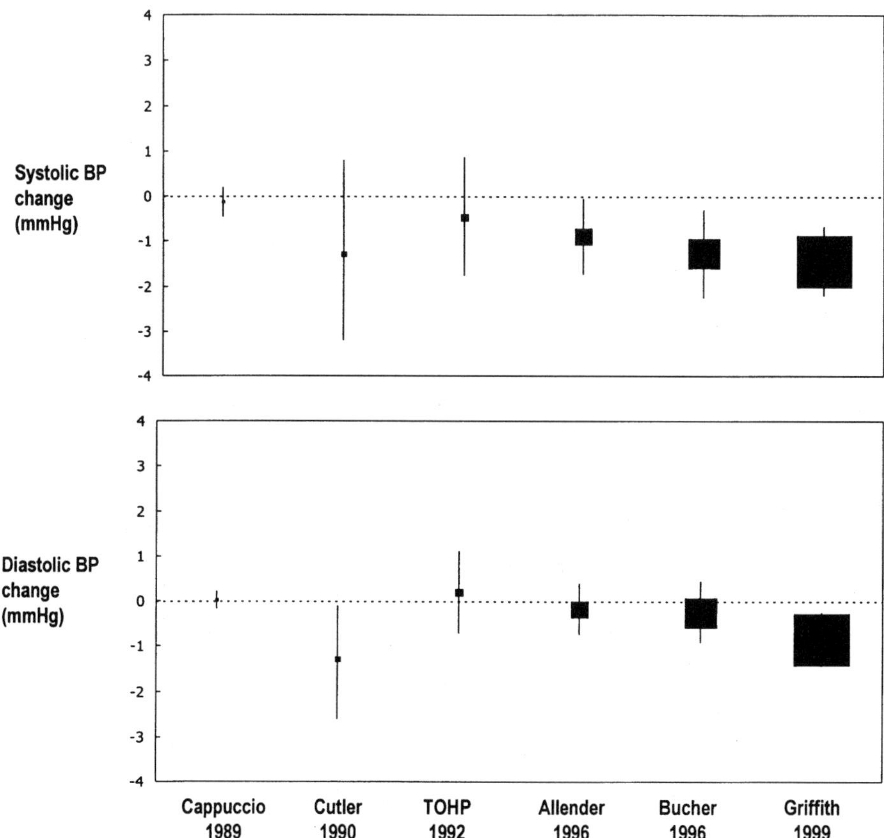

FIGURE 2 Effect of calcium supplementation on blood pressure in clinical trials: summary of the pooled results of quantitative overviews of controlled clinical trials of oral calcium supplementation and changes in blood pressure and the results of a large trial (TOHP). The size of the square is proportional to the total sample size. Bars indicate 95% confidence intervals. *Source*: Redrawn from Refs. 18,40.

their results justify the use of calcium supplementation for patients with mild hypertension. Updating their meta-analysis [16] 3 years later, the same authors obtained comparable results but modified their conclusions, avoiding making statements about the use of calcium supplements for the treatment of hypertension.

Unlike previous meta-analyses, Griffith et al. [16] also presented for the first time a pooled analysis of dietary interventions in which the effects on blood pressure of "experimental" diets were studied. The calcium content of such experimental diets was higher than control diets, but so were a number of other nutrients known to affect blood pressure, such as potassium and fiber [18]. It is therefore difficult to attribute any beneficial effect to any specific nutrient.

The "Calcium Antihypertension Theory"

Why is the evidence about the effect of calcium intake on blood pressure subject to such distortion in interpretation? In 1982, a campaign to release the pressure on the sodium–blood pressure issue was undertaken by a snack food giant. Part of its strategy was the idea that it should encourage and support the calcium antihypertension theory despite the admission of its own experts that an increase in dietary calcium would be unlikely to have an effect on hypertension. Since then, the campaign has progressed and many of the studies purporting the wisdom of the calcium antihypertension theory have been funded by the National Dairy Council [15,16] and the food industry [19].

Calcium Supplementation in Pregnancy and Preeclampsia

In the early 1980s Belizan et al. were the first to describe an inverse relationship between calcium intake and gestational hypertension and pre-eclampsia [20,21]. Studies in animal models have also suggested that severe calcium depletion may induce pregnancy-related hypertension [22]. Early randomized clinical trials of calcium supplementation in pregnant women suggested that the epidemiological inverse relationship between calcium intake and maternal blood pressure could be a causal one [23–25]. Small sample sizes, however, limited the assessment of the effects on important maternal and neonatal outcomes in the highly selected populations in South America. They were high-risk young women of low socioeconomic background and low calcium intake (known to have a disproportionately high incidence of pre-eclampsia). Therefore it is difficult to generalize to the wider population of pregnant women in Europe and the United States. Since then several small and larger randomized controlled clinical trials have been carried out, and their results were recently reviewed in a quantitative meta-analysis [26]. The objective of this systematic overview was to examine the impact of calcium supplementation in pregnancy on systolic and diastolic blood pressure and on maternal and neonatal outcomes. The review looked at 14 trials involving 2459 women. More than half of these trials, however, had been carried out in South America. The majority of them had sample sizes of less than 100 and only one had a large enough sample size to be able to look at maternal and neonatal outcomes [25]. The amount of calcium given as a supplement varied between 375 and 2000 mg per day. The duration of the intervention also varied substantially, from 10 to 22 weeks. The results on the effects of calcium supplementation on blood pressure are summarized in Fig. 3. The majority of trials showed a significant reduction in both systolic and diastolic blood

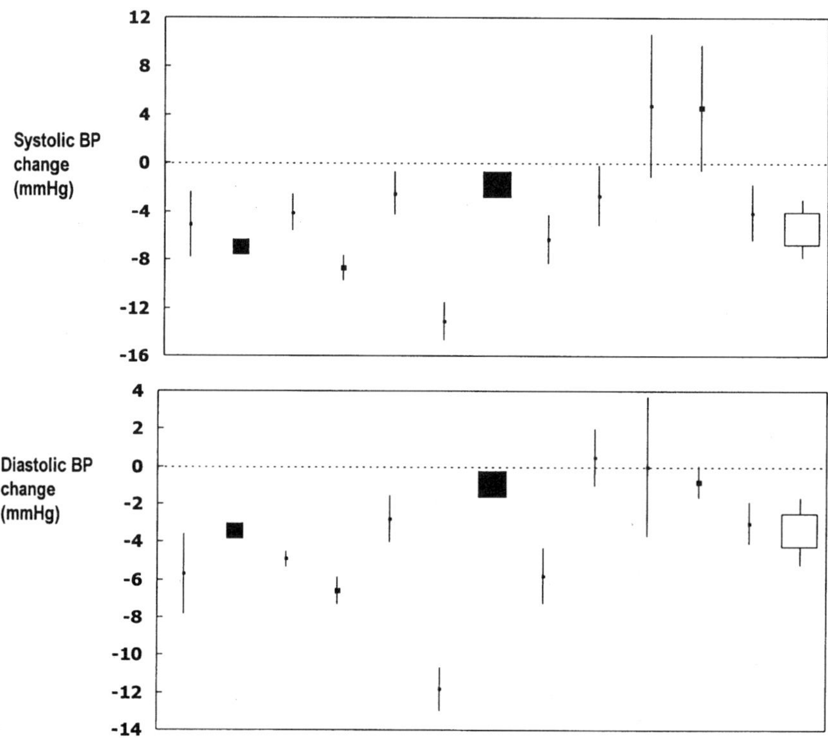

FIGURE 3 Effect of calcium supplementation on blood pressure in pregnancy: changes in systolic and diastolic blood pressure in randomized controlled trials of calcium supplementation in pregnancy. Results are shown as average change in each study and 95% confidence intervals. The size of the square is proportional to the sample size. An open square indicates the pooled estimate (95% CI). *Source*: Redrawn from Ref. 26.

pressure with calcium supplementation, leading to a pooled estimate of effect of −5.4 mmHg (95% CI −7.8 to −3.0) for systolic and −3.4 mmHg (−5.2 to −1.7) for diastolic blood pressure. Furthermore, some of these trials also determined the incidence of hypertension. The odds ratios of the effect of calcium supplementation on the incidence of hypertension in pregnancy varied, with a pooled effect of 0.30 (0.17 to 0.54) (Fig. 4). The definition of hypertension was not clearly stated in the overview, but some studies used different definitions of hypertension, so the comparison between studies is somewhat arbitrary. The effect of calcium supplementation on the incidence of pre-eclampsia is shown in Fig. 5. Only two studies indicated a significant reduction in the occurrence of pre-eclampsia following calcium supplemen-

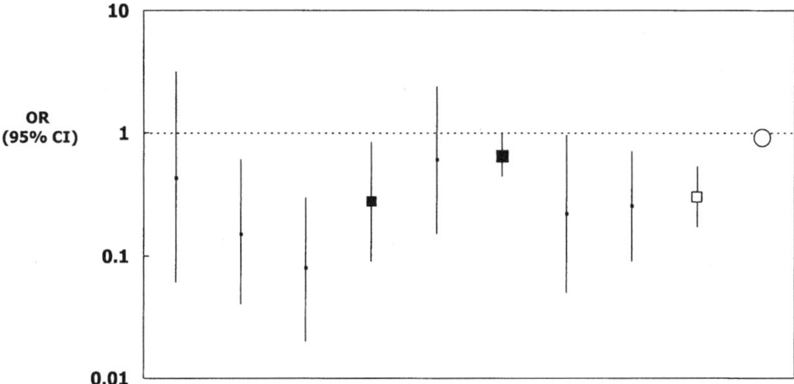

FIGURE 4 Incidence of hypertension after calcium supplementation in pregnancy: overview of the effect of calcium supplementation in pregnancy, and effect on the incidence of hypertension. Results are shown as odds ratios and 95% confidence intervals. The size of the square is proportional to the sample size. An open square indicates the pooled estimate (95% CI). *Note*: the open circle indicates the effect in the CPEP trial [RR=0.90 (0.81–1.00)][27]. *Source*: Redrawn from Ref. 26.

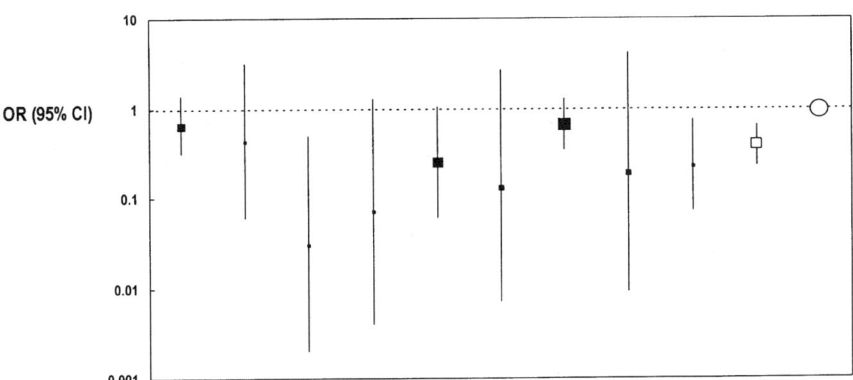

FIGURE 5 Incidence of pre-eclampsia after calcium supplementation in pregnancy: overview of the effect of calcium supplementation in pregnancy, and effect on the incidence of pre-eclampsia. Results are shown as odds ratios and 95% confidence intervals. The size of the square is proportional to the sample size. An open square indicates the pooled estimate (95% CI). The open circle indicates the effect in the CPEP trial [RR=0.94 (0.76–1.16)][27]. *Source*: Redrawn from Ref. 26.

tation. The pooled estimate of effect showed a reduction in risk [OR: 0.38 (0.22 to 0.65)], however, Bucher's meta-analysis [26] also reported inconsistent effects of calcium supplementation on other maternal and neonatal outcomes [pooled odds ratio for preterm delivery 0.69 (0.48 to 1.01), for intrauterine growth retardation 0.77 (0.51 to 1.16), and for cesarian section 0.80 (0.60 to 1.07)]. Based on these results, it was concluded that "calcium supplementation results in an important reduction in systolic and diastolic blood pressure and preeclampsia in pregnant women and that the current evidence supports a policy of offering calcium supplementation to all pregnant women in whom there is a concern about the development of preeclampsia" [26]. These statements imply that the results are fully generalizable to *all* pregnant women. Concerns have been raised that the underlying dietary calcium intake of the participants in the earlier trials was too little compared to the average calcium intake of a pregnant woman in Europe or in the United States, and also that more than a reduction in blood pressure, the most important outcomes to consider in pregnancy would be the major maternal and neonatal outcomes. In response to the need for a more definitive evaluation of calcium supplementation to prevent pre-eclampsia, a large, multicenter randomized clinical trial was undertaken in the United States [27]. The calcium for pre-eclampsia prevention (CPEP) trial was carried out in 4589 healthy nulliparous women who were 13 to 21 weeks pregnant. They were randomized to receive either 2000 mg of elemental calcium per day or placebo for the remainder of their pregnancy. Outcomes of interest were pregnancy-associated hypertension, pregnancy-associated proteinuria, pre-eclampsia, eclampsia, obstetrical complications, and perinatal outcomes such as growth retardation, neonatal distress, and perinatal deaths. Calcium supplementation did not reduce the incidence or severity of pre-eclampsia (Fig. 5) or delay its onset. There were no differences between treatment groups in the prevalence of pregnancy-associated hypertension without pre-eclampsia or of all hypertensive disorders (Fig. 4). The mean systolic and diastolic pressures during pregnancy were similar in both groups. Calcium supplementation did not reduce the numbers of preterm deliveries, small-for-gestational-age births, or fetal and neonatal deaths. The conclusions of the CPEP trial were that calcium supplementation during pregnancy does not prevent pre-eclampsia, pregnancy-associated hypertension, or adverse perinatal outcomes in healthy nulliparous women in the United States, therefore not supporting the earlier claims of a policy of calcium supplementation in pregnancy.

While there is no doubt that it is premature to advocate a widespread use of calcium supplements in prenancy, it is still open to debate whether a high dietary calcium intake in the mother (whether as a diet or as a supplement) might have a beneficial effect on the blood pressure of the offspring. In support of this view there are reports of an inverse association between maternal dietary calcium and infant blood pressure [28,29] and the results of a follow-up of the offspring of those women who took part in a large intervention trial of calcium supplementation during pregnancy [25]. At ages 5 to 9, children whose mother had been randomized to the calcium supplement group tended to have a lower systolic blood pressure than children from control mothers [−1.4 mmHg (95% CI −3.2 to +0.05)]. This effect was more evident in overweight children [−5.8 mmHg (−9.8 to −1.7)]. These results are intriguing. They are in support of the hypothesis that there may be a fetal programming for future blood pressure and that a nutritional intervention during pregnancy may directly interfere with mechanisms leading to high blood pressure. Yet again, however, the trial was carried out in women whose habitual dietary calcium intake is much lower than that seen in European and American women. Before we could generalize these findings, similar evidence should be provided in women with normal dietary calcium intake.

MAGNESIUM

Association Between Magnesium Intake and Blood Pressure in Observational Studies

The possible association between dietary magnesium intake and blood pressure has been also intensively studied. A recent overview of observational epidemiological studies identified at least 29 studies relating dietary magnesium intake to blood pressure [30]. As for the studies with dietary calcium, the majority were cross-sectional, employing a wide variety of tools for assessing dietary magnesium (24-hr dietary recalls, food-frequency questionnaires, food records). They had been carried out in different parts of the world and included young, middle-aged, and old populations, as well as children. Individual estimates are either negative or null (Fig. 6). A pooled estimate of effect suggests a −0.81 (95% CI −0.91 to −0.72) mmHg change in systolic blood pressure and −0.60 (−0.67 to −0.53) mmHg change in diastolic blood pressure per 100-mg change in dietary magnesium, pointing to a possible negative association between dietary magnesium intake and blood pressure. As mentioned earlier, however, great caution should be used in interpreting and generalizing pooled results from observational studies.

Effect of Magnesium Supplementation on Blood Pressure in Clinical Trials

A few clinical trials on the effects of magnesium supplementation on blood pressure have been reported, mostly with small sample sizes. (See Ref. 5 for a review.) Some were carried out in hypertensive patients either on treatment with diuretics [31–33], which lead to magnesium wasting, or in conjunction

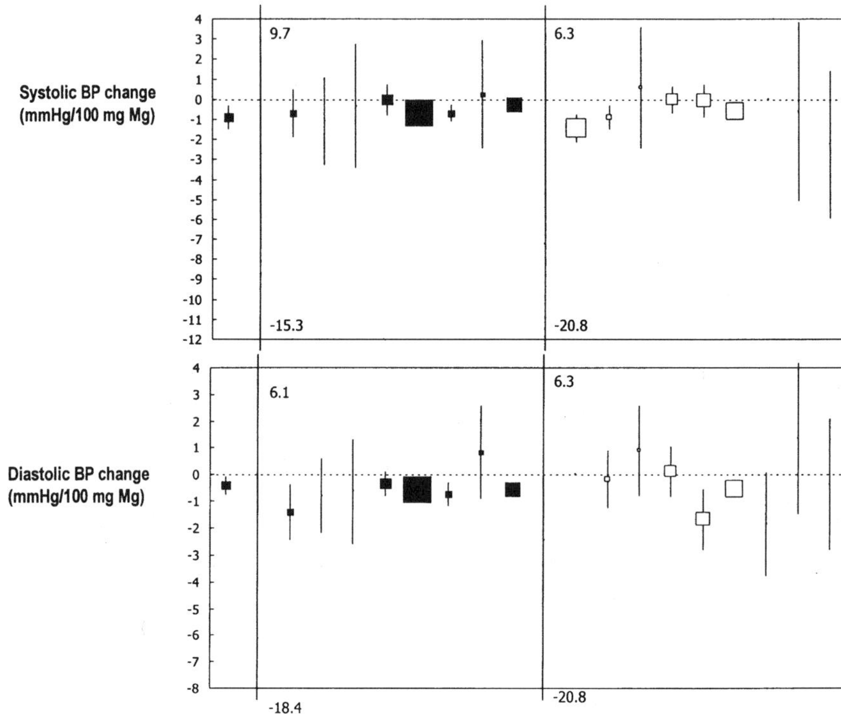

FIGURE 6 Association between magnesium intake and blood pressure in observational studies: overview of population-based studies of dietary magnesium intake and blood pressure, and average regression coefficients (mmHg/100 mg magnesium) and 95% confidence intervals. The size of the square is proportional to the sample size. *Note*: Closed squares = men; open squares = women; closed circles = men and women combined. *Source*: Redrawn from Ref. 30.

with potassium supplementation [34] or sodium restriction [35]. There are two controlled trials, one small with a crossover design [36] and one larger with a parallel-group design [17]. Both these controlled trials did not detect any effect of magnesium supplementation on blood pressure. In the small trial the average blood pressure of 17 untreated patients with mild-to-moderate hypertension rose from 151/97 to 154/98 mmHg after 4 weeks of treatment with magnesium aspartate (15 mmol of magnesium per day). The significant increase in both plasma and 24-hr urinary magnesium supported the adherence to the supplementation. In the TOHP trial, 227 patients with normal to high blood pressure (diastolic 80 to 89 mmHg) were randomized to 6 months' treatment with 15 mmol per day of magnesium as a supplement. Their blood pressure was compared with that of 234 similar patients given placebo for

6 months. No blood pressure-lowering effect due to magnesium supplement was detected [−0.20 mmHg (95% CI −1.47 to +1.07) for systolic and −0.05 mmHg (−0.94 to +0.84) for diastolic]. There is therefore no useful implication as yet for the nonpharmacological management of hypertension.

DIETARY CALCIUM AND MAGNESIUM

"Dietary" Calcium and Magnesium and Blood Pressure

People eat food rather than individual nutrients. There is a high degree of association of nutrients in many types of foods (e.g., potassium, magnesium, and fiber in fruit and vegetables). It can therefore be very difficult to isolate the effects of one food component from another and to attribute specificity to any one association in observational studies of diet and blood pressure. Furthermore, randomized clinical trials often do not help clarify this specificity when effect sizes are rather small and inconsistent, as for calcium and magnesium. As individual components of a "healthy" diet may exert small but additional effects on the outcome of interest, and since a population strategy would aim at achieving healthy dietary patterns, it is of greater interest to test the effectiveness and efficacy of dietary changes rather than individual nutrients' effects on blood pressure. This is what the Dietary Approaches to Stop Hypertension (DASH) diet has successfully attempted in recent years [37,38]. The DASH trials have established that a diet rich in fruit and vegetables and low in fat significantly reduces blood pressure and that the effect is additive to the effect of dietary salt intake on blood pressure. (The lower the salt in the diet, the lower the blood pressure.)

CONCLUSION

To establish whether the evidence is sufficient to warrant recommendations to hypertensive patients and to the population at large, it is worth considering the possible benefits and risks of implementing a policy including either calcium and/or magnesium supplementation, or increasing dietary calcium and/or magnesium, as tools for the prevention and management of hypertension. In accordance with the recommendations of the American Heart Association nutrition committee [39], there is insufficient evidence to recommend high intake of calcium (and the use of calcium supplements) for prevention or treatment of hypertension [40]. Calcium deficiency should be avoided, however. This is particularly important during pregnancy, as contrary to earlier evidence of a benefit of calcium supplementation in high-risk pregnancy, calcium supplementation during pregnancy does not prevent pre-eclampsia or pregancy-associated hypertension in healthy nulliparous women whose calcium intake is not low. There is even less evidence to consider magnesium supplements at all for the prevention and treatment of hypertension. A diet that is rich in calcium and magnesium, however, as well as in such other nutrients as potassium and fiber, and that is low in both saturated fat and salt, produces benefits to the blood pressure levels that if sustained would be associated with significant reductions in cardiovascular events.

REFERENCES

1. Schroeder HA. Relation between mortality from cardiovascular disease and treated water supplies: variations in states and 163 largest municipalities of the United States. JAMA 1960;172:1902–1908.
2. Stitt FW, Crawford MD, Clayton DG, Morris JN. Clinical and biochemical indicators of cardiovascular disease among men living in hard and soft water areas. Lancet 1973;i:122–126.
3. Neri LC, Johnsen HL. Water hardness and cardiovascular mortality. Ann NY Acad Sci 1978;304:203–219.
4. Folsom AR, Prineas RJ. Drinking water composition and blood pressure: a review of the epidemiology. Am J Epidemiol 1982;115:818–832.
5. Cappuccio FP. Electrolyte intake and human hypertension—Calcium and magnesium. In: Swales JD, ed. Textbook of Hypertension. Oxford: Blackwell Scientific, 1994:551–566.
6. Cappuccio FP, Elliott P, Allender PS, Pryer J, Follman DA, Cutler JA. Epidemiologic association between dietary calcium intake and blood pressure: a meta-analysis of published data. Am J Epidemiol 1995;142:935–945.
7. Pryer J, Cappuccio FP, Elliott P. Dietary calcium and blood pressure: a review of the observational studies. J Human Hypertens 1995;9:597–604.
8. Freudenheim JL. Dietary assessment in nutritional epidemiology. Nutr Metab Cardiovasc Dis 1991;1:207–212.
9. Cappuccio FP. The epidemiology of diet and blood pressure. Circulation 1992;86:1651–1653.
10. Birkett NJ. Comments on a meta-analysis of the relation between dietary calcium intake and blood pressure. Am J Epidemiol 1998;148:223–228.
11. Cappuccio FP, Elliott P, Follman DA, Cutler JA. Authors' response to "Comments on a meta-analysis of the relation between dietary calcium intake and blood pressure." Am J Epidemiol 1998;148:232–233.
12. Cappuccio FP, Siani A, Strazzullo P. Oral calcium supplementation and blood pressure: an overview of randomized controlled trials. J Hypertens 1989;7:941–946.
13. Cutler JA, Brittain E. Calcium and blood pressure: an epidemiologic review. Am J Hypertens 1990;3:137S–146S.
14. Allender PS, Cutler JA, Follman DA, Cappuccio FP, Pryer J, Elliott P. Dietary calcium and blood pressure: a meta-analysis of randomized clinical trials. Ann Intern Med 1996;124:825–831.

15. Bucher HC, Cook RJ, Guyatt GH, Lang JD, Cook DJ, Hatala R, Hunt DL. Effects of dietary calcium supplementation on blood pressure: a meta-analysis of randomized controlled trials. JAMA 1996;275:1016–1022.
16. Griffith LE, Guyatt GH, Cook RJ, Bucher HC, Cook DJ. The influence of dietary and nondietary calcium supplementation on blood pressure: an updated metaanalysis of randomized controlled trials. Am J Hypertens 1999; 12:84–92.
17. TOHP Collaborative Research Group. The effects of nonpharmacological interventions on blood pressure of persons with high normal levels. JAMA 1992;267:1213–1220.
18. Cappuccio FP. The "calcium antihypertension theory." Am J Hypertens 1999; 12:93–95.
19. McCarron DA, Oparil S, Chait A, Haynes B, Kris-Etherton P, Stern JS, Resnick LM, Clark S, Morris CD, Hatton DC, Metz JA, McMahon M, Holcomb S, Snyder GW, Pi-Sunyer X. Nutritional management of cardiovascular risk factors: a randomized clinical trial. Arch Int Med 1997; 157:169–177.
20. Belizan JM, Villar J. The relationship between calcium intake and edema, proteinuria and hypertension-gestosis: an hypothesis. Am J Clin Nutr 1980;33:2202–2210.
21. Villar J, Belizan JM, Fischer PJ. Epidemiologic observations on the relationship between calcium intake and eclampsia. Int J Gynaecol Obstet 1983;21: 271–278.
22. Prada JA, Richardus R, Clark KE. Hypocalcemia and pregancy-induced hypertension produced by maternal fasting. Hypertension 1992;20:620–626.
23. Villar J, Repke J, Belizan JM, Pareja G. Calcium supplementation reduces blood pressure during pregnancy: results of a randomised controlled clinical trial. Obstet Gynaecol 1987;70:317–322.
24. Lopez-Jaramillo P, Narvaez M, Weigel RM, Yepez R. Calcium supplementation reduces the risk of pregnancy-induced hypertension in an Andes population. Br J Obstet Gynaecol 1989;96:648–655.
25. Belizan JM, Villar J, Gonzalez L, Campodonico L, Bergel E. Calcium supplementation to prevent hypertensive disorders of pregnancy. N Engl J Med 1991; 325:1399–1405.
26. Bucher HC, Guyatt GH, Cook RJ, Hatala R, Cook DJ, Lang JD, Hunt D. Effect of calcium supplementation on pregnancy-induced hypertension and preeclampsia: a meta-analysis of randomized controlled trials. JAMA 1996;275: 1113–1117.
27. Levine RJ, Hauth JC, Curet LB, Sibai BM, Catalano PM, Morris CD, DerSimonian R, Esterlitz JR, Raymond EG, Bild DE, Clemens JD, Cutler JA. Trial of calcium to prevent preeclampsia. N Engl J Med 1997;337:69–76.
28. McGarvey S, Zimmer S, Willett W, Rosner B. Maternal prenatal dietary potassium, calcium, magnesium and infant blood pressure. Hypertension 1991;17: 218–224.
29. Gillman M, Oliveria S, Moore L, Ellison C. Inverse association of dietary calcium with systolic blood pressure in young children. JAMA 1992;267:2343

30. Mizushima S, Cappuccio FP, Nichols R, Elliott P. Dietary magnesium intake and blood pressure: a qualitative overview of the observational studies. J Hum Hypertens 1998;12:447–453.
31. Dyckner T, Wester PO. Effect of magnesium on blood pressure. Br Med J 1983;286:1847–1849.
32. Henderson DG, Scherys J, Schott T. Effect of magnesium supplementation on blood pressure and electrolyte concentrations in hypertensive patients receiving long-term diuretic treatment. Br Med J 1986;293:664–665.
33. Saito K, Hattori K, Omatsu T, Hirouchi H, Sano H, Fukuzaki H. Effects of oral magnesium on blood pressure and electrolyte concentrations in hypertensive patients receiving long-term thiazide diuretics for hypertension. Am J Hypertens 1988;1:71s–74s.
34. Patki PS, Singh J, Gokhale SV, Bulakh PM, Shrotri DS, Patwardhan B. Efficacy of potassium and magnesium in essential hypertension: a double-blind, placebo controlled, crossover study. Br Med J 1990;301:521–523.
35. Nowson CA, Morgan TO. Magnesium supplementation in mild hypertensive patients on a moderately low sodium diet. Clin Exp Pharmacol Physiol 1989; 16:299–302.
36. Cappuccio FP, Markandu ND, Beynon GW, Shore AC, Sampson B, MacGregor GA. Lack of effect of oral magnesium on high blood pressure: a double blind study. Br Med J 1985;291:235–238.
37. Appel LJ, Moore TJ, Obarzanek E, Vollmer WM, Svetkey LP, Sacks FM, Bray GA, Vogt TM, Cutler JA, Windhauser MM, Lin P-H, Karanja N. A clinical trial of the effects of dietary patterns on blood pressure. N Engl J Med 1997;336:1117–1124.
38. Sacks FM, Svetkey LP, Vollmer WM, Appel LJ, Bray GA, Harsha D, Obarzanek E, Conlin PR, Miller ER III, Simons-Morton DG, Karanja N, Lin P-H, for the DASH-Sodium Collaborative Research Group. Effects on blood pressure of reduced dietary sodium and the Dietary Approaches to Stop Hypertension (DASH) diet. N Engl J Med 2001;344:3–10.
39. Kotchen TA, McCarron DA. Dietary electrolytes and blood pressure: a statement for healthcare professionals from the American Heart Association Nutrition Committee. Circulation 1998;98:613–617.
40. Cappuccio FP. Dietary calcium supplementation and blood pressure. JAMA 1996;276:1385–1386.

11

Macronutrients, Fiber, Cholesterol, and Dietary Patterns

Lawrence J. Appel
Johns Hopkins University School of Medicine,
Baltimore, Maryland, U.S.A.

Paul Elliott
Imperial College of Science, Technology, and Medicine,
London, England

INTRODUCTION

The available data strongly support the hypothesis that multiple dietary factors influence blood pressure (BP) and that modification of the diet can have powerful, beneficial effects. A persuasive body of evidence has documented that weight and dietary intakes of sodium, potassium, and alcohol influence BP. The objective of this chapter is to summarize evidence on other aspects of diet that might also affect BP, specifically macronutrients, fiber, cholesterol, and dietary patterns. In the process, the strengths and limitations of available evidence will be highlighted.

FAT

In view of the well-recognized changes in BP that occur during migration to economically developed societies and the high prevalence of elevated BP in these societies, researchers have focused on aspects of lifestyle, particularly diet, that might account for these changes. Of those dietary factors that might be responsible for these changes, modification of dietary fat has considerable appeal, in part because of concurrent associations of dietary fat with atherosclerosis and dyslipidemia.

A wide variety of studies have investigated the relationship between BP and types of fat. These studies include cross-sectional studies that assess the association of fat intake and tissue levels of fat with BP, longitudinal observational studies that assess the effects of fat intake on incident hypertension or BP change, and controlled trials that tested whether or not modifications of dietary fat intake affect BP. An excellent review article by Morris [1] summarizes this exceedingly complex literature.

The complexity of the literature results in part from methodologic issues that are inherent to the evaluation of nutrient–disease relationships. These issues include random and systematic errors in measuring nutrient intake, differential measurement error by nutrient, colinearity of nutrient intake, and the scientific and logistic challenges of conducting controlled trials. The challenge of studying macronutrients is heightened by the fundamental interdependence of macronutrient intake. Specifically, under steady state or eucaloric conditions, a change in intake of one macronutrient (e.g., an increase in monounsaturated fat) must be accompanied by an opposite change in other macronutrients (i.e., a reduction in carbohydrate, protein, and/or other fats).

Total Fat

Total fat includes saturated fat, omega-3 polyunsaturated fat, omega-6 polyunsaturated fat, and monounsaturated fat. While early studies focused on the effects of total fat intake on BP, there is a plausible biological basis to hypothesize that certain types of fats (e.g., omega-3 polyunsaturated fat) might reduce BP and that other types of fats (e.g., saturated fat) might raise BP; hence the net effects of total fat intake likely depend on the distribution of component types. Because the direction of net effect might be direct (positive) or inverse, depending on the distribution of fats, this chapter will examine the effects of each type of fat rather than total fat.

Saturated Fat

Several observational studies and a few clinical trials have assessed the impact of saturated fat on BP. In the vast majority of studies, including two prospective observational studies, the Nurses Health Study and the Health Professional Follow-up Study, saturated fat intake (percentage kcal as determined by a food-frequency questionnaire) was not associated with incident hypertension over 4 years of follow-up [2,3]. In contrast, in observational analyses from the Multiple Risk Factor Intervention Trial (MRFIT) trial cohort, there was significant direct association between saturated fat intake (as determined by a replicated 24-hr dietary recalls) and diastolic BP, as well as a significant inverse association between the P/S ratio and diastolic BP [4].

In clinical trials, diets reduced in saturated fat had no significant effect on BP. Some trials tested diets that were reduced in both saturated and total fat; other trials held total fat constant by increasing polyunsaturated fat and reducing saturated fat. Overall, diets reduced in saturated fat had no significant effect on BP. Initial trials were large, enrolled nonhypertensive individuals, and had comparatively long duration of follow-up. Over the course of a year, the National Diet Heart Study (n = 1007) tested four diets (total fat: 30–37% kcal) that varied in P/S ratio (0.3, 1.5, 2.0, 4.5) [5]. A Medical Research Council (MRC)-supported trial (n = 393) with 5 years of follow-up tested two diets that differed in P/S ratio (0.2 versus 2.0) but had similar (45% kcal) total fat intake [6]. In these two large trials and several much smaller trials, diets reduced in saturated fat had no significant impact on BP [1]. Because most trials tested diets that were reduced in saturated fat and increased in polyunsaturated fat, the absence of an effect on BP also suggests no benefit from polyunsaturated fat.

Still, there are several potential limitations that might lead to a spurious null finding in these trials. First, if the effect of saturated fat on BP results from long-term effects on arterial compliance (stiffness) rather than short-term effects on vasomotor function or blood volume, the duration of the trials, even the trial of 5 years, was too brief. Other major limitations of these trials are small sample size, enrollment of nonhypertensives, and inadequate number of BP measurements. Hence it remains uncertain whether a sustained reduction in saturated fat can lower BP.

Omega-6 Polyunsaturated Fat

Changes in consumption of omega-6 polyunsaturated fat (mainly linoleic acid in Western diets) appear to have little effect on BP. In an overview of cross-sectional studies that correlated BP with tissue or blood levels of omega-6 polyunsaturated fat [1], there was no apparent relationship (no association in eight studies, inverse association in four studies, and one positive association). As highlighted above, prospective observational studies and clinical trials, have likewise been unsupportive of a relationship [2,3].

Omega-3 Polyunsaturated Fat

The effects of increased omega-3 polyunsaturated fat consumption are discussed in Chap. 12. In brief, evidence from laboratory investigations, observational epidemiologic studies, and clinical trials indicates that regular consumption of fish or supplementation of diet with high doses of omega-3 polyunsaturated fatty acids (commonly termed "fish oil") can reduce BP. Plausible mechanisms by which omega-3 polyunsaturated fat might reduce BP include an increase in vasodilatory prostaglandins (e.g., prostacyclin), an increase in endothelial nitric oxide release, a reduction in vasoconstrictor prostaglandins (e.g., thromboxane A2), and a reduction in blood viscosity.

The most convincing evidence of the effects of omega-3 polyunsaturated fat supplementation comes from several predominantly small clinical trials In the early 1990s, two meta-analyses aggregated data across these trials and reached the same conclusion; namely, that high doses of omega-3 polyunsaturated fat, typically 3 or more g of fish oil per day, can reduce BP [7,8]. Significant BP reduction was documented in hypertensive individuals but not in nonhypertensive individuals.

Since those reports, additional studies have suggested that regular consumption of fish may also reduce BP [9], that the effects of fish oil with weight loss is additive [10], and that the most effective omega-3 polyunsaturated fat might be docosahexaenoic acid rather than eicosapentanoic acid [11]. Still, the high dose of omega-3 polyunsaturated fat with its attendant side effects precludes recommendations for its routine use as a means to lower BP.

Monounsaturated Fat

The effect of monounsaturated fatty acid intake on BP is uncertain, primarily because few studies have tested this relationship. Five of seven cross-sectional studies did not detect a relationship [1], and neither of two prospective studies conducted in the United States documented an effect of monounsaturated fat intake on subsequent hypertension [2,3]. Until recently, evidence from clinical trials did not support a relationship between monounsaturated fat and BP [1]. Early trials were small studies, conducted in nonhypertensive individuals. Accordingly, the lack of significant findings can reasonably be attributed to inadequate power.

Recent trials have tended to support an inverse relationship between monounsaturated fat and BP. In a trial that enrolled individuals with type II diabetics, replacement of carbohydrate with monounsaturated fat significantly reduced both systolic and diastolic daytime ambulatory BP [12]. Recently, another trial documented that replacing saturated fat with olive oil significantly lowered BP and the need for antihypertensive medications, in comparison to sunflower oil, which is rich in linoleic acid [13].

PROTEIN

Until recently, it has often been assumed, especially by investigators from Western countries, that there is either no association [14] or a direct association of protein intake (or intake of animal foods and protein of animal origin) with BP [15–17]. The evidence for a direct effect includes observations on people with protein malnutrition in whom BP is often low [18], while diets low in protein content improve the prognosis in people with renal insufficiency [19], an important secondary cause of hypertension [20]. Furthermore, the rice diet—characterized by its low protein (20 g/day), low sodium (150 mg/day), and high carbohydrate content (420–570 g/day)—was an effective treatment of severe and malignant hypertension before the advent of pharmacologic therapy [21,22]. In addition, vegetarians tend to have lower BPs in comparison with meat eaters, although factors other than animal protein intake also differ between these two groups. (See below.)

Recently, an alternative view has been espoused; namely, that there is an inverse association of protein intake with BP [23–25]. This reassessment of the evidence has been stimulated by recent epidemiologic and clinical trial data, reviewed below. It builds on observations from the 1970s and 1980s in Asian countries, especially Japan and China, that implicated low protein intake as one of the factors underlying traditionally high rates of hypertension and high stroke rates in some regions of those countries [26,27]. In addition, experimental data have shown that protein-rich diets can slow the rise in BP and reduce stroke rates in laboratory animals; for example, in response to sodium load in salt-sensitive rats [26].

One potential set of mechanisms whereby protein intake could influence BP is through the actions of the constituent amino acids. For example, consumption of tyrosine and phenylalanine affects synthesis of catecholamines in the central nervous system [28], and both tryptophan [29] and tyrosine [30] lower BP when injected intraperitoneally in animal models. Histidine is a precursor for the synthesis of histamine, which has regulatory activity on the sympathetic nervous system [31] and dilates peripheral vessels [32]. Arginine is the metabolic precursor of nitric oxide, which is a potent vasodilator acting on the endothelium [33]. It has been hypothesized that increased ingestion of arginine may reverse vascular reactivity changes and reduce intimal thickness in atherosclerosis, reduce the excessive proliferation of smooth-muscle cells in hypertension, and lower BP [33].

Epidemiologic Studies of Protein Intake

The epidemiologic studies of the relation of protein intake with BP among adults are summarized in Table 1. The studies were identified from previous reviews [23–25] and through bibliometric searches, reference lists from cited papers, and the authors' own knowledge. Studies have been listed by year of publication, except insofar that reports from the same study have been listed sequentially. The first part of Table 1 gives results of studies that have examined cross-sectional relationships between protein intake and BP; there was one ecologic study [34], while the remainder were analyzed at the level of

TABLE 1 Epidemiologic Studies of Dietary Protein and Blood Pressure in Adults

Author and study	Population	Dietary method (protein)	Confounders	Main findings[a]	Comment
Cross-sectional studies					
Dawber et al., 1967; Framingham diet study	912 M&W, 37–69 yr	Not specified	None	No association	
Yamori et al., 1981; Kihara et al., 1984	1120 M&W, >30 yr Japanese villagers	Spot urine sulfate:urea N ratio	Age, obesity, urinary Na/K, hct, chol, TG, fasting glucose	Inverse association of sulphate:urea N ratio to SBP (M only)	Indicative of inverse association of % animal (to total) prot with SBP
Fehily et al., 1982; Caerphilly Heart Study	134 M, 44–60 yr	7–day weighed dietary record	Age, BMI, fiber, macronutrients (stepwise)	No association	
Elliott et al., 1987; Caerphilly Heart Study	387 M, 45–59 yr	7-day weighed dietary record	Age, BMI, alc	No association with BP. Inverse association (g/d) with HTN.	HTN = SBP ≥ 160 and/or DBP ≥ 95 mm Hg
Pellum and Madeiros, 1983	61 M&W, 22–25 yr NTN university students and staff	3-day food record	Sex, fat, exercise, chol (SBP model) or urinary K (PP model; stepwise)	Inverse association (g/d) with SBP and PP (stepwise)	Positive association with DBP (inverse with PP) in M (univariate)
McCarron et al., 1984; NHANES-I	10,372 M&W, 18–74 yr	24-hr dietary recall	Age, race, sex +/- alc, macro- and micronutrients (discriminant analysis)	Inverse association (g/d) with HTN & top vs bottom BP decile. Discriminant NS	HTN = SBP ≥ 160. Lower energy intake in HTN vs NTN
Harlan et al., 1984; NHANES-I	2055 M&W, 25–74 yr	24-hr dietary recall and 3-month FFQ	Age, BMI, serum biochemistry, macro- and micronutrients (stepwise)	No association	
Gruchow et al., 1985; NHANES-I	9553 M&W, 18–74 yr	24-hr dietary recall	Age; and age, race, BMI, alc, macro- and micronutrients (stepwise)	Inverse association (g/d) with HTN. Stepwise NS	HTN = SBP ≥ 160. Lower energy intake in HTN vs NTN
Reed et al., 1985; Honolulu Heart Program	6496 M, 46–68 yr Japanese ancestory	24-hr dietary recall	Age, BMI, phys, alc	Inverse association (g/d) with SBP and DBP	Energy not reported

Joffres et al., 1987; Honolulu Heart Program	615 M, 61–82 yr Japanese ancestory	24-hr dietary recall	Age, BMI, alc	Inverse association of veg prot (g/d) with SBP and DBP	Borderline inverse association for animal prot with SBP, DBP. Energy not reported
Slattery et al., 1988	330 M&W, 22–66 yr twins	FFQ	None	No association	
Zhou et al., 1989	2672 M&W, 35–59 yr 10 Chinese populations	3× 24-hr dietary recall	Age, sex, BMI, Na, Ca, K	Inverse association of mean animal prot (% kcal) with mean SBP	Ecologic analysis across 10 population samples
Havlik et al., 1990	402 M, 42–56 yr monozygotic twins	FFQ	Wt, TG, chol, +/- energy (stepwise)	Direct association (g/d and % kcal) with DBP (twin-pair differences)	SBP differences NS
Elliott et al., 1992 (abst.); British dietary and nutritional survey	1,922 M&W, 16–64 yr	7-day weighed dietary record	Age, alc, Na, K, BMI +/- energy	Inverse association (g/d and % kcal) with SBP and DBP	
Zhou et al., 1994	705 M&W, 40–59 yr, 3 Chinese populations	3× 24-hr dietary recall	Age, BMI, sex, center, pulse, Na, alc (stepwise)	Inverse association (% kcal) with SBP and DBP	Inverse association with BP also found for sulfur containing amino acids
He et al., 1995; Yi Migrant Study	827 M; mean age 31.6–45.1 yr, 3 Chinese populations	3× 24-hr dietary recall	Age, BMI, alc, energy, urinary Na +/- location	Inverse association of total and veg prot (g/day) with SBP and DBP	NS with location added to model (except total prot and SBP)
Stamler et al., 1996; MRFIT	11,342 M, 35–57 yr, SI and UC groups combined.	4 or 5× 24-hr dietary recall	Age, race, education, alc, smok, HBP-med, BMI +/- serum chol, caffeine, Na, K, other macronutrients	Inverse association (% kcal) with SBP and DBP	SBP NS in macronutrient models
Stamler et al., 1996; INTERSALT	10,020 M&W, 20–59 yr, 52 population samples	24-hr urinary N, urea-N, and sulfate excretion	Age, sex +/- BMI, alc, urinary Na, K, Ca, Mg	Inverse association of urinary N, urea-N (g/day) with SBP, DBP (multivariate)	Direct association with SBP (DBP NS age, sex adj)
Liu et al., 1996; CARDIA	4146 M&W, 18–30 yr at baseline; 4 race-sex groups (analyzed separately)	FFQ at baseline and yr 7	Age, education, hostility, K, Ca, HBP-med, yr & BMI, alc, phys, smok (baseline and)	Inverse association (% kcal) for white W, DBP	

(*continued on next page*)

TABLE 1 (continued)

Author and study	Population	Dietary method (protein)	Confounders	Main findings[a]	Comment
Rafie et al., 1998 (abst.)	950 M&W	FFQ	None	Direct association of veg prot (g/day) with HTN	Higher energy intake in HTN vs. NTN
Liu et al., 2000; CARDIAC study	619 M&W, 4 Chinese population samples	24-hr urine collection	Age, sex +/- BMI +/- alc, urinary K, Na (not on HBP-med)	Inverse association of urinary 3-methyl histidine with SBP, DBP	
Liu et al., 2000; CARDIAC study	1681 Japanese M&W, 1151 Chinese M&W	24-hr urine collection	Age +/- sex, center, BMI, urinary Na, Mg (stepwise) (not on HBP-med)	Inverse association of urinary 3-methyl histidine to create ratio with SBP, DBP for Chinese W (age adj) & for Chinese (SBP, DBP) and Japanese (DBP, (stepwise)	Also inverse association of taurine to create ratio for Chinese M, DBP (age adj.)
Liu et al., 2001; CARDIAC study	1614 M&W, 4 ethnic Chinese populations	24-hr urine collection	Age, sex +/-urinary K (not on HBP-med)	Inverse association of urinary 3-methyl histidine to create ratio with SBP, DBP for 3 (of 4) ethnic samples	DBP significant for both age, sex and age, sex, K adj.
He et al., 1998 (abst.); NHANES-III	13,977 M&W, ≥ 18 yr, not on HBP-med	24-hr dietary recall	Age, sex, ethnicity, energy	No association	
Hajjar et al., 2001; NHANES-III	17,030 M&W, ≥ 20 yr	24-hr dietary recall	Age, sex, ethnicity, BMI +/- Na, K, Na/K, Mg, Ca, alc (stepwise)	Direct association (g/kcal or g/kcal/m^2) with SBP and PP (full model only)	
Longitudinal studies					
Liu et al., 1996; CARDIA	4146 M&W, 18–30 yr at baseline; 7 yr follow-up	FFQ at baseline and yr 7	Not specified	No association	Prot (% kcal) vs. Δ BP at 7 years
Ludwig et al., 1999; CARDIA	2731 M & W, 18–30 yr at baseline; 10 yr BP follow-up	FFQ at yr 7	Age, sex, center, education, energy, vits, smok, alc, phys +/- insulin	No association	Prot (% kcal) at 7 years vs. BP at 10 years

Stamler et al., 1996; MRFIT	11,342 M, 35–57 yr years; 1–6 vs. baseline separately for SI and UC	4 or 5× 24-hr dietary recall	Age, race, education, smok, special diet, baseline BP, HBP-med & alc, wt, smok	Inverse association of Δ prot (% kcal) with Δ SBP (SI) and DBP (UC)	
Vupputuri et al., 1998 (abst.); NHANES I follow-up	5727 M & W, mean age 47.9 yr at baseline, average 10 yr follow-up	24-hr dietary recall	Age, race, sex, BMI, energy, Na, K	Inverse association with incidence of HTN (univariate). NS (multiple)	
Morris et al., 2001; Calcium for Preeclampsia Prevention Study	4,157 pregnant W; Intervention and control trial arms combined	24-hr dietary recall	Energy	No association	Outcome = pre-eclampsia or HTN in pregnancy
Stamler et al., 2002; Western Electric Study	1714 men, 40–55 yr at baseline, up to 9 yr follow-up	Usual intake in preceding 28 days	Age, ht, education, smok, alc, wt +/- macro- and micronutrients	Inverse association for veg prot (% kcal) with Δ SBP, DBP (direct for animal prot with SBP)	Animal prot (and in some models veg prot) and BP NS in macro/micro nutrient analyses

Note: Abst abstract; M men; W women; yr year; SBP systolic blood pressure; DBP diastolic blood pressure; PP pulse pressure; HTN hypertension (or hypertensive); NTN normotension (or normotensive); HBP-med antihypertensive medication; BMI body mass index; wt weight; ht height; hr hour; FFQ food frequency questionnaire; % kcal protein as % energy; NS not significant; adj adjusted; veg vegetable; prot protein; alc alcohol; smok smoking; phys physical activity; vits vitamin supplements; Na sodium; K potassium; Ca calcium; N nitrogen; hct hematocrit; TG triglyceride; chol cholesterol; creat creatinine; SI special intervention, UC usual care (MRFIT trial); change.

[a] Findings relate to total protein intake and to statistically significant associations with BP unless otherwise stated.

individuals. The second part of Table 1 gives findings from longitudinal studies that have examined baseline or subsequent diet [35–37] or diet change [4,38,39] in relation to change in BP or incident hypertension.

Overall, 26 reports of cross-sectional analyses were identified from 18 different studies, while there were six reports of longitudinal analyses from five studies (three of which were also reported cross-sectionally). Of the 18 cross-sectional studies, two found no association between protein intake and BP [40,41]. Eight studies reported a significant inverse association in at least one analysis [42–45,34,46–52] and two reported a direct association [53,54], while different reports from four studies variously found either an inverse association [55–58] or no association [59–61]. One further study, INTERSALT, found a significant inverse association of systolic and diastolic BP with both total and urea nitrogen (measured in 24–hr urine collections as a biomarker for total protein intake) in fully adjusted models, although a direct association in analyses adjusted only for age and sex [62]. Another study [63] found inverse associations with systolic BP and pulse pressure in multiple regression analyses, but both a direct (diastolic BP) and an inverse (pulse pressure) association in males in univariate analysis.

One important issue is the degree to which studies allowed for variations in reported energy intakes [64]. One problem is that people with high BP tend to be overweight, and overweight people tend to underreport energy intake [65], so that a spurious inverse association between low protein intake (an important contributor to total energy intake) and BP might result. There was indication that such an effect may have been operating in a number of studies cited in Table 1, including NHANES-I [56,57], the Honolulu Heart Program [44,45], and to a lesser extent the Caerphilly Heart Study [55]. In contrast, Rafie et al. [54] reported a direct association of vegetable protein with BP, but also reported *higher* energy intake among hypertensive compared with normotensive people. Most of the other studies either adjusted for energy or included protein as a percentage of kcal in the regression models.

Among the longitudinal studies, Stamler et al. [4,66] reported a significant inverse association of change in protein intake (as a percentage of kcal) with change in BP in both the special intervention group (systolic) and the usual care group (diastolic) among over 11,000 men with 6-year follow-up as part of the MRFIT trial cohort. Men in both arms of the trial had 24-hr dietary recall information collected four or five times, thus enabling more precise estimation of usual dietary intake (over 5 to 6 years) than would be the case with a single 24-hr record or single urine collection (used in many of the other studies reported in Table 1). Analyses of the Western Electric Study [37] showed an inverse association of vegetable protein with change in BP at up to 9 years of follow-up (and suggestion of direct association with animal protein), while 10-year follow-up of the NHANES-I cohort [35] showed an inverse association with the incidence of hypertension, although only in univariate analysis. In contrast, follow-up of the coronary artery risk development in young adults (CARDIA) cohort [38,39] showed no association between protein and BP change over 7 to 10 years of follow-up. Likewise, there was no association in another study that examined diet and BP in pregnancy [36].

In addition to these studies in adults, four studies in children have been reported [67–70]. Boulton found small BP differences between groups with contrasting protein, fat, and carbohydrate intakes, but these seemed to be accounted for by body size and maturity rather than nutritional variables [68]. Jenner et al. reported an inverse association of protein intake with diastolic BP among 9-year-old children, but this was of borderline significance once energy intake was added to the model [69]. In a 3-year follow up of 7 to 10-year-old children, Simons-Morton et al. found an inverse association of protein intake (measured from three 24-hr dietary recalls) with both systolic and diastolic BP, although this was no longer significant when other dietary variables were added to the regression models [70]. The remaining study in children found no association between protein and BP [67].

Clinical Trials of Protein Intake

A number of trials of protein supplementation, protein restriction, or substitution of meat for vegetarian products have been undertaken, with varying and inconsistent results. Sacks et al. [15] and Obarzanek et al. [24] provide reviews of the earlier literature. In a series of randomized controlled studies, Sacks and co-workers investigated the short-term (2 to 6 weeks) effects on BP of different combinations of added beef, low vs. high protein, soy protein, and the addition of an egg per day to the diet [71–74]. Apart from an increase in systolic BP with added beef in one trial [71], these studies failed to find a significant effect of dietary protein manipulation on BP.

Very recently, a number of trials of soy protein supplementation [75–81] have been undertaken, which, despite some inconsistencies, tend to demonstrate a BP-lowering effect (Table 2). For example, using a 2 × 2 factorial design that tested the effects on BP of high vs. low fiber and high vs. low protein, Burke et al. [81] reported significant reductions in systolic and diastolic BP of 5.9 and 2.6 mmHg from a 66 g/day supplement of soy protein. Most of this benefit was found in the high-fiber, high-protein arm and only a minor effect on BP in the low-fiber, high-protein arm. He et al. [77] and Teede et al. [80] also reported significant falls in BP with soy supplements of 40 g/day. While the supplements used in these studies also provided an increased intake of isoflavones, two recent trials have found that isoflavones alone, without soy supplementation, had no effect on BP [82,83].

Alteration of protein intake is also a feature of complex interventions that test, for example, vegetarian or lactovegetarian diets [73,84,85] or the

TABLE 2 Recent Clinical Trials of Soy Protein Supplementation and Blood Pressure (Published Since 1999)

Author	N	Baseline BP	Protein intervention	Design	Duration	Net SBP (mmHg)	P value	Net DBP (mmHg)	P value
Washburn et al., 1999	51 W	132/82	Soy 20 g/day with 34 mg phytoestrogen (twice/day)	X-over	6 weeks	−1.3	NS	−4.9	<0.01
			Soy 20 g/day with 34 mg phytoestrogen (once/day)			−2.4	NS	−2.3	NS
Crouse et al., 1999	156 M&W	127/71	Soy 25 g/day, with 62, 37, 27, or 3 mg isoflavones	Parallel gp	9 weeks	–	NS	−3 (W) (higher vs. lower isoflavones)	<0.04 (trend)
He et al., 2000 (abstract)	150	135/83	Soy 40 g/day	Parallel gp	3 months	−3	0.05	−1.7	0.07
Williams et al., 2000 (abstract)	22 M&W	149/93	W: soy 38 g/day with 73 mg isoflavones M: soy 35 g/day with 162 mg isoflavones	X-over	4 weeks	−0.4	NS	+1	NS
Hermansen et al., 2001	20 M&W	130/78	Soy 50 g/day with >165 mg isoflavones and 20 g soy cotyledon fiber	X-over	6 weeks	+1	NS	0	NS
Teede et al., 2001	213 M&W	130/76	Soy 40 g/day with 118 mg isoflavones	Parallel gp	3 months	−3.9	<0.05	−2.4	<0.05
Burke et al., 2001	36 M&W	134/77	Soy 66 g/day (~25% kcal protein)	Parallel gp	8 weeks	−5.9	0.001	−2.6	0.006

Note: Change; M men; W women; X-over crossover; gp group.

DASH diet [86]. Compared to a control diet, the DASH diet significantly lowered BP. As displayed in Table 3, there were several differences in nutrients between these two diets, including the higher protein content of the DASH diet (17.9% vs. 13.8% kcal from protein).

In summary, despite some inconsistencies, recent data from both epidemiologic studies and clinical trials support the concept that protein

TABLE 3 Nutrient Targets, Composite Meal Analyses, and Average Daily Servings of Food Groups by Diet in DASH

	Control		Fruits and vegetables		Combination	
	Nutrient target	Composited menus[a]	Nutrient target	Composited menus[a]	Nutrient target	Composited menus[a]
I. Nutrients						
Fat (% kcal)	37	35.7	37	35.7	27	25.6
Saturated fat	16	14.1	16	12.7	6	7.0
Monounsaturated fat	13	12.4	13	13.9	13	9.9
Polyunsaturated fat	8	6.2	8	7.3	8	6.8
Carbohydrates (% kcal)	48	50.5	48	49.2	55	56.5
Protein (% kcal)	15	13.8	15	15.1	18	17.9
Cholesterol (mg/day)	300	233	300	184	150	151
Fiber (g/day)	9	n/a	31	n/a	31	n/a
Potassium (mg/day)	1700	1752	4700	4101	4700	4415
Magnesium (mg/day)	165	176	500	423	500	480
Calcium (mg/day)	450	443	450	534	1240	1265
Sodium (mg/day)	3000	3028	3000	2816	3000	2859
II. Servings of Food Groups (number of servings/day)						
Fruits and juices	1.6		5.2		5.2	
Vegetables	2.0		3.3		4.4	
Grains	8.2		6.9		7.5	
Low-fat dairy	0.1		0.0		2.0	
Regular-fat dairy	0.4		0.3		0.7	
Nuts, seeds, and legumes	0.0		0.6		0.7	
Beef, pork, and ham	1.5		1.8		0.5	
Poultry	0.8		0.4		0.6	
Fish	0.2		0.3		0.5	
Fat, oils, and salad dressing	5.8		5.3		2.5	
Snacks and sweets	4.1		1.4		0.7	

For 2100-Kcal energy level.
Note: n/a = not available.
[a] Nutrient analyses of menus prepared during validation phase and during trial.
Source: Adapted with permission, NEJM, 1997;336:1117–24.

intake is inversely associated with BP, although which component of dietary protein might be involved is at present uncertain. Of interest in this regard, the INTERMAP study (International Co-operative Study of Macronutrients, Other Factors and Blood Pressure) found that vegetable (but not animal or total) protein was inversely associated with both systolic and diastolic BP in multivariate models that included extensive control for potential confounding (unpublished observations). The new findings on protein and BP potentially have important implications for public health and clinical (nonpharmacologic) recommendations for BP control at both individual and population levels [62].

CARBOHYDRATE

Carbohydrate includes such simple sugars as monosaccharides (glucose and fructose) or disaccharides (sucrose—comprising glucose and fructose—maltose, and lactose) and complex carbohydrates (polysaccharides), especially starch found in cereal grains, legumes, and potatoes. Much less attention has focused on carbohydrate intake in relation to BP than on fat or protein intake, except insofar as both carbohydrate and BP are associated with insulin resistance, metabolic syndrome, and obesity [87,88]. It is of note that no mention was made of the possible effects on BP of carbohydrate intake in relation to chronic diseases in a major review undertaken by the National Research Council in 1989 [89]. An earlier review [90] as well as more recent reviews [23,88] focused on the intake of simple sugars in relation to glucose tolerance, and the well-established acute pressor effect of sucrose and fructose ingestion reported in animal models [91–94]. Suggested mechanisms for this acute direct BP effect include increased catecholamine production or release with stimulation of the sympathetic nervous system [95–98], interactions with salt intake, and promotion of salt retention [99,100].

In contrast to the direct association found in animal studies, the rice diet used to treat severe hypertension was *high* in carbohydrate (as well as being low in sodium and protein), as noted in the section on protein above [21,22].

Epidemiologic Studies of Carbohydrate Intake

Sixteen of the studies (21 reports) listed in Table 1 [34–37,41,44,45,47–49,53–57,59–61,63,66] examined carbohydrate intake in relation to BP in addition to protein (as well as fat and other nutrients). Of the 16 studies, eight found no significant association of carbohydrate intake with BP. While reports from the National Health and Nutrition Examination Survey (NHANES) I study [56,57] and the Honolulu Heart Program [44,45] found inverse associations with BP, these again could be artefactual, due to lower energy intakes among hypertensive people in those studies. In energy-adjusted analyses, however, reports from the Yi Migrant Study (diastolic BP only) [48], NHANES-III (systolic and diastolic BP) [61], and NHANES-I follow-up study (incident hypertension) [35] also showed inverse associations of BP with carbohydrate intake. In contrast, Stamler et al. [66] found *direct* associations of dietary starch with both systolic and diastolic BPs in the MRFIT trial cohort (although there was an inverse association of 6-year change in total carbohydrate with change in diastolic BP in the special intervention group). Pellum and Madeiros [63] and Rafie et al. [54] also reported direct associations of carbohydrate intake with either BP or prevalent hypertension.

In children, Simons-Morton et al. [70] reported an inverse association of energy-adjusted carbohydrate with diastolic BP over up to 3 years of follow-up, although this did not persist when other nutrients were added to the regression model.

Clinical Trials of Carbohydrate Intake

In contrast to the large number of experimental studies of carbohydrate and BP carried out in animal models, data from human experimental studies are sparse [23,88]. Rebello et al. [100] tested BP response after ingestion of solutions of five simple sugars using a Latin square design among 20 healthy normotensive men. Both glucose and sucrose ingestion were associated with significant increases in systolic BP at 1 hr (+9 to10 mmHg), as well as significant antinatriuresis. In a crossover study of 24 men and women classified as "carbohydrate-sensitive" on the basis of exaggerated insulin response to a sucrose load, diastolic BP was significantly increased after 6 weeks of a diet containing 33% of calories as sucrose [101]. Kraikitpanitch et al. [102], however, found no correlation between BP and sodium retention secondary to glucose loading, and Sacks et al found no effect on BP of a diet that replaced saturated fat with carbohydrate [103].

In summary, the direct effect of simple sugars on BP found in animal studies and the human epidemiologic data are inconsistent. While a direct association with starch intake was reported from the MRFIT trial cohort [66], several epidemiologic studies showed inverse associations of carbohydrate intake with BP. Further high-quality epidemiologic and human trial data are needed to clarify these issues.

FIBER

Though there are various definitions of dietary fiber, none is entirely satisfactory [23]. Trowell [104] defined dietary fiber as those components of the plant cell wall—including cellulose, hemicelluloses, pectin, and lignin—that resist digestion by secretions of the human alimentary tract, but the definition was later extended to include indigestible plant materials that are not cell-wall components, such as gums and mucilages [105]. Differences in definition and characterization of fiber intakes among investigators has complicated interpretation of findings from different studies [23].

Fiber can be either soluble or insoluble in water. Soluble fibers include pectins, gums, mucilages, and some hemicelluloses, while lignins and most hemicelluloses are insoluble [106]. Soluble fibers affect gastrointestinal function, slowing digestion and absorption of nutrients, and indirectly affecting metabolism of glucose and lipids [23]. Animal studies have found that increased fiber can reduce the BP rise associated with a sucrose load [107] or a fat-enriched diet [108].

As with diets high in complex carbohydrate or simple sugars, there has been considerable interest in the effect of high-fiber diets on insulin sensitivity and glucose metabolism, with potential impact on BP through its association with insulin resistance [87,88]. Other possible mechanisms include the absorption of short-chain fatty acids in the large bowel from fermentable fiber components, which in themselves may have a beneficial effect on BP [109].

Epidemiologic Studies of Fiber Intake

Several of the studies listed in Table 1 with respect to protein intake also examined fiber intake in relation to BP. Cereal fiber was inversely associated with systolic BP in two reports from the Caerphilly Heart Study [59,110], but not in a third [55], while in the Honolulu Heart Program [45], the Yi Migrant Study [48], the MRFIT trial cohort [4,66], and NHANES-III [61], inverse associations of dietary fiber with both systolic and diastolic BPs were reported. One other cross-sectional study found no association [63]. In longitudinal studies, Stamler et al. [4,66] reported inverse association of change in fiber intake (g/1000 kcal) with change in BP in the MRFIT trial cohort. In CARDIA there was inverse association of fiber intake at year 7 with 10-year change in systolic and diastolic BP (in white men and women) [39], and in the NHANES-I follow-up study, fiber was inversely associated with incident hypertension [35].

The relation of fiber to BP and incident of hypertension was also studied among U.S. male health professionals [2], U.S. female nurses [3,111], and in cross-sectional [112] and longitudinal [113] surveys of men in Boston and Baltimore. Among over 50,000 U.S. male health professionals, dietary fiber (adjusted for energy) had inverse association with 4-year cumulative risk of self-reported hypertension and with systolic BP change after adjustment for other dietary variables [2]. In the U.S. nurses' study, a 1989 report found an inverse association between energy-adjusted fiber intake and 4-year cumulative risk of self-reported hypertension, but this was no longer significant with inclusion of calcium and magnesium in the regression models [111]. A further study, however, covering a later 4-year follow-up period, found an inverse association (adjusted for calcium, magnesium, and potassium) of dietary fiber with subsequent systolic and diastolic BP [3]. The other two studies noted above also reported an inverse association of energy-adjusted fiber intake with diastolic BP [112] and with both systolic and diastolic pressure over an average 8 years of follow-up [113].

In children, Jenner et al. [69] reported an inverse association of energy-adjusted fiber intake and diastolic pressure in 9-year-old boys, while Simons-Morton et al. [70] reported inverse associations with both systolic and diastolic BPs over up to 3 years of follow-up, which persisted for diastolic pressure after adjustment for other dietary variables.

Clinical Trials of Fiber Intake

In a sequential, nonrandomized study (without a control group) Wright et al. [114] examined the effects of either reduced or increased fiber intakes on BP. They found BP falls of 3.9/3.7 mmHg (systolic/diastolic) with an increase in dietary fiber from 16.2 g/day to 24.5 g/day over a 4-week period ($n = 17$), and in a separate trial ($n = 14$) falls of 1.8/2.7 mmHg with an increase in fiber intake from 16.8 to 28.6 g/day. A third trial found an increase in BP (systolic/diastolic) of 7.7/2.8 mmHg following reduction in fiber intake from 30.8 to 14.8 g/day.

Subsequently, a large number of randomized controlled trials of dietary fiber supplementation have been carried out, although most did not have BP as their primary outcome [25]. An overview of the trials in humans published in the English language has been carried out by He et al. [115] utilizing a random effects model to obtain a summary of effect because of significant between-trial differences. Twenty (of 47 identified trials) were included, with average 14 g/day fiber intake. Exclusion of studies was done mainly because of concomitant changes in dietary sodium, potassium, or fat intake in the active treatment arm. The summary net changes in BP (mmHg) were −1.6 (95% CI: −0.4 to −2.7) systolic and −2.0 (−1.1 to −2.9) diastolic (both $p < 0.01$) [115].

As noted above in the discussion of protein trials, recently Burke et al. [81] examined the effects of protein and fiber intake in a trial with a 2×2 factorial design. There was a significant inverse effect of added dietary fiber (15 g psyllium/day) on 24-hr systolic BP [−5.9 mmHg (−8.1 to −3.7)], though the effect on diastolic pressure was not significant. Most of the fiber (and protein) effect was found in the high fiber, high-protein arm of the trial.

In summary, there is consistent evidence from both epidemiologic studies and clinical trials of an inverse association of dietary fiber with BP or incident hypertension. Uncertainties in the definitions and quantification of dietary fiber, concomitant dietary changes, and possible confounding in the epidemiologic studies, however, mean that the evidence of an inverse association with BP, though suggestive, is not yet persuasive. Further high-quality epidemiologic studies and clinical trials are needed.

CHOLESTEROL

Few studies have examined the effect of dietary cholesterol intake on BP. In the MRFIT trial cohort, there were significant, direct (positive) relationships between cholesterol intake (mg/day) and both systolic and diastolic BP [4,66]. The Keys score was also associated with diastolic BP but not systolic BP in the MRFIT study. In longitudinal, multivariate analyses from the Western Electric Study, there were significant positive relationships of change in systolic BP over 8 years with both dietary cholesterol and Keys score [37]. Still, despite these consistent reports from two studies, the paucity of evidence precludes any conclusion about a relationship between dietary cholesterol intake and BP.

DIETARY PATTERNS

Vegetarian Diets

Certain dietary patterns, particularly vegetarian diets, have been associated with low BP. In industrialized countries, in which high BP is commonplace, individuals who consume a vegetarian diet have markedly lower BP than nonvegetarians. Vegetarians also experience a markedly lower, age-related rise in BP [16,74]. Some of the lowest BPs observed in industrialized countries have been documented in strict vegetarians ("macrobiotics") living in Massachusetts. (See Fig. 1.)

Aspects of a vegetarian lifestyle that might affect BP include nondietary factors (e.g., physical activity), well-established dietary risk factors for elevated BP (e.g., salt, potassium, weight, alcohol), and other aspects of a vegetarian diet (e.g., high fiber, no meat). To a very limited extent, these observational studies have controlled for the well-established determinants of BP. For instance, in a study of Seventh Day Adventists, analyses were adjusted for weight but not dietary sodium or potassium [16].

Two trials, one in nonhypertensive individuals [81] and another in hypertensive persons [84], documented that a vegetarian diet can reduce BP. In the trial of nonhypertensive individuals, consumption of a vegetarian

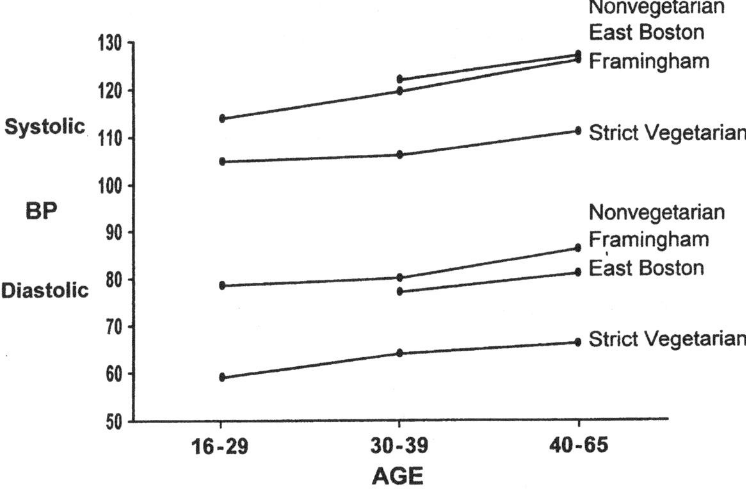

FIGURE 1 Blood pressure by age in a strict vegetarian population in Boston and in nonvegetarian populations in East Boston and Framingham, Massachusetts. *Source*: Adapted with permission, *American Journal of Clinical Nutrition*, 1988;48: 795–800.

diet, similar in nutrient composition to a ovolactovegetarian diet, led to significant reductions in systolic BP (5 to 6 mmHg) and diastolic BP (2 to 3 mmHg), compared to a nonvegetarian diet. In the other trial, an ovolacto-vegetarian diet compared to a nonvegetarian diet reduced systolic BP by 5 mmHg but not diastolic BP. Sodium and potassium intakes appeared similar in the vegetarian and nonvegetarian diets. Still, neither trial tightly controlled these aspects of the diets, which might have differed across randomized groups and partially account for the observed benefit of the vegetarian diet.

"Mediterranean-Style" Diets

In view of the heterogeneous cultures and agricultural patterns of the Mediterranean region, the Mediterranean diet is a not a single diet; rather, this term applies to dietary patterns that emphasize fruits, vegetables, bread, cereals, potatoes, beans, nuts, and seeds; that include olive oil, dairy products, fish, poultry, wine, and eggs; and that are reduced in red meat [116]. Despite the difficulties of characterizing a Mediterranean-style diet, interest in such diets is considerable because of the apparent health benefits, particularly a reduced risk of heart disease.

The Seven Countries Study provides indirect evidence that a Mediterranean-style diet may reduce BP. Specifically, in parts of Greece in which traditional diets are eaten, the prevalence of hypertension was half that of Western Europe and the United States [117]. The few trials that tested the effects of Mediterranean-style diets on BP have been equivocal, however. In one small-scale study that enrolled nonhypertensive adults residing in southern Italy, replacement of their usual diet with a diet increased in saturated fats and reduced in monounsaturated fat and carbohydrate led to a rise in BP [118]. However, in the Lyon Diet Heart Study Mediterranean-style diet with increased linolenic acid had no effect on BP [119,120].

The DASH (Dietary Approaches to Stop Hypertension) Dietary Pattern

In the early 1990s, when the DASH research effort was initiated, the well-established, dietary determinants of BP were salt, weight, and alcohol. Several lines of evidence suggested that other dietary factors likely affect BP, however. As highlighted above, vegetarian diets were associated with lower BP in both observational and experimental studies. In other observational studies, an increased intake of potassium, calcium, magnesium, fiber, and protein had each been associated with lower BP. Still, in clinical trials in which these nutrients were tested separately, reductions in BP were typically small and/or inconsistent.

In this setting, the DASH trial tested whether modification of whole dietary patterns might affect BP [82]. The DASH trial tested two hypotheses: (1) that increased intake of fruits and vegetables lowers BP, and (2) that an overall healthy dietary pattern (originally termed the "combination" diet, now termed the DASH diet) lowers BP.

In contrast to most diet–BP trials, the DASH trial was a feeding study in which participants received all of their food for 11 weeks. After a 3-week run-in on a control diet that is typical of what many Americans eat, participants were randomized to eat for 8 weeks one of the following three diets: (1) the control diet, (2) the "fruits and vegetables" diet, or (3) the DASH diet. The DASH diet emphasized fruits, vegetables, and low-fat dairy products; included whole grains, poultry, fish, and nuts; and was reduced in fats, red meat, sweets, and sugar-containing beverages (Table 3). This diet was rich in potassium, magnesium, calcium, and fiber, and was reduced in total fat, saturated fat, and cholesterol. It was also slightly increased in protein. The control diet had a nutrient composition that is typical of that consumed by many Americans. Its potassium, magnesium, and calcium levels were comparatively low, while its macronutrient profile and fiber content corresponded to average U.S.-consumption. The fruits and vegetables diet was rich in potassium, magnesium, and fiber, but was otherwise similar to the control diet.

All three diets contained similar amounts of sodium (approximately 3000 mg/day). Energy intake was adjusted to maintain the initial body weight of each participant. Permissible alcohol intake during the trial was ≤2 drinks per day. In this fashion, the study directly controlled the major established dietary determinants of BP.

DASH participants were 459 adults with untreated systolic BP < 160 mmHg and diastolic BP 80 to 95 mmHg. The mean age was 45 years, average BP was 131/85 mmHg, and 29% had stage 1 hypertension (systolic BP 140 to 159 mmHg and/or diastolic BP 90 to 95 mmHg). By design, African Americans comprised 60% of the population.

Among all participants, the DASH diet significantly lowered mean systolic BP by 5.5 mmHg and mean diastolic BP by 3.0 mmHg. The fruits and vegetables diet also significantly reduced BP, but to a lesser extent, about 50% of the effect of the DASH diet. The effect was relatively rapid; the full effect was apparent after only 2 weeks. (See Fig. 2.) In subgroup analyses, the

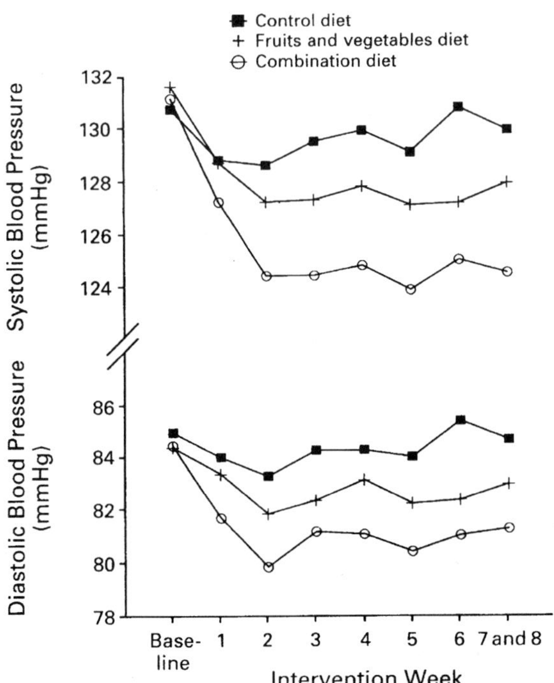

FIGURE 2 Blood pressure by week during the DASH trial, according to diet. *Source*: Adapted with permission, *New England Journal of Medicine*, 1997;336: 1117–1124.

DASH diet significantly lowered BP in all major subgroups (men, women, African Americans, non-African-Americans, hypertensives, and nonhypertensives). The effects of the DASH diet in the African-American participants (6.9/3.7 mmHg), however, were significantly greater than corresponding effects in white participants (3.3/2.4 mmHg). The effects in hypertensive individuals (11.6/5.3 mmHg) were striking, and were significantly greater than the effects in nonhypertensive (3.5/2/2 mmHg) individuals [121].

Results from the DASH trial have important public health and clinical implications. The effect of the DASH diet in hypertensive individuals is similar in magnitude to drug monotherapy for hypertension, hence in combination with the established lifestyle factors, the DASH diet should be an effective initial treatment for hypertension before prescription of drug therapy. Although the DASH diet was not tested in medication-treated individuals, the DASH diet, similar to other effective lifestyle changes, should also be effective as adjuvant therapy.

From a public health perspective, the DASH diet may be an effective means to prevent hypertension. In addition, adoption of the DASH diet could shift the population BP distribution downward, thereby reducing the risk of BP-related cardiovascular disease. It has been estimated that a population-wide reduction in BP of the magnitude observed in DASH could reduce stroke incidence by 27% and coronary heart disease by 15%.

Speculation about the effective components of the DASH diet has been considerable. The diet that emphasized fruits and vegetables resulted in BP reductions that were approximately half of the total effect of the DASH diet. Fruits and vegetables are rich in potassium, magnesium, fiber, and many other nutrients. Of these nutrients, potassium is best established as a means to lower BP, particularly in persons with low intake, in persons with hypertension, and in blacks [122].

Aside from testing fruits and vegetables, the DASH trial was not designed to identify the specific nutrients and foods responsible for the observed reductions in BP. Compared to the fruits and vegetables diet, the combination diet had more vegetables, low-fat dairy products, fish, calcium, protein, and complex carbohydrate, and was lower in saturated fat, monounsaturated fat, total fat, cholesterol, and red meat. Inferences about the effects of specific nutrients and foods thus are largely speculative and rely more on the interpretation of data from other studies than on results of the DASH trial itself.

Results from the DASH trial led some individuals to inappropriately question the importance of the established dietary risk factors for elevated BP. To this end, the subsequent DASH-sodium trial provides convincing empiric support for recommendations to simultaneously implement sodium reduction with the DASH diet. The DASH-sodium trial tested the effects of sodium reduction and the DASH diet, alone and combined, on BP. While sodium reduction alone and the DASH diet alone each lowered BP, the combination of sodium reduction with the DASH diet led to the largest BP reductions [123]. Overall, adoption of the DASH diet should supplement rather than supplant established lifestyle changes to reduce BP.

CONCLUSION

Available evidence is sufficiently persuasive to conclude that certain dietary patterns can lower BP (Table 4). Specifically, consumption of the DASH diet or vegetarian diets can reduce BP. A high intake of omega-3 polyunsaturated fat can also reduce BP. Other factors may also affect BP. Specifically, an escalating body of evidence suggests that increased protein intake, particularly protein intake from vegetable sources, may lower BP. Whether increased fiber intake lowers BP remains an appealing but as yet unproven hypothesis.

TABLE 4 Effects of Macronutrients, Fiber, Cholesterol, and Dietary Patterns on Blood Pressure: A Summary of the Evidence

	Hypothesized effect	Evidence
Fat		
Saturated fat	Direct	+/-
Omega-3 polyunsaturated fat	Inverse	++
Omega-6 polyunsaturated fat	Inverse	+/-
Monounsaturated fat	Inverse	+/-
Protein		
Total protein	Inverse	+
Vegetable protein	Inverse	+
Animal protein	Uncertain	+/-
Carbohydrate		
Total	Uncertain	+/-
Simple sugars	Direct	+/-
Starch	Uncertain	+/-
Fiber	Inverse	+
Cholesterol	Direct	+/-
Dietary patterns		
Vegetarian diets	Inverse	++
Mediterranean-style diets	Inverse	+/-
DASH diet	Inverse	++

Note: +/- = limited or equivocal evidence; + = suggestive evidence, typically from observational studies and some clinical trials; + + = persuasive evidence, typically from clinical trials.

For other macronutrients and for cholesterol, corresponding evidence is either limited or equivocal.

REFERENCES

1. Morris MC. Dietary fats and blood pressure. J Cardio Risk 1994;1: 21–30.
2. Ascherio A, Rimm EB, Giovannucci EL, Colditz GA, Rosner B, Willett WC, Sacks FM, Stampfer MJ. A prospective study of nutritional factors and hypertension among US men. Circulation 1992;86:1475–1484.
3. Ascherio A, Hennekens CH, Willett WC, Sacks FM, Rosner B, Manson J, Witteman J, Stampfer MJ. A prospective study of nutritional factors, blood pressure, and hypertension among US women. Hypertension 1996; 27:1065–1072.
4. Stamler J, Caggiula A, Grandits GA, Kjelsberg M, Cutler JA, for the MRFIT Research Group. Relationship to blood pressure of combinations of dietary macronutrients: findings of the Multiple Risk Factor Intervention Trial (MRFIT). Circulation 1996;94:2417–2423.
5. National Diet Heart Study Research Group. The national diet and heart study final report. Circulation 1968; 37–38 (suppl. 1): 1228–30.
6. Research Committee to the Medical Research Council. Controlled trial of soya-bean oil in myocardial infarction. Lancet 1968; 11: 693–699.
7. Appel LJ, Miller ER, Seidler AJ, Whelton PK. Does supplementation of diet with "fish oil" reduce blood pressure? a meta-analysis of controlled clinical trials. Arch Int Med 1993;153:1429–1438.
8. Morris MC, Sacks FM, Rosner B. Does fish oil reduce blood pressure? a meta-analysis of controlled trials. Circulation 1993; 88:523–533.
9. Pauletto P, Puato M, Caroli MG, et al. Blood pressure and atherogenic lipoprotein profiles of fish diet and vegetarian villagers in Tanzania: the Lugalawa study. Lancet 1996;348: 784–788.
10. Bao DQ, Mori TA, Burke V, Puddey IB, Beilin LJ. Effects of dietary fish and weight reduction on ambulatory blood pressure in overweight hypertensives. Hypertension 1998; 32: 710–717.
11. Mori TM, Bao DQ, Burke V, Puddey IP, Beilin LJ. Docosahexaenoic acid but not eicosapentaenoic acid lowers ambulatory blood pressure and heart rate in humans. Hypertension 199; 34: 253–260.
12. Rasmussen OW, Thomsen C, Hansen KW, et al. Effects on blood pressure, glucose and lipid levels of a high-monounsaturated fat diet compared with a high-carbohydrate diet in NIDDM subjects. Diabetes Care 1993;16:1565–1571.
13. Ferrara LA, Raimondi AS, d'Episcopa L, et al. Olive oil and reduced need for antihypertensive medications. Arch Int Med 2000;160:837–842.
14. Meyer TW, Anderson S, Brenner BM. Dietary protein intake and progressive glomerular sclerosis: the role of capillary hypertension and hyperperfusion in the progression of renal disease. Ann Int Med 1983; 98 (part 2): 832–838.
15. Sacks FM, Rosner B, Kass EH. Blood pressure in vegetarians. Am J Epidemiol 1974;100:390–398.

16. Armstrong B, van Merwyk AJ, Coates H. Blood pressure in Seventh-Day Adventists. Am J Epidemiol 1977; 105: 444–449.
17. McCarron DA, Henry HJ, Morris CD. Human nutrition and blood pressure regulation: an integrated approach. Hypertension 1982; 4 (suppl. III): III-2–III-13.
18. Viart P. Hemodynamic findings in severe protein-calorie malnutrition. Am J Clin Nutr 1977;30:334–348.
19. Ihle BU, Becker GJ, Whitworth JA, Charlwood RA, Kincaid-Smith PS. The effect of protein restriction on the progression of renal insufficiency. New Engl J Med 1989; 321: 1773–1777.
20. Brod J, Bahlmann J, Cachovan M, Pretschner P. Development of hypertension in renal disease. Clin Sci 1983; 64: 141–152.
21. Kempner W. Treatment of hypertensive vascular disease with rice diet. Am J Med 1948; 4: 545–577.
22. Watkin DM, Froeb HF, Hatch FT, Gutman AB. Effect of diet in essential hypertension. II. Results with unmodified Kempner rice diet in fifty hospitalized patients. Am J Med 1950; 9: 441–493.
23. Burke V, Beilin LJ, Sciarrone S. Vegetarian diets, protein and fibre. In: Swales JD, ed. Textbook of Hypertension. Oxford: Blackwell, 1994: 619–632.
24. Obarzanek E, Velletri Pa, Cutler JA. Dietary protein and blood pressure. JAMA 1996; 275: 1598–1603.
25. He J, Whelton PK. Effect of dietary fiber and protein intake on blood pressure: a review of epidemiologic evidence. Clin Exper Hypertens 1999; 21: 785–796.
26. Yamori Y, Horie R, Nara Y, Kihara M, Ikeda K, Mano M, Fujiwara K. Dietary prevention of hypertension in animal models and its applicability to human. Ann Clin Res 1984; 16 (suppl. 43): 28–31.
27. Liu L. Hypertension studies in China. Clin Exper Hypertens A 1989; 11: 859–868.
28. Anderson GH. Proteins and aminoacids: effects on the sympathetic nervous system and blood pressure regulation. Can J Physiol Pharmacol 1986; 64: 863–870.
29. Sved AF, van Itallie CM, Fernstrom JD. Studies on the antihypertensive action of L-tryptophan. J Pharmacol Exp Ther 1982; 221: 329–333.
30. Sved AF, Fernstrom JD, Wurtman RJ. Tyrosine administration reduces blood pressure and enhances brain norepinephrine release in spontaneously hypertensive rats. Proc Natl Acad Sci 1979; 76: 3511–3514.
31. Akins VF, Bealer SL. Central nervous system histamine regulates peripheral sympathetic activity. Am J Physiol 1991; 260: H218–H224.
32. Bender DA. Histidine. In: Bender DA, ed. Aminoacid Metabolism. 2nd ed. Chichester, UK: Wiley, 1985: 188–200.
33. Moncada S, Higgs A. The L-arginine–nitric oxide pathway. New Engl J Med 1993; 329: 2003–2012.
34. Zhou B, Wu Z, Tao S, et al. Dietary patterns in 10 groups and the relationship with blood pressure. Chinese Med J 1989; 102(4): 257–261.
35. Vupputuri S, He J, Ogden LG, Loria C, Whelton PK. Dietary intake of macronutrients and risk of hypertension: a prospective study using the First

National Health and Nutrition Examination Survey (NHANES) cohort. Circulation 1998; 98 (suppl. 1): 859.
36. Morris CD, Jacobson S-L, Anand R, Ewell MG, Hauth JC, Curet LB, Catalano PM, Sibai BM, Levine RJ. Nutrient intake and hypertensive disorders of pregnancy: evidence from a large prospective cohort. Am J Obstet Gynecol 2001; 184(4): 643–651.
37. Stamler J, Liu K, Ruth KJ, Pryer J, Greenland P. Eight-year blood pressure change in middle-aged men: relationship to multiple nutrients. Hypertension 2002; 39:1000–1006.
38. Liu K, Ruth KJ, Flack JM, Jones-Webb R, Burke G, Savage PJ, Hulley SB. Blood pressure in young blacks and whites: relevance of obesity and lifestyle factors determining differences. the CARDIA Study. Circulation 1996; 93: 60–66.
39. Ludwig DS, Pereira MA, Kroenke CH, Hilner JE, Van Horn L, Slattery ML, Jacobs DR. Dietary fiber, weight gain, and cardiovascular disease risk factors in young adults. JAMA 1999; 282(16):1539–1546.
40. Dawber TR, Kannel WB, Kagan A, Donabedian RK, McNamara PM, Pearson G. Environmental factors in hypertension. In: Stamler J, Stamler R, Pullman TN, eds. The Epidemiology of Hypertension. New York: Grune & Stratton, 1967: 255–288.
41. Slattery ML, Bishop DT, French TK, Hunt SC, Meikle AW, Williams RR. Lifestyle and blood pressure levels in twins in Utah. Genet Epidemiol 1988; 5(4): 277–287.
42. Yamori Y, Kihara M, Nara Y, Ohtaka M, Horie R, Tsunematsu T, Note S. Hypertension and diet: multiple regression analysis in a Japanese farming community. Lancet 1981; 1: 1204–1205.
43. Kihara M, Fujikawa J, Ohtaka M, Mano M, Nara Y, Horie R, Tsunematsu T, Note S, Fukase M, Yamori Y. Hypertension 1984; 6: 736–742.
44. Reed D, McGee D, Yano K, Hankin J. Diet, blood pressure, and multicollinearity. Hypertension 1985; 7: 405–410.
45. Joffres MR, Reed DM, Yano K. Relationship of magnesium intake and other dietary factors to blood pressure: the Honolulu heart study. Am J Clin Nutr 1987; 45: 469–475.
46. Elliott P, Freeman J, Pryer J, Brunner E, Marmot M. Dietary protein and blood pressure: a report from the Dietary and Nutritional Survey of British Adults. J Hypertens 1992; 109(suppl. 1): S141 (abstract).
47. Zhou B, Zhang X, Zhu A, Zhao L, Zhu S, Ruan L, Zhu L, Liang S. The relationship of dietary animal protein and electrolytes to blood pressure: a study on three Chinese populations. Int J Epidemiol 1994; 23(4): 716–722.
48. He J, Klag MJ, Whelton PK, Chen J-Y, Qian M-C, He G-Q. Dietary macronutrients and blood pressure in southwestern China. J Hypertens 1995; 13: 1267–1274.
49. Stamler J, Caggiula A, Grandits GA, Kjelsberg M, Cutler JA for the MRFIT Research Group. Relationship to blood pressure of combinations of dietary macronutrients: findings of the Multiple Risk Factor Intervention Trial (MRFIT). Circulation 1996; 94: 2417–2423.

50. Liu LJ, Ikeda K, Yamori Y. Twenty-four hour urinary sodium and 3-methylhistidine excretion in relation to blood pressure in Chinese: results from the China–Japan cooperative research for the WHO-CARDIAC Study. Hypertens Res 2000: 23(2): 151–157.
51. Liu LJ, Mizushima S, Ikeda K, Hattori H, Miura A, Gao M, Nara Y, Yamori Y. Comparative studies of diet-related factors and blood pressure among Chinese and Japanese: results from the China–Japan Cooperative Research of the WHO-CARDIAC Study. Hypertens Res 2000; 23(5): 413–420.
52. Liu LJ, Liu LS, Ding Y, Huang ZD, He BX, Sun SF, Zhao GS, Zhang HX, Miki T, Mizushima S, Ikeda K, Nara Y, Yamori Y. Ethnic and environmental differences in various markers of dietary intake and blood pressure among Chinese Han and three other minority peoples of China: results from the WHO Cardiovascular Diseases and Alimentary Comparison (CARDIAC) Study. Hypertens Res 2001; 24(3): 315–322.
53. Havlik RJ, Fabsitz RR, Kalousdian S, Borhani NO, Christain JC. Dietary protein and blood pressure in monozygotic twins. Prev Med 1990; 19(1):31–39.
54. Rafie M, Boshtam M, SarrafZadegan N, Abdar N, Sedigheh K, Asgary S, Naderi G. The impact of macro and micronutrients daily intake on blood pressure. Atherosclerosis 1998; 136 (suppl. 1): S62 (abstract).
55. Elliott P, Fehily AM, Sweetnam PM, Yarnell JWG. Diet, alcohol, body mass, and social factors in relation to blood pressure: the Caerphilly Heart Study. J Epidemiol Commun Health 1987; 41: 37–43.
56. McCarron DA, Morris CD, Henry HJ, Stanton JL. Blood pressure and nutrient intake in the United States. Science 1984; 224: 1392–1398.
57. Gruchow HW, Sobocinski KA, Barboriak JJ. Alcohol, nutrient intake, and hypertension in US adults. JAMA 1985; 253(11): 1567–1570.
58. Hajjar I, Grim CE, Varghese G, Kotchen TA. Impact of diet on blood pressure and age-related changes in blood pressure in the US population: analysis of NHANES III. Arch Int Med 2001; 161(4): 589–593.
59. Fehily AM, Milbank JE, Yarnell JWG, Hayes TM, Kubiki AJ, Eastham RD. Dietary determinants of lipoproteins, total cholesterol, viscosity, fibrinogen, and blood pressure. Am J Clin Nutr 1982; 36: 890–896.
60. Harlan WR, Hull AL, Schmouder RL, Landis JR, Thompson FE, Larkin FA. Blood pressure and nutrition in adults: the National Health and Nutrition Examination Survey. Am J Epidemiol 1984; 120(1): 17–28.
61. He J, Loria C, Vupputuri S, Whelton PK. Dietary macronutrient intake and level of blood pressure: results from the Third National Health and Nutrition Examination Survey (NHANES III). Circulation 1998; 98 (suppl. 1): 858 (abstract).
62. Stamler J, Elliott P, Kesteloot H, Nichols R, Claeys G, Dyer AR, Stamler R, for the INTERSALT Cooperative Research Group. Inverse relation of dietary protein markers with blood pressure: findings for 10 020 men and women in the INTERSALT Study. Circulation 1996; 94: 1629–1634.
63. Pellum LK, Madeiros DM. Blood pressure in young adult normotensives: effect of protein, fat, and cholesterol intakes. Nutr Rep Int 1983; 27(6): 1277–1285.

64. Willett W, Stampfer M. Implications of total energy intake for epidemiologic analyses. In: Willett W, ed. Nutritional Epidemiology. 2nd ed. Oxford: Oxford University Press, 1998: 273–301.
65. Pryer JA, Vrijheid M, Nichols R, Kiggins M, Elliott P. Who are the "low energy reporters" in the Dietary and Nutritional Survey of British Adults? Int J Epidemiol 1997; 26: 146–153.
66. Stamler J, Caggiula AW, Grandits GA. Relation of body mass and alcohol, nutrient, fiber, and caffeine intakes to blood pressure in the special intervention and usual care groups in the Multiple Risk Factor Intervention Trial. Am J Clin Nutr 1997; 65(suppl.): 338S–365S.
67. Frank GC, Berenson GS, Webber F. Dietary studies and the relationship of diet to cardiovascular disease risk factor variables in 10-year old children—the Bogalusa Heart Study. Am J Clin Nutr 1978; 31: 328–340.
68. Boulton TJC. Nutrition in childhood and its relationship to early somatic growth, body fat, blood pressure and physical fitness. Acta Paediatr Scand 1981; 284 (suppl.): 68–79.
69. Jenner DA, English DR, Vandongen R, Beilin L, Armstrong BK, Miller MR, Dunbar D. Diet and blood pressure in 9-year-old Australian children. Am J Clin Nutr 1988; 47: 1052–1059.
70. Simons-Morton DG, Hunsberger SA, van Horn L, Barton BA, Robson AM, McMahon RP, Muhonen LE, Kwiterovich PO, Lasser NL, Kimm SYS, Greenlick MR. Nutrient intake and blood pressure in the Dietary Intervention Study in Children. Hypertension 1997; 29: 930–936.
71. Sacks FM, Donner A, Castelli WP, Gronemeyer J, Pletka P, Margolius HS, Landsberg L, Kass EH. Effect of ingestion of meat on plasma cholesterol of vegetarians. JAMA 1981; 246: 640–646.
72. Sacks FM, Marais GE, Handysides GH, Salazar J, Miller L, Foster JM, Rosner B, Kass EH. Lack of an effect of dietary saturated fat and cholesterol on blood pressure in normotensives. Hypertension 1984; 6: 193–198.
73. Sacks FM, Wood PG, Kass EH. Stability of blood pressure in vegetarians receiving dietary protein supplements. Hypertension 1984; 6: 199–201.
74. Sacks FM, Kass EH. Low blood pressure in vegetarians: effects of specific foods and nutrients. Am J Clin Nutr 1988; 48:795–800.
75. Washburn S, Burke GL, Morgan T, Anthony M. Effect of soy protein supplementation on serum lipoproteins, blood pressure, and menopausal symptoms in perimenopausal women. Menopause 1999; 6(1): 7–13.
76. Crouse JR, Morgan T, Terry J, Ellis J, Vitolins M, Burke G. A randomizing trial comparing the effect of casein with that of soy protein containing varying amounts of isoflavones on plasma concentrations of lipids and lipoproteins. Arch Int Med 1999; 159(17): 2070–2076.
77. He J, Wu XG, Gu DF, Duan XF, Whelton PK. Soybean protein supplementation and blood pressure: a randomized, controlled clinical trial. Circulation 2000; 101(6): 711 (abstract).
78. Williams JL, McCoy RA, Martin DS, Albers JE. Effects of a soy diet on blood pressure and vascular reactivity in hypertensive men and postmenopausal

women. Third International Symposium on the Role of Soy in Preventing and Treating Chronic Disease, Washington, DC, Oct. 31–Nov. 3, 1999 (abstract).
79. Hermansen K, Sondergaard M, Hoie L, Carstensen M, Brock B. Beneficial effects of a soy-based dietary supplement on lipid levels and cardiovascular risk markers in type 2 diabetic subjects. Diabetes Care 2001; 24(2): 228–233.
80. Teede HJ, Dalais FS, Kotsopoulos D, Liang Y-L, Davis S, McGrath BP. Dietary soy has both beneficial and potentially adverse cardiovascular effects: a placebo-controlled study in men and postmenopausal women. J Clin Endocrinol Metab 2001; 86: 3053–3060.
81. Burke V, Hodgson JM, Beilin LJ, Giangiulioi N, Rogers P, Puddey IB. Dietary protein and soluble fiber reduce ambulatory blood pressure in treated hypertensives. Hypertension 2001; 38: 821–826.
82. Nestel PJ, Yamashita T, Takayuki S, Pomeroy S, Dart A, Komesaroff P, Owen A, Abbey M. Soy isoflavones improve systemic arterial compliance but not plasma lipids in menopausal and perimenopausal women. Arteriosclerosis Thromb Vasc Biol 1997; 17: 3392–3398.
83. Hodgson JM, Puddey I, Beilin LJ, Mori TA, Burke V, Croft KD, Rogers PB. Effects of isoflavonoids on blood pressure in subjects with high-normal ambulatory blood pressure levels: a randomized controlled trial. Am J Hypertens 1999; 12: 47–53.
84. Rouse IL, Beilin LJ, Armstrong BK, Vandongen R. Blood pressure-lowering effect of a vegetarian diet: controlled trial in normotensive subjects. Lancet 1983; i : 5–10.
85. Margetts BM, Beilin LJ, Vandongen R, Armstrong BK. Vegetarian diet in mild hypertension: a randomised controlled trial. Br Med J 1986; 293: 1468–1471.
86. Appel LJ, Moore TJ, Obarzanek E, Vollmer WM, Svetkey LP, Sacks FM, Bray GA, Vogt TM, Cutler JA, Windhauser MM, Lin P-H, Karanja N, for the DASH Collaborative Research Group. A clinical trial of the effect of dietary patterns on blood pressure. N Engl J Med 1997; 336:1117–1124.
87. Reaven GM, Hoffman BB. Hypertension as a disease of carbohydrate and lipoprotein metabolism. Am J Med 1989; 87 (suppl. 6A): 6A-2S–6A-6S.
88. Preuss HG, Gondal JA, Lieberman S. Association of macronutrients and energy intake with hypertension. J Am Coll Nutr 1996; 15: 21–35.
89. National Research Council. Diet and Health. Washington, DC: National Academy Press, 1989: 273–290.
90. Hodges RE, Rebello T. Carbohydrates and blood pressure. Ann Int Med 1983; 98 (part 2): 838–841.
91. Hwang I-S, Ho H, Hoffman BB, Reaven GM. Fructose-induced insulin resistance and hypertension in rats. Hypertension 1987; 10: 512–516.
92. Martinez FJ, Rizza RA, Romero JC. High-fructose feeding elicits insulin resistance, hyperinsulinism, and hypertension in normal mongrel dogs. Hypertension 1994; 23: 456–463.
93. Preuss HG, Knapka JJ, MacArthy P, Yousufi AK, Sabnis SG, Antonovych TT. High sucrose diets increase blood pressure of both salt-sensitive and salt-resistant rats. Am J Hypertens 1992; 5: 585–591.

94. Zein M, Areas JL, Knapka J, MacCarthy P, Yousufi AK, DiPette D, Holland B, Goel R, Preuss HG. Excess sucrose and glucose ingestion acutely elevate blood pressure in spontaneously hypertensive rats. Am J Hypertens 1990; 3: 380–386.
95. Bunag RD, Tomita T, Sasaki S. Chronic sucrose ingestion induces mild hypertension and tachycardia in rats. Hypertension 1983; 5: 218–225.
96. Fournier RD, Chiueh CC, Kopin IJ, Knapka JJ, DiPette D, Preuss HG. Refined carbohydrate increases blood pressure and catecholamine excretion in SHR and WKY. Am J Physiol 1986; 250: E381–E385.
97. Young JB, Landsberg L. Stimulation of the sympathetic nervous system during sucrose feeding. Nature 1977; 269: 615–617.
98. Gradin K, Nissbrand H, Ehrenstom F, Henning M, Persson B. Adrenergic mechanisms during hypertension induced by sucrose and/or salt in the spontaneously hypertensive rat. Arch Pharmacol 1988; 337: 47–52.
99. Preuss HG. Interplay between sugar and salt on blood pressure in spontaneously hypertensive rats. Nephron 1994; 68: 385–387.
100. Rebello T, Hodges RE, Smith JL. Short-term effects of various sugars on antinatriuresis and blood pressure changes in normotensive men. Am J Clin Nutr 1983; 38: 84–94.
101. Israel KD, Michaelis OE, Reiser S, Keeney M. Serum uric acid, inorganic phosphorus, and glutamic-oxalacetic transaminase and blood pressure in carbohydrate-sensitive adults consuming three different levels of sucrose. Ann Nutr Metab 1983; 27: 425–435.
102. Kraikitpanitch S, Chrysant SG, Lindenmann RD. Natriuresis and carbohydrate induced antinatriuresis in fasted, hydrated, hypertensives. Proc Soc Exp Biol Med 1975; 149: 319–324.
103. Sacks FM, Rouse IL, Stampfer MJ, Bishop LM, Lenherr CF, Walther RJ. Effect of dietary fats and carbohydrate on blood pressure of mildly hypertensive patients. Hypertension 1987; 10: 452–460.
104. Trowell H. Crude fibre, dietary fibre and atherosclerosis. Atheroscerosis 1972; 16: 138–140.
105. Trowell H, Southgate DAT, Wolever TMS, Leeds AR, Gassull MA, Jenkins DJA. Dietary fiber redefined. Lancet 1976; i: 967.
106. National Research Council. Diet and Health. Washington, DC: National Academy Press, 1989: 291–309.
107. Gondal JA, MacArthy P, Myers AK, Preuss HG. Effects of dietary sucrose and fibers on blood pressure in hypertensive rats. Clin Nephrol 1996; 45: 163–168.
108. Burstyn BG, Husbands DR. Fat induced hypertension in rabbits: effects of dietary fibre on blood pressure and blood lipid concentration. Cardiovasc Res 1980; 14: 185–191.
109. MacIver DH, McNally PG, Ollerenshaw JD, Sheldon TA, Heagerty AM. The effect of short chain fatty acid supplementation on membrane electrolyte transport and blood pressure. J Hum Hypertens 1990; 4: 485–490.
110. Lichtenstein MJ, Burr ML, Fehilly AM, Yarnell JWG. Heart rate, employment status, and prevalent ischaemic heart disease confound the relation

between cereal fibre and blood pressure. J Epidemiol Comm Health 1986; 40: 330–333.

111. Witteman JCM, Willett WC, Stampfer MJ, Colditz GA, Sacks F, Speizer FE, Rosner B, Hennekens CH. A prospective study of nutritional factors and hypertension among US women. Circulation 1989; 80: 1320–1327.
112. Ascherio A, Stampfer MJ, Colditz GA, Willett WC, McKinlay J. Nutrient intakes and blood pressure in normotensive males. Int J Epidemiol 1991; 20: 886–891.
113. Hallfrisch J, Tobin JD, Muller DC, Andres R. Fiber intake, age, and other coronary risk factors in men of the Baltimore Longitudinal Study (1959–1975). J Gerontol 1988; 43: M64–M68.
114. Wright A, Burstyn PG, Gibney MJ. Dietary fibre and blood pressure. BMJ 1979;2:1541–1543.
115. He J, Whelton P, Klag MJ. Dietary fiber supplementation and blood pressure reduction: a meta-analysis of controlled clinical trials. Am J Hypertens 1996; 9: 74A (abstract).
116. Kris-Etherton P, Eckel R, Howard B, et al. Lyon Diet Heart Study: benefits of a Mediterranean style, national cholesterol education program/American Heart Association step I dietary petter on cardiovascular disease. Circulation 2001; 103: 1823–1825.
117. Keys A. Seven Countries Study. Cambridge, MA: Harvard University Press, 1980.
118. Struzzullo P, Ferro-Luzzi A, Siani A, et al. Changing the Mediterranean diet: effect on blood pressure. J Hypertens 1986;4:407–412.
119. de Lorgeril M, Renaud S, Mamelle N, et al. Mediterranean alpha-linolenic acid-rich diet in secondary prevention of coronary heart disease. Lancet 1994; 343: 1454–1459.
120. de Lorgeril M, Salen P, Martin J, et al. Mediterranean diet traditional risk factors, and the rate of cardiovascular complications after myocardial infarction. Circulation 1999: 779–785.
121. Svetkey LP, Simons-Morton D, Vollmer WM, Appel LJ, Conlin PR, Ryan DH, Ard J, Kennedy BM, for the DASH research group. Effects of dietary patterns on blood pressure: subgroup analysis of the Dietary Approaches to Stop Hypertension (DASH) randomized clinical trial. Arch Int Med 1999;159:285–293.
122. Brancati FL, Appel LJ, Seidler AJ, Whelton PK. Effect of potassium supplementation on blood pressure in African-Americans on a low potassium diet: a randomized, souble-blind, placebo-controlled trial. Arch Int Med 1996; 156: 61–67.
123. Sacks FM, Svetkey LP, Vollmer WM, Appel LJ, Bray GA, Harsha D, Obarzanek E, Conlin PR, Miller ER, Simons-Morton DG, Karanja N, Lin PH, for the DASH-sodium collaborative research group. A clinical trial of the effects on blood pressure of reduced dietary sodium and the DASH dietary pattern (the DASH-sodium trial). N Engl J Med 2001;344:3–10.

12

Dietary ω3 Fatty Acids

Lawrence J. Beilin and Trevor A. Mori
The University of Western Australia and the West Australian Heart Research Institute, Perth, Australia

INTRODUCTION

Hypertension is a powerful risk factor for cardiovascular disease (CVD) and stroke, affecting up to 20% of the adult population [1]. The control of high blood pressure is a keystone of primary and secondary prevention of CVD and stroke in the population. The higher the level of systolic or diastolic blood pressure, the greater the risk of CVD [2]. In addition to genetic predisposition, diet, stress, body weight, alcohol, inadequate physical activity, and smoking all influence blood pressure [3]. Hypertension is seldom an isolated condition, and population studies have shown that it clusters with hyperlipidemia [4], obesity, diabetes, hyperinsulinemia, and insulin resistance [5]. Nutritional factors appear to be of significant importance in the pathogenesis of hypertension [6]. Dietary modification in the treatment of hypertension has gained attention in an effort to reduce the cost burden to the individual and society, as well as the undesirable side effects of antihypertensive drug therapy. The possibility of the simultaneous correction of more than one risk factor with a dietary approach is therefore appealing and worthy of careful evaluation.

In this regard, there is considerable evidence from clinical, experimental, and some epidemiological observations that the omega-3 (ω3) fatty acids, derived primarily from fish and fish oils, are protective against atherosclerotic heart disease and sudden coronary death [7,8]. The ω3 fatty acids have a wide range of biological effects leading to improvements in blood pressure [9,10] and cardiac function [11], arterial compliance [12], endothelial function and vascular reactivity [13], lipid and lipoprotein metabolism [14–16], reduced neutrophil and monocyte cytokine formation [17], and potent antiplatelet and anti-inflammatory effects [7]. Moreover, recent evidence has demonstrated that in humans, the two principal ω3 fatty acids, eicosapentaenoic acid (EPA, 20:5 ω3) and docosahexaenoic acid (DHA, 22:6 ω3), have differential effects on lipids and lipoproteins [18,19], blood pressure [20] and heart rate [20], and vascular reactivity [21].

This review will focus on the antihypertensive effects of ω3 fatty acids in fish and fish oil supplements and the possible mechanisms through which they lower blood pressure, and will also address some of the other biological properties of these compounds that are relevant to cardiovascular disease.

OBSERVATIONAL STUDIES

Interest in the cardiovascular effects of ω3 fatty acids first arose from the observation of the low incidence of coronary deaths in Greenland Eskimos, whose high-fat diet was mainly derived from seal and whale blubber compared with their mainland Denmark counterparts, who ate a more typical Western diet [22]. It was subsequently recognized that the ω3 fatty acids EPA [23] and DHA [24] were the active components of the diet that accounted for the prolonged bleeding time, decreased platelet adhesiveness, and low triglyceride levels in those eating marine oil products. These observations led to further studies of the role of dietary fish and ω3 fatty acids on the incidence of CVD and such risk factors as hypertension.

Several prospective population studies have confirmed a relationship between increased fish consumption and a lower rate of coronary mortality and/or sudden death. The Zutphen study from Holland found that men eating as little as more than one fish meal a week had a greater than 50% lower coronary death rate than those who never or rarely ate fish [25]. A subsequent study by the same authors extended these findings to demonstrate that a small amount of fish protected against coronary heart disease mortality in an elderly population in Rotterdam, Holland [26]. An inverse association between fish consumption and coronary heart disease mortality was demonstrated in studies from Sweden [27] and North America [28–31], and in heavy smoking Japanese-American men in the Honolulu Heart Program [32]. Dolecek [28] showed that when the 6250 men making up the control group of the large Multiple Risk Factor Intervention Trial (MRFIT) were divided into quintiles according to their mean consumption of ω3 fatty acids, there were significant inverse correlations among ingestion of fish oils and coronary heart disease, all cardiovascular diseases, and all-cause mortality, with the highest quintile having the lowest mortality rates of some 40–50%. In the Chicago Western Electric study of 1822 middle-aged men, those who at outset consumed 35 g or more of fish daily showed a 38% reduced risk of death from coronary heart disease at 30-year follow-up, with a dose-dependant effect of increasing fish consumption [30]. In the 20,551 male patients who took part in the U.S. Physicians' Health Study, consumption of more than one fish meal per week conferred a 52% risk-adjusted reduction in sudden cardiac death compared with men that consumed fish less than monthly [29]. In the same cohort, however, no significant association was observed between fish consumption and overall cardiovascular endpoints [33]. In a case control study of 334 patients with primary cardiac arrest, Siscovick et al. [31] found evidence suggesting that eating the equivalent of one fatty fish meal per week in the month prior to the event was equivalent to a 50% reduction in risk of a primary event. This risk reduction was associated with increased levels of ω3 fatty acids in red cell membrane phospholipids in blood specimens collected from 82 cases and 108 controls. Burchfiel et al. [32] reported that consumption of fish at least twice a week was associated with a 65% risk reduction in Japanese-American men who were heavy smokers. Not all studies have shown any association between fish consumption and cardiovascular events [34], however, possibly due to the relative crudity of estimation of usual dietary fish consumption, failure to distinguish fatty from low-fat fish, and the complex correlation between diet and other lifestyle factors. In a systematic review, Marckmann et al. [35] concluded that the discrepancy among studies may also be related to differences in the populations studied, with only high-risk individuals benefiting from increasing their fish consumption. The authors proposed that in high-risk populations, an optimum fish intake (estimated at 40 to 60 g daily) would lead to an approximately 50% reduction in death from coronary heart disease.

Comparisons of different populations also indirectly support a cardioprotective effect of dietary fish. For example, the Japanese, who consume relatively large amounts of fish, have the lowest rates of coronary heart disease despite being heavy smokers. They have until recently also had much lower intakes of saturated fats and hence of blood cholesterol levels, however, which are likely to be major contributors to their paucity of coronary disease.

Perhaps the strongest evidence for a protective effect of ω3 fatty acids comes from two randomized controlled trials in patients who had had heart attacks. The first, a study in 2033 patients in Wales who had recovered from a myocardial infarction, randomized the men to either a "usual care" group or they were advised to increase their ω3 fatty acid intake by eating two to three servings of fatty fish weekly [36]. Those men who increased dietary fish consumption and/or took fish oil supplements had a 29% reduction over 2 years in sudden cardiac death. The second and larger GISSI Prevenzione study [37] involved 11,324 patients who had survived a myocardial infarction within the previous 3 months. Patients were randomized in a factorial, open-label, controlled design to either fish oil (1 g daily), or vitamin E (300 mg daily), both interventions, or no treatment. After 3.5 years, fish oil supplementation was associated with a 30% reduction in cardiac mortality, a 20% reduction in total mortality, and a 45% decrease in sudden death, whereas vitamin E had no significant effect. Interestingly, the combination of fish oil with vitamin E did not increase the benefit compared with fish oil alone.

There is less evidence for benefits of fish on blood pressure from population studies, although again this may be largely due to methodologic issues. Estimates of ω3 fatty acid consumption from diet records or food frequency records have been relatively crude and have not been part of most dietary studies on population blood pressure and hypertension. One of the more convincing population studies associating dietary fish and blood pressure comes from a cross-sectional comparison of Bantu fisherman compared with non-fish-eating Bantu farmers, in which the former showed a much lower increase in blood pressure with aging and lower serum triglycerides [38]. Even this finding was potentially confounded by the higher levels of alcohol consumption in the farmers, however, paradoxically, the high incidence of hypertension in Japan occurs despite their high fish intake, but this phenomenon may be due to their very high level of salt consumption. Some other—but not all—regional population studies are, however, in keeping with lower blood pressures in areas of higher fish consumption, although the methodology is such as to make it difficult to exclude the influence of other confounding factors.

Interestingly, a recent study by Iso et al. [39], showed an inverse association between increasing intakes of ω3 fatty acids and risk of stroke in the Nurses' Health Study during 16 years of follow-up. The effect was primarily observed for ischemic stroke, and no association was seen for hemorrhagic stroke.

CLINICAL TRIALS AND META-ANALYSIS

Randomized controlled trials of fish oil supplements or increased dietary fish consumption provide unequivocal evidence for a blood pressure-lowering effect of ω3 fatty acids. Early meta-analyses of such trials have shown such an effect in hypertensives [9,10]. In a meta-analysis of 31 placebo-controlled trials of effects of fish oils on blood pressure in 1356 subjects who averaged 4.8 g/day ω3 fatty acids, Morris et al. [10] found a fall in pressure overall of

−3.0/−1.5 mmHg, with a significant dose response effect estimated at −0.66/ −0.35 mmHg/g ω3 fatty acid. The hypotensive effect was strongest in hypertensive (treated and untreated) subjects (−3.4/−2.0 mmHg) and not clinically significant in a subgroup of eight studies of normotensives (−0.4/ −0.7). Similarly, Appel et al. [9] estimated that blood pressure fell 1.0/0.5 mmHg in normotensives (11 trials) and 5.5/3.5 mmHg in untreated hypertensives (six trials), with the average intake being more than 3 g/day of ω3 fatty acids.

One well-designed and adequately powered clinical trial is probably more relevant than a host of small studies of variable design, and in this respect the trial by Bonaa et al. [40] is most conclusive. This population-based study from Norway involved 156 men and women with untreated mild hypertension screened from the community and randomized to 10 weeks supplementation with either 6 g/day of 85% EPA and DHA, or 6 g/day corn oil. Relative to the corn oil group pressures fell with fish oil supplementation by 6.4/2.8 mmHg. Blood pressure reductions were inversely related to baseline levels of plasma phospholipid ω3 fatty acids. A number of other placebo-controlled studies have demonstrated significant benefits of dietary ω3 fatty acids on blood pressure in hypertensive populations [41–45]. More recently, Prisco et al. [46] showed that 24-hr ambulatory blood pressure in mild essential hypertensive, normolipidaemic men was reduced by 6/5 mmHg after taking 3.44 g/day of ω3 fatty acids for 2 months. Subsequent trials of fish oil supplementation confirming these findings in hypertensives include a study from Toft et al. [47], in which they were also able to show an absence of effect of fish oils on glucose metabolism in essential hypertensives whose blood pressures fell by 3.8/2.0 mmHg more than controls after 16 weeks of 4 g/day of fish oil containing 85% EPA plus DHA.

The hypotensive effects of ω3 fatty acids may be potentiated by sodium restriction [48] and the concomitant administration of antihypertensive drugs. While fish oil amplified the hypotensive action of the β-adrenergic receptor blocker propranolol, in mild-to-moderate hypertensives [49], there was no additional blood pressure-lowering benefit in those hypertensives on ACE inhibition [50]. Fish oil supplementation, however, may be a useful adjunct to antihypertensive therapy with β-blockers or diuretics [51]. Lungershausen et al. [51] showed that blood pressure was reduced by 3.1/1.8 mmHg in treated hypertensives who were taking either β-blockers or diuretics alone or a combination of the two.

In a study comparing the effects of increasing the intake of ω3 fatty acids by fish feeding or fish oil supplements, Vandongen et al. [52] compared the effects of 12 weeks of either fish or fish oil supplements providing ω3 fatty acids in doses ranging from 2.2 to 6.3 g/day (mean intake 3.65 g/day) in the setting of a high- or low-fat diet in 120 men with cardiovascular risk factors, including high-normal blood pressure. Although individual subgroups showed no significant falls in blood pressure, in the combined groups there was a significant inverse correlation between the falls in systolic and diastolic blood pressure and heart rate, and increases in ω3 and decreases in ω6 fatty acids in platelet phospholipids. This again suggests that the extent of incorporation of ω3 fatty acids into tissue phospholipids largely determines their blood pressure-lowering efficacy.

More recent studies from Perth have sought to establish whether increasing dietary ω3 fatty acid consumption in the form of dietary fish would cause independent and additive effect to weight control on blood pressure and blood lipids [53]. It was postulated that the effects on blood pressure might be additive because of the known disturbance of endothelial dilator function in obese hypertensives and the effects of ω3 fatty acids on vascular endothelial function. Sixty-three overweight treated hypertensives were randomized to one of four groups for 4 months using a factorial design: weight loss alone by calorie restriction, a daily fish meal containing approximately 3.65 g/day ω3 fatty acids, the two combined, or a control diet. The last 4 weeks involved weight stabilization for the weight control groups, whose weight fell on average 5.6 kg. Changes in 24-hr ambulatory blood pressure recordings from the beginning to the end of the study showed significant independent and additive effects of dietary fish and weight loss (Fig. 1). Compared with controls, daytime blood pressures fell by 6.0/3.0 mmHg in the fish group, 5.5/2.2 in the weight loss group, and 13.0/9.3 with the combination. Interestingly, fish consumption was also associated with significant reductions in the heart rate- 3 to 4 beats per min—suggesting an autonomic/cardiac component to the blood pressure reduction (Fig. 2). In addition to the substantial blood pressure reduction seen when fish was incorporated into a weight-reducing regimen, this group showed the greatest improvement in lipid profile in terms of reducing triglycerides and increasing in HDL_2-cholesterol level, and the greatest in improvement in glucose tolerance (Fig. 3) [54]. Although platelet adhesiveness was not measured in this study this would also be expected to decrease with the amount of ω3 fatty acids consumed [55]. Together these changes are likely to substantially reduce long-term cardiovascular risk in overweight hypertensives.

The issue of potential adverse effects of ω3 fatty acids on glucose homeostasis was raised in some of the earlier studies, in which up to 20 g/day of fish oils were administered, often without adequate controls. As mentioned above, Toft et al. [47] were unable to show any effects of fish oils in essential hypertensives using both oral glucose tolerance tests and a euglycemic hyperinsulinemic clamp. Similarly, in 57 hypertriglyceridemic subjects randomized to 4 g/day corn oil or fish oil containing 85% ω3 fatty acids for 12 weeks, there were no changes in plasma glucose or insulin

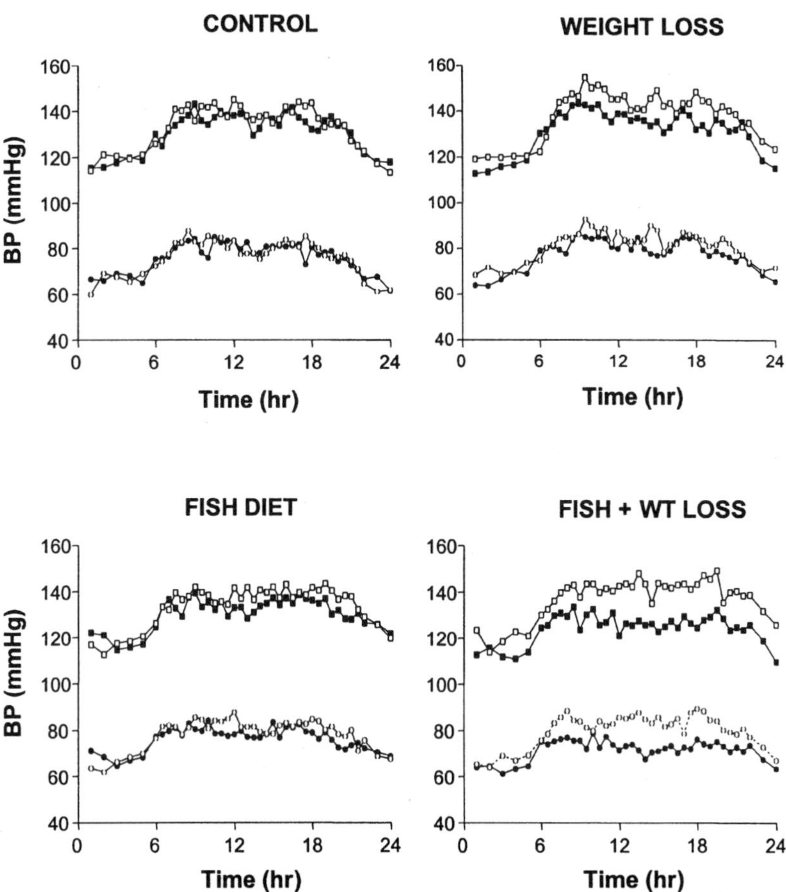

FIGURE 1 Twenty-four-hr ambulatory mean unadjusted systolic blood pressure (SBP) and diastolic blood pressure (DBP) at baseline and postintervention in the four treatment groups: □, baseline SBP; ■, postintervention SBP; ○, baseline DBP; ●, postintervention DBP. *Source*: From Ref. 53.

levels, despite expected falls in triglycerides with the fish oil [56]. The situation maybe different in non-insulin-dependent diabetes, however, Dunstan et al. [57] conducted a study in which 49 men with type 2 diabetes enrolled in a randomized, controlled trial of the effects of exercise training, a daily fish meal containing 3.6 g/day ω3 fatty acids, or the two modalities combined. The authors found increased fish consumption resulted in significant increases in home blood sugar levels and a small increase in

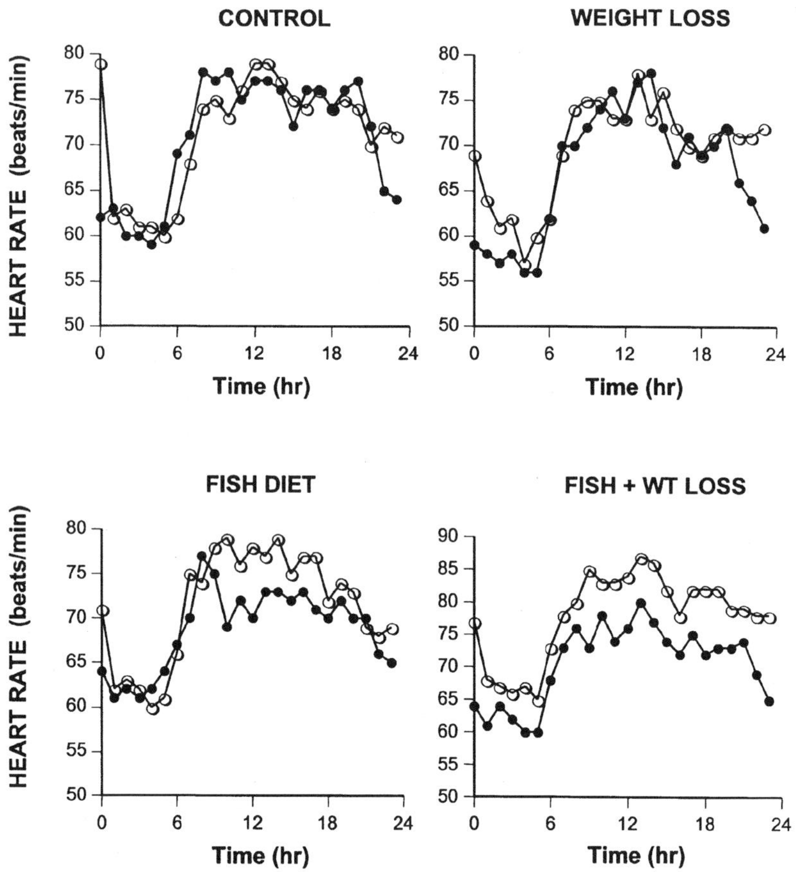

FIGURE 2 Twenty-four-hr ambulatory mean unadjusted heart rate at baseline and postintervention in the four treatment groups: ○, baseline heart rate; ●, post-intervention heart rate. *Source*: From Ref. 53.

HbA1c after 8 weeks. These effects on glucose were prevented by the concomitant exercise program while retaining beneficial effects on the lipid profile. Similarly, in a 6-week trial of highly purified EPA or DHA versus olive oil control in non-insulin-dependent diabetic patients who were on treatment for hypertension, there were significant increases in fasting glucose with both EPA and DHA and an increase in home blood sugars, which appeared to peak at 3 weeks and normalize thereafter [57a]. In that study there were no changes in insulin resistance or secretion as estimated

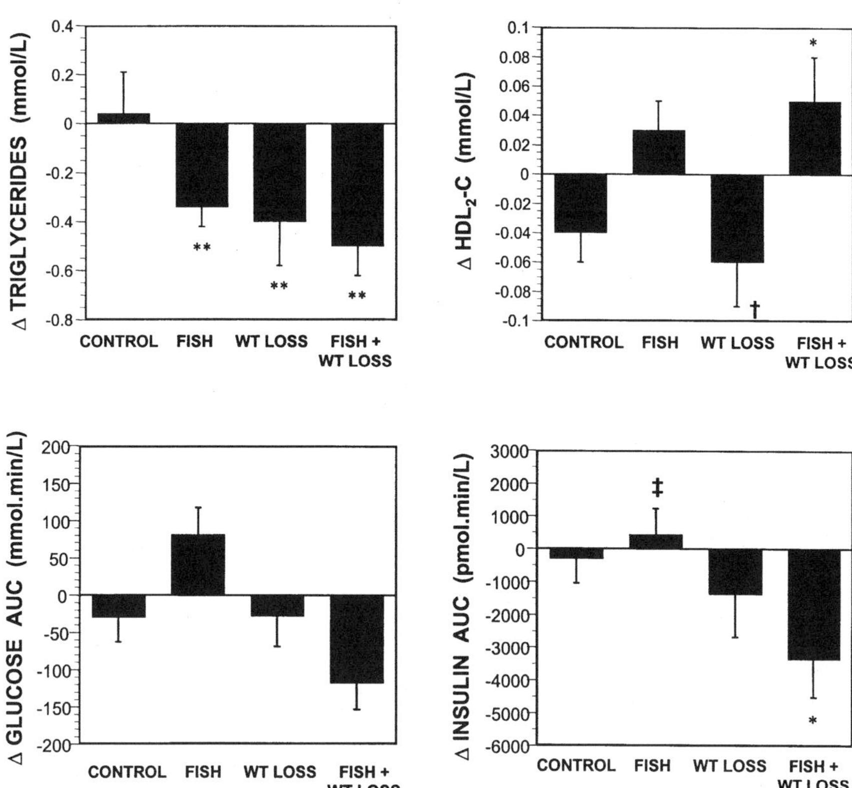

FIGURE 3 Changes from baseline to end of intervention in serum triglycerides, HDL_2-C, and glucose and insulin area under the curve (AUC), by group. Values expressed as mean ± SEM. General linear modeling (GLM) was used to assess treatment effects, main and interactive effects on postintervention values, adjusted for baseline values. There were no significant interactions for postintervention parameters after adjustment for baseline values: Δ triacylglycerols, treatment effect ($P=0.0001$), weight loss main effect ($P=0.002$), fish main effect ($P<0.001$); Δ HDL_2-C, treatment effect ($P=0.036$), fish main effect ($P=0.004$); Δ glucose AUC: weight loss main effect ($P=0.047$); Δ insulin AUC: treatment effect ($P=0.018$), weight loss main effect ($P= 0.003$). *Note*: * $P<0.05$; ** $P<0.001$ relative to the control group; † $P<0.05$ relative to fish and fish + weight loss groups; ‡ $P<0.05$ relative to weight loss and fish + weight loss groups; control group (n=16), fish group (n=17), weight loss group (n=16), and fish + weight loss group (n=14). *Source*: Adapted from Ref. 54.

by the LDIGIT clamp test. At this stage, therefore, it would seem advisable that diabetic hypertensives should be carefully monitored for glucose control if substantially increasing their intake of ω3 fatty acids by dietary means or oil supplements.

ANIMAL STUDIES

In general, a hypotensive effect of ω3 fatty acids has been demonstrated in various animal models of hypertension. Results from studies in the spontaneously hypertensive rat (SHR) have shown that dietary ω3 fatty acids attenuated the development of hypertension [58–64]. In most instances, however, systolic blood pressure of the rats remained in the hypertensive range (i.e., ≥ 150 mmHg), thus Singer et al. [60] showed that fish oil fed to 4-week-old SHR until 22 weeks of age was more effective than evening primrose oil in attenuating hypertension development. The systolic blood pressure of SHR fed fish oil was reduced by 32 mmHg compared with the control animals. Karanja et al. [61] fed SHR with 18% of the diet (36% of the calories) as fat, containing butterfat, fish oil, or corn oil, from 3 to 26 weeks of age. Fish oil consumption resulted in significantly lower blood pressures compared with butterfat or corn oil. Yin et al. [62] demonstrated that after 4 weeks of a diet supplemented with 10% by weight fish oil (Max EPA), systolic blood pressure in adult SHR was attenuated by 9 mmHg, compared with a diet supplemented with hydrogenated coconut oil. In a subsequent study, the same authors showed that 4 weeks' feeding 10% or 20% fish oil attenuated systolic blood pressure by 9 mmHg and 15 mmHg, respectively [63]. Systolic blood pressure of SHR decreased by an average of 24 mmHg after 8 weeks' treatment with EPA (100 mg/kg/day s.c.), compared to saline-injected animals [64].

The influence of fish oils in modulating the development of hypertension in the stroke-prone spontaneously hypertensive rat (SHRSP) was examined by Head et al. [65]. The authors found that 4-week-old rats placed for 13 weeks on diets containing fish oil (at a total dietary fat level of either 5% or 15%) had mean blood pressures approximately 20 to 25 mmHg lower than other SHRSP rats maintained on diets containing olive oil, safflower oil, or beef fat. Similarly, Howe et al. [66] showed that feeding diets containing 5% fish oil to young SHRSP resulted in a small but consistent suppression of the development of hypertension. Furthermore, this effect could be counteracted by increasing dietary sodium intake, as had been described in SHR by Codde et al. [67]. In a subsequent study, Howe et al. [68] examined the effects of fish oil combined with dietary sodium restriction on blood pressure in adult normotensive Wistar-Kyoto (WKY) and SHRSP rats. Rats were fed normal or low-sodium diets containing fish oil, olive oil, or safflower oil. Small but significant reductions of blood pressure were seen in SHRSP but not in WKY after 8 weeks on a fish oil/low sodium diet, compared with rats fed olive or safflower oil diets with normal sodium content. Subcutaneous injection of fish oil reduced blood pressure in adult SHRSP on a normal sodium diet. There was a further fall in blood pressure when sodium intake was reduced, however, the results indicated that the antihypertensive effect of fish oil could be enhanced by restricting sodium intake. Rayner et al. [69], fed synthetic diets containing 2% sodium (wt:wt) and either 5% olive oil or 4.5% γ-linolenic acid, EPA or DHA, to SHRSP aged 1 or 4 months, for 12 weeks. The authors reported that blood pressure was lower in those rats fed DHA or EPA than in the γ-linolenic acid or olive oil groups. In addition, adult rats (aged 4 months) fed the DHA also had significantly lower proteinuria, suggesting that ω3 fatty acids, but not ω6 fatty acids, were able to retard the development of proteinuria, caused by salt-induced hypertension in SHRSP. Other studies have shown that in borderline hypertensive rats (backcross of SHR and WKY), dietary supplementation with fish oil or sunflower oil attenuated the increase in blood pressure as a result of salt loading [70].

Others studies have shown that fish oils prevented dexamethasone-induced hypertension in SHR and Sprague-Dawley rats [71,72]. Codde et al. [71] demonstrated that a combination of cod liver oil/linseed oil rich in ω3 fatty acids prevented the development of glucocorticoid-induced hypertension in SHR fed for 4 weeks. Similarly, Yin et al. [72] showed that blood pressure was not increased in Sprague-Dawley rats treated with dexamethasone and fed a semisynthetic diet containing 10% by weight fish oil for 5 weeks. In contrast, Codde et al. [73] showed no blood pressure differences in Goldblatt 1-kidney, 1-clip hypertensive rats fed safflower oil or cod liver oil–linseed oil.

THE ANTIHYPERTENSIVE EFFECT OF EPA VS. DHA

In vitro, animal and human studies have shown that EPA and DHA are differentially incorporated into plasma, platelets, and tissue lipids [74–76]. These differences may play an important role in the utilization and metabolism of the two fatty acids. For example, there is evidence that in vitro, DHA, but not EPA, decreased cytokine-induced expression of endothelial leukocyte adhesion molecules [77]. Recent reports have also described differences in lipid metabolism [18,19,78] and platelet aggregation [79]. Blood pressure control is also differentially affected by EPA and DHA. McLennan et al. [80] reported that DHA was more effective than EPA at retarding hypertension development in SHR, but not in adult SHR with already established hypertension. Other studies have shown DHA prevented the development of hypertension in SHRSP [81] and that when compared with γ-linolenic acid, EPA reduced the elevation of blood pressure in the SHR [82]. In humans, Mori et al. [20] recently showed that in overweight, mildly hyperlipidaemic, but otherwise healthy men, purified DHA, but not EPA, resulted in a significant reduction in ambulatory blood pressure. Patients were given 4 g daily of highly purified EPA, DHA, or olive oil (placebo) capsules while continuing their usual diets for 6 weeks. Relative to the placebo group, 24-hr blood pressure fell 5.8/3.3 (systolic/diastolic) mmHg and awake blood pressure fell 3.5/2.0 mmHg with DHA. EPA had no effect on blood pressure. The study also demonstrated that DHA, but not EPA, significantly reduced 24-hr awake and asleep ambulatory heart rates. The latter finding on heart rate supported differences previously shown in rats, whereby DHA but not EPA inhibited ischaemia-induced cardiac arrhythmias in Hooded Wistar rats [80].

MECHANISMS FOR THE ANTIHYPERTENSIVE EFFECTS OF ω3 FATTY ACIDS

There are a number of possible mechanisms to explain the antihypertensive effects of ω3 fatty acids. Among others, these include improvements in endothelial and smooth muscle vasodilator function, enhanced production or the release of nitric oxide, increased vascular compliance, improved cardiac function, reduced plasma noradrenaline, alterations in vasodilator and vasoconstrictor prostanoids, and improved membrane function as a result of increased membrane fluidity. Each of these potential mechanisms will be addressed below.

Vascular Function and the Role of Nitric Oxide

Improvements in blood pressure following dietary ω3 fatty acids are most likely related to changes in vascular function, which have been demonstrated in animals and humans. Fish oil feeding to hypertensive rats leads to increased endothelial relaxation in response to acetylcholine in aortic rings [63] and decreased pressor reactivity of perfused mesenteric resistance vessels [83]. Yin et al. [63] produced evidence that the increased endothelial relaxant effects were due at least in part to suppression of thromboxane A_2 (TXA_2) or cyclic endoperoxides, with the possible additional effect of enhanced endothelial nitric oxide (NO) synthesis. Studies in humans have shown that fish oil feeding leads to reduced forearm vascular reactivity to angiotensin II and noradrenaline [84–86]. Furthermore, it was possible to antagonize the blunting effect of fish oils on responses to both noradrenaline and angiotensin II in human forearm resistance arteries by oral administration of indomethacin, suggesting that ω3 fatty acids exert their suppressive effects at least in part by modifying cyclo-oxygenase-derived prostanoids [87]. At the dose given, indomethacin per se did not effect responses to the two agonists.

Fish oils have a minimal effect on the vasodilation induced by either acetylcholine or reactive hyperemia in forearm resistance arteries of healthy subjects [87]; that is, they do not influence the function of the intact endothelium of healthy subjects. Omega-3 fatty acids, however, are able to restore impaired responses to endothelium-dependent vasodilators in patients with coronary artery disease [88,89], as well as in animal models, including the SHR [63], the glucocorticoid-induced hypertensive rat [72], and the hypercholesterolemic and atherosclerotic pig [90], all characterized by some form of endothelial damage. Vasodilatory responses to acetylcholine in hypercholesterolemic subjects have also been enhanced by dietary fish oil (Max EPA) without a change in total cholesterol levels [91].

Patients with type 2 diabetes fed fish oil have shown improved forearm vasodilator responses to acetylcholine, but not to glyceryl trinitrate, suggesting that fish oils may protect against vasospasm and thrombosis by enhancing NO release and suppressing thromboxane [92]. Other studies have provided evidence that fish oils may affect production or release of NO by demonstrating enhanced responses to such endothelium-dependent vasodilators as bradykinin, serotonin, adenosine diphosphate (ADP), and thrombin in rings of coronary arteries taken from pigs fed cod liver oil [93]. Furthermore, EPA has been shown in vitro to potentiate NO release evoked by IL-1β in vascular smooth muscle cells [94] and in endothelial cells in response to ADP and bradykinin [95].

There is evidence of a beneficial role of ω3 fatty acids to improve endothelial function in systemic large arteries in humans. Goodfellow et al. [96] recently showed a significant improvement in flow-mediated dilatation of the brachial artery following a 4-month treatment with 4 g daily of ω3 fatty acids in subjects with hyperlipidemia. The improvement was confined to endothelial-dependent responses.

Several studies in rats have demonstrated differential effects of EPA and DHA on vascular function [80,97]. These may be related to the differential effects on blood pressure control described above. Engler et al. [97] reported that in aortic rings from SHR and WKY rats, EPA- and DHA-induced endothelium-dependent and independent vasodilation, respectively. McLennan et al. [80] have also demonstrated that DHA was also more effective than EPA at inhibiting thromboxane-like vasoconstrictor responses in the aortas from SHR. They postulated that DHA prevented thromboxane-induced contraction and perhaps restored the vasoconstrictor/vasodilator balance following impairment of the normal NO-related processes. It remains uncertain whether or not DHA inhibits thromboxane synthetase or thromboxane A_2/prostaglandin H_2 receptor function.

In humans, Harris et al. [98] provided indirect evidence, based on the urinary excretion of NO metabolites, that DHA may enhance endothelial function compared with EPA. Mori et al. [21], recently reported that DHA, but not EPA, improved vasodilator responses to endogenous and exogenous NO donors and attenuated vasoconstrictor response to noradrenaline in the forearm microcirculation of overweight subjects with hyperlipidaemia. The mechanisms appeared to be predominantly endothelium-independent, based on enhanced vasodilatory responses following coinfusion of acetylcholine with L-NMMA and also infusion of nitroprusside, both of which are endothelium-independent. The results, however, did not preclude some endothelial component in the dilatory responses associated with DHA. These findings were thought to explain in part the reduction in blood pressure observed in these patients following supplementation with DHA but not EPA [20]. The finding of an endothelial-independent vasodilatory effect has not previously been reported in humans or animals following dietary ω3 fatty acids. An exception is the study of Yin et al. [63], in which enhanced relaxation to sodium nitroprusside but not to acetylcholine was demonstrated in perfused mesenteric resistance vessels from SHR fed fish oils.

The favorable effects of DHA on vasoreactivity [21] may have been attributable to direct and indirect effects of DHA on the arterial wall. For example, selective DHA incorporation into endothelial membranes could increase membrane fluidity, calcium influx, and endogenous synthesis and release of NO. Additional mechanisms may have included a direct effect of DHA on receptor-stimulated NO release, enhanced release of vasodilator prostanoids, and/or endothelial-derived hyperpolarizing factor (EDHF), consistent with experimental evidence [72]. The enhanced vasodilator response to sodium nitroprusside may be explained by increased biotransformation to NO or increased reactivity of smooth muscle cells to vasorelaxation as a result of decreased calcium influx, as previously reported [99]. The increased release of a vasodilatory cyclo-oxygenase metabolite may also have accounted for the decreased vasoconstrictor response to noradrenaline following DHA [21]. Additionally, the vasodilator effects of DHA could be related to increased basal production of NO in smooth muscle cells as a consequence of decreased release of platelet-derived growth factor (PDGF) from platelets [100]. Induction of nitric oxide synthase (NOS) in vascular smooth muscle cells is inhibited by PDGF [101].

Increased Vascular Compliance

The blood pressure-lowering effect of ω3 fatty acids may be related to improved vascular compliance. In a double-blind, placebo-controlled study, McVeigh et al. [102] examined the effects of dietary fish oil supplementation on arterial wall characteristics in patients with type 2 diabetes. Estimates reflecting compliance values in the large arteries and more peripheral vasculature, as measured by pulse-contour analysis, improved significantly after 6 weeks of fish oil therapy compared with values recorded at baseline and after 6 weeks administration of olive oil. No changes occurred in arterial blood pressure, cardiac output, stroke volume, or systemic vascular resistance with either intervention. These results supported the hypothesis that fish oils alter vascular reactivity and favorably influence arterial wall characteristics.

Alterations in Vasodilator and Vasoconstrictor Prostanoids

It has been proposed that the antihypertensive effect of ω3 fatty acids is in part related to the modulation of vasodilator and vasoconstrictor prostanoids. Omega-3 fatty acids have been shown to suppress the production of thromboxane B_2 (TXB_2), a metabolite of the vasoconstrictor and potent aggregator TXA_2 [103]. Diets rich in ω3 fatty acids resulted in decreased TXA_2 production, with concomitant increased TXA_3, the analogous but significantly less biologically active EPA-derived metabolite, in patients with severe atherosclerosis [104]. Increased prostaglandin I_3 (prostacyclin, PGI_3), which is derived from EPA, was also reported following ω3 fatty acids [104,105]. This was not always accompanied by a suppression in the formation of prostaglandin I_2 (PGI_2), which derives from arachidonic acid. PGI_2 and PGI_3 are equipotent in their vasodilatory and antiaggregatory activities [106], thus it was suggested that a significant increase in total prostacyclin (PGI_2 and PGI_3) formation, together with reduced total thromboxane (TXA_2 and TXA_3), might explain the altered endothelial and vascular responses observed following dietary ω3 fatty acids.

Reduced Plasma Noradrenaline and Increased ATP Levels

Hashimoto et al. [107] have recently reported that the antihypertensive effects of DHA may be related to reduced plasma noradrenaline and increased adenosine triphosphate (ATP) levels. The authors showed that rats fed DHA intragastrically had reduced plasma noradrenaline levels. In addition, increased adenyl purines, such as ATP, released both spontaneously and in response to noradrenaline from segments of caudal artery, were significantly inversely associated with blood pressure. It is known that ATP causes vasodilation by stimulating the release of NO from endothelial cells [108] by a direct action on vascular smooth muscle cells [109] and by hyperpolarizing smooth muscle cells [110]. It was therefore suggested that DHA altered membrane fatty acid composition and accelerated ATP release from vascular endothelial cells, which in conjunction with reduced plasma noradrenaline, may have been responsible for the fall in blood pressure [107].

Improved Membrane Function/Membrane Fluidity

It is feasible that the incorporation of ω3 fatty acids into plasma and cellular membranes may alter the physicochemical structure of the membrane. This could lead to changes in fluidity, flexibility, permeability, and function of the membrane and membrane-bound proteins. The structure of the membrane also affects enzyme activity, receptor affinity, and transport capacity of the cell. These alterations could also affect the synthesis and/or release of NO. In this regard, Hashimoto et al. [111], showed that DHA had a greater effect than EPA in increasing membrane fluidity of endothelial cells cultured from rat thoracic aortas. These findings may be significant, in view of the greater effect of DHA than EPA on maintaining vascular function and reducing blood pressure in humans [20,21].

Improved Cardiac Function

The reduction in heart rate observed in animals [112,113] and humans [20,52,53,114] following dietary ω3 fatty acid intake suggests that there may be a significant cardiac component associated with the antihypertensive effects. This is possibly mediated by effects on autonomic nerve function or β-adrenoreceptor activity. Studies in humans have also shown that ω3 fatty acids decreased heart rate variability, which is a powerful predictor of mortality, sudden cardiac death, and arrhythmic events in postmyocardial infarction patients [115]. Christensen et al. [116] reported significantly increased heart rate variability in human survivors of myocardial infarction, suggesting an antiarrhythmic effect. In a subsequent report, the same authors demonstrated a beneficial dose-dependent effect of ω3 fatty acids on heart rate variability in healthy men and women randomized to either ω3 fatty acids or olive oil for 12 weeks [117].

In humans, Mori et al. [20] recently demonstrated that heart rate reduction following ω3 fatty acids was due to DHA and not EPA. The authors showed that in overweight, mildly hyperlipidemic, but otherwise healthy men given 6 g daily EPA, DHA, or olive oil for 6 weeks, 24-hr awake and asleep heart rates fell 3.5, 3.7, and 2.8 bpm, respectively [20]. Interestingly, EPA resulted in an insignificant rise in heart rates. These differential effects of EPA and DHA on heart rate were substantiated by the findings of Grimsgaard et al. [114].

Conceivably, incorporation of ω3 fatty acids into myocardial cells results in metabolic and functional changes allied to those implicated in the antiarrhythmic effects of fish oils in experimental animal, human, and cell culture studies [11,118]. Such studies suggest that ω3 fatty acids are incorporated into myocardial cells and alter electrophysiological function in a manner that reduces the vulnerability to ventricular fibrillation. The antiarrhythmic effects of ω3 fatty acids are considered to be related to their ability to inhibit myocardial Ca^{2+} overload [119], thromboxane production [120], ischaemic acidosis, and ischaemic K^+ loss [121]. Moreover, it has been shown that the free fatty acids and not phospholipid-bound fatty acids conferred the inhibitory effect [122,123]. McLennan et al. [80] have also shown that DHA, but not EPA, prevented ischemia-induced cardiac arrhythmias in Hooded Wistar rats fed purified oils for 5 weeks, confirming the differential effects demonstrated in humans [20,114].

PRACTICAL RECOMMENDATIONS

Most populations prone to hypertension have a very low intake of dietary ω3 fatty acids. Increasing fish consumption to at least four serving a week is most likely to have cardiovascular benefits that may help protect against hypertension, coronary disease, and ischemic stroke. Smaller amounts providing around 1 to 1.5 g/ day ω3 fatty acids appear to provide secondary prevention against coronary death. The importance of increased dietary ω3 fatty acids has recently been highlighted by the American Heart Association as an optimal approach to the prevention of coronary artery disease [124], with the nutrition committee of the AHA advising that a healthy eating pattern for desirable blood lipids and blood pressure management should include, among other nutrients, increasing fish consumption to at least two servings per week [125]. Moreover, eating fish rather than fish oil supplements has the advantage of avoiding increased total fat calories, and at the same time substituting ω3 fatty acids for saturated fat in meat products while maintaining protein and other nutrient intake. In hypertensives some modest blood pressure reduction may be seen with 3 to 4 g/day ω3 fatty acids, an effect that can become substantial when increased fish consumption is part of a broader dietary change along with increased fruit and vegetable consumption and moderation of salt intake [126], and fish is incorporated into weight-reducing regimens [53]. In hypertensive diabetics recommended to increase ω3 fatty acid intake, closer monitoring of glycemic control is advisable initially while randomized controlled trials of the effects of increasing ω3 fatty acid consumption on cardiovascular outcome may be justified in these high-risk subjects.

REFERENCES

1. Kannel WB, Higgins M. Smoking and hypertension as predictors of cardiovascular risk in population studies. J Hypertens 1990; 8(5):S3–8.
2. Stamler J, Stamler R, Neaton JD. Blood pressure, systolic and diastolic, and cardiovascular risks. US population data. Arch Int Med 1993; 153(5):598–615.

3. 1999 World Health Organization–International Society of Hypertension Guidelines for the Management of Hypertension. Guidelines Subcommittee. J Hypertens 1999; 17(2):151–183.
4. Bonaa KH, Thelle DS. Association between blood pressure and serum lipids in a population: the Tromso Study. Circulation 1991; 83(4):1305–1314.
5. DeFronzo RA, Ferrannini E. Insulin resistance: a multifaceted syndrome responsible for NIDDM, obesity, hypertension, dyslipidemia, and atherosclerotic cardiovascular disease. Diabetes Care 1991; 14(3):173–194.
6. Beilin LJ. Lifestyle and hypertension—an overview. Clin Exper Hypertens 1999; 21(5–6):749–762.
7. Health effects of ω3 polyunsaturated fatty acids in seafoods. In: Simopoulos AP, Kifer RR, Martin RE, Barlow SM., eds. World Review of Nutrition and Dietetics. Basel: Karger, 1991.
8. von Schacky C. n-3 Fatty acids and the prevention of coronary atherosclerosis. Am J Clin Nutr 2000; 71(1 suppl.):224S–227S.
9. Appel LJ, Miller ER III, Seidler AJ, Whelton PK. Does supplementation of diet with "fish oil" reduce blood pressure? Arch Int Med 1993; 153: 1429–1438.
10. Morris MC, Sacks F, Rosner B. Does fish oil lower blood pressure? A meta-analysis of controlled trials. Circulation 1993; 88:523–533.
11. Leaf A, Kang JX. Prevention of cardiac sudden death by N-3 fatty acids: a review of the evidence. J Int Med 1996; 240(1):5–12.
12. McVeigh GE, Brennan GM, Cohn JN, Finkelstein SM, Hayes RJ, Johnston GD. Fish oil improves arterial compliance in non-insulin-dependent diabetes mellitus. Arterioscler Thromb 1994; 14(9):1425–1429.
13. Chin JP. Marine oils and cardiovascular reactivity. Prost Leuk Essent Fatty Acids 1994; 50:211–222.
14. Harris WS. Fish oils and plasma lipid and lipoprotein metabolism in humans: a critical review. J Lipid Res 1989; 30:785–807.
15. Harris WS. n-3 Fatty acids and lipoproteins: comparison of results from human and animal studies. Lipids 1996; 31(3):243–252.
16. Harris WS. n-3 fatty acids and serum lipoproteins: human studies. Am J Clin Nutr 1997; 65(5 suppl.):1645S–1654S.
17. Alexander JW. Immunonutrition: the role of omega-3 fatty acids. Nutrition 1998; 14(7–8):627–633.
18. Mori TA, Bao DQ, Burke V, Puddey IB, Watts GF, O'Neal DN, Best JD, Beilin LJ. Purified eicosapentaenoic acid and docosahexaenoic acid have differential effects of on serum lipids and lipoproteins, LDL—particle size, glucose and insulin, in mildly hyperlipidaemic men. Am J Clin Nutr 2000; 71:1085–1094.
19. Grimsgaard S, Bonaa KH, Hansen JB, Nordoy A. Highly purified eicosapentaenic acid and docosahexaenic acid in humans have similar triacylglycerol-lowering effects but divergent effects on serum fatty acids. Am J Clin Nutr 1997; 66:649–659.
20. Mori TA, Bao DQ, Burke V, Puddey IB, Beilin LJ. Docosahexaenoic acid but

not eicosapentaenoic acid lowers ambulatory blood pressure and heart rate in humans. Hypertension 1999; 34:253–260.
21. Mori TA, Watts GF, Burke V, Bao DQ, Hilme E, Beilin LJ, Puddey IB. Differential effects of eicosapentaenoic acid and docosahexaenoic acid on forearm vascular reactivity of the microcirculation in hyperlipidaemic, overweight men. Circulation 2000; 102:(11):1264–1269.
22. Bang HO, Dyerberg J, Nielsen AB. Plasma lipid and lipoprotein pattern in Greenlandic west-coast Eskimos. Lancet 1971;1(7710):1143–1145.
23. Dyerberg J, Bang HO, Stoffersen E, Moncada S, Vane JR. Eicosapentaenoic acid and prevention of thrombosis and atherosclerosis? Lancet 1978;2(8081): 117–119.
24. Sanders TA, Vickers M, Haines AP. Effect on blood lipids and haemostasis of a supplement of cod-liver oil, rich in eicosapentaenoic and docosahexaenoic acids, in healthy young men. Clin Sci 1981;61(3):317–324.
25. Kromhout D, Bosschieter EB, de Lezenne Coulander C. The inverse relation between fish consumption and 20-year mortality from coronary heart disease. N Engl J Med 1985;312(19):1205–1209.
26. Kromhout D, Feskens EJ, Bowles CH. The protective effect of a small amount of fish on coronary heart disease mortality in an elderly population. Int J Epidemiol 1995;24(2):340–345.
27. Norell SE, Ahlbom A, Feychting M, Pedersen NL. Fish consumption and mortality from coronary heart disease. BMJ 1986;293(6544):426.
28. Dolecek TA. Epidemiological evidence of relationships between dietary polyunsaturated fatty acids and mortality in the multiple risk factor intervention trial. Proc Soc Exper Biol Med 1992;200(2):177–182.
29. Albert CM, Hennekens CH, O'Donnell CJ, Ajani UA, Carey VJ, Willett WC, Ruskin JN, Manson JE. Fish consumption and risk of sudden cardiac death. JAMA 1998;279(1):23–28.
30. Daviglus ML, Stamler J, Orencia AJ, Dyer AR, Liu K, Greenland P, Walsh MK, Morris D, Shekelle RB. Fish consumption and the 30-year risk of fatal myocardial infarction. N Engl J Med 1997;336(15):1046–1053.
31. Siscovick DS, Raghunathan TE, King I, Weinmann S, Wicklund KG, Albright J, Bovbjerg V, Arbogast P, Smith H, Kushi LH, et al. Dietary intake and cell membrane levels of long-chain n-3 polyunsaturated fatty acids and the risk of primary cardiac arrest. JAMA 1995;274(17):1363–1367.
32. Burchfiel CM, Reed DM, Strong JP, Sharp DS, Chyou PH, Rodriguez BL. Predictors of myocardial lesions in men with minimal coronary atherosclerosis at autopsy: the Honolulu heart program. Ann Epidemiol 1996; 6(2):137–146.
33. Morris MC, Manson JE, Rosner B, Buring JE, Willett WC, Hennekens CH. Fish consumption and cardiovascular disease in the physicians' health study: a prospective study. Am J Epidemiol 1995;142(2):166–175.
34. Ascherio A, Rimm EB, Stampfer MJ, Giovannucci EL, Willett WC. Dietary intake of marine n-3 fatty acids, fish intake, and the risk of coronary disease among men. N Engl J Med 1995;332(15):977–982.

35. Marckmann P, Gronbaek M. Fish consumption and coronary heart disease mortality: a systematic review of prospective cohort studies. Eur J Clin Nutr 1999;53(8):585–590.
36. Burr ML, Fehily AM, Gilbert JF, Rogers S, Holliday RM, Sweetnam PM, Elwood PC, Deadman NM. Effects of changes in fat, fish, and fibre intakes on death and myocardial reinfarction: diet and reinfarction trial (DART). Lancet 1989;2(8666):757–761.
37. GISSI-Prevenzione Investigators. Dietary supplementation with n-3 polyunsaturated fatty acids and vitamin E after myocardial infarction: results of the GISSI-Prevenzione trial. Gruppo Italiano per lo Studio della Sopravvivenza nell'Infarto miocardico. Lancet 1999;354(9177):447–455.
38. Pauletto P, Puato M, Caroli MG, Casiglia E, Munhambo AE, Cazzolato G, Bittolo Bon G, Angelli MT, Galli C, Pessina AC. Blood pressure and atherogenic lipoprotein profiles of fish-diet and vegetarian villagers in Tanzania: the Lugalawa study. Lancet 1996;348:784–788.
39. Iso H, Rexrode KM, Stampfer MJ, Manson JE, Colditz GA, Speizer FE, Hennekens CH, Willett WC. Intake of fish and omega-3 fatty acids and risk of stroke in women. JAMA 2001;285(3):304–312.
40. Bonaa KH, Bjerve, KS, Straume B, Gram IT, Thelle D. Effect of eicosapentaenoic acid and docosahexaenoic acid on blood pressure in hypertension: a population based intervention trial from the Tromso study. N Engl J Med 1990;322:795–801.
41. Knapp HR, FitzGerald GA. The antihypertensive effects of fish oil: a controlled study of polyunsaturated fatty acid supplements in essential hypertension. N Engl J Med 1989;320(16):1037–1043.
42. Radack K, Deck C, Huster G. The effects of low doses of n-3 fatty acid supplementation on blood pressure in hypertensive subjects: a randomized controlled trial. Arch Int Med 1991;151(6):1173–1180.
43. Norris PG, Jones CJ, Weston MJ. Effect of dietary supplementation with fish oil on systolic blood pressure in mild essential hypertension. BMJ 1986; 293(6539):104–105.
44. Singer P, Berger I, Luck K, Taube C, Naumann E, Godicke W. Long-term effect of mackerel diet on blood pressure, serum lipids and thromboxane formation in patients with mild essential hypertension. Atherosclerosis 1986; 62(3):259–265.
45. Levinson PD, Iosiphidis AH, Saritelli AL, Herbert PN, Steiner M. Effects of n-3 fatty acids in essential hypertension. Am J Hypertens 1990;3(10): 754–760.
46. Prisco D, Paniccia R, Bandinelli B, Filippini M, Francalanci I, Giusti B, Giurlani L, Gensini GF, Abbate R, Neri Serneri GG. Effect of medium-term supplementation with a moderate dose of n-3 polyunsaturated fatty acids on blood pressure in mild hypertensive patients. Thromb Res 1998;91(3):105–112.
47. Toft I, Bonna KH, Ingebretsen OC, Nordoy A, Jenssen T. Effects of n-3 polyunsaturated fatty acids on glucose homeostasis and blood pressure in essential hypertension: a randomized, controlled trial. Ann Int Med 1995;123:911–918.

48. Cobiac L, Nestel PJ, Wing LM, Howe PRC. A low sodium diet supplemented with fish oil lowers blood pressure in the elderly. J Hyperten 1992;10:87–92.
49. Singer P, Melzer S, Goschel M, Augustin S. Fish oil amplifies the effect of propranolol in mild essential hypertension. Hypertension 1990;16(6):682–691.
50. Howe PR, Lungershausen YK, Cobiac L, Dandy G, Nestel PJ. Effect of sodium restriction and fish oil supplementation on BP and thrombotic risk factors in patients treated with ACE inhibitors. J Human Hypertens 1994;8(1):43–49.
51. Lungershausen YK, Abbey M, Nestel PJ, Howe PR. Reduction of blood pressure and plasma triglycerides by omega-3 fatty acids in treated hypertensives. J Hypertens 1994;12(9):1041–1045.
52. Vandongen R, Mori TA, Burke V, Beilin LJ, Morris J, Ritchie J. Effects on blood pressure of ω3 fats in subjects at increased risk of cardiovascular disease. Hypertension 1993;22:371–379.
53. Bao DQ, Mori TA, Burke V, Puddey IB, Beilin LJ. Effects of dietary fish and weight reduction on ambulatory blood pressure in overweight hypertensives. Hypertension 1998; 32: 710–717.
54. Mori TA, Bao, Burke V, Puddey IB, Watts GF, Beilin LJ. Dietary fish as a major component of a weight reducing diet: impact on serum lipids, glucose and insulin metabolism in overweight hypertensive subjects. Am J Clin Nutr 1999;70(5):817–825.
55. Mori TA, Beilin LJ, Burke V, Morris J, Ritchie J. Interractions between dietary fat, fish and fish oils, on platelet function in men at risk of cardiovascular disease. Arterioscler Thromb Vasc Biol 1997;17 (2):279–286.
56. Grundt H, Nilsen DWT, Hetland O, Aarsland T, Baksaas I, Grande T, Woie L. Improvement of serum lipids and blood pressure during intervention with n-3 fatty acids was not associated with changes in insulin levels in subjects with combined hyperlipidemia. J Int Med 1995;237:249–259.
57. Dunstan DW, Mori TA, Puddey IB, Beilin LJ, Burke V, Morton AR, Stanton KG. The independent and combined effects of aerobic exercise and dietary fish on serum lipids and glycemic control in non-insulin-dependent diabetes mellitus: a randomised, controlled study. Diabetes Care 1997;20(6): 913–921.
58. Woodman RJ, Mori TA, Burke V, Puddey IB, Watts GF, Beilin LJ. Effects of purified eicosapentaenoic and docosahesaenoic acids on glycemic control, blood pressure, and serum lipids in type 2 diabetic patients with treated hypertension. Am J Clin Nutr 2002; 76:1007–1015.
59. Schoene NW, Fiore D. Effect of a diet containing fish oil on blood pressure in spontaneously hypertensive rats. Prog Lipid Res 1981; 20:569–570.
60. Singer P, Moritz V, Wirth M, Berger I. Forster D. Blood pressure and serum lipids from SHR after diets supplemented with evening primrose, sunflowerseed or fish oil. Prost Leuk Essent Fatty Acids 1990; 40(1):17–20.
61. Karanja N, Phanouvong T, McCarron DA. Blood pressure in spontaneously hypertensive rats fed butterfat, corn oil, or fish oil. Hypertension 1989; 14(6):674–679.

62. Yin K, Chu ZM, Beilin LJ. Effects of fish oil feeding on blood pressure and vascular reactivity in spontaneously hypertensive rats (SHR). Clin Exper Pharmacol Physiol 1990; 17(3):235–239.
63. Yin K, Chu ZM, Beilin LJ. Blood pressure and vascular reactivity changes in spontaneously hypertensive rats fed fish oil. Br J Pharmacol 1991; 102: 991–997.
64. Bayorh MA, McGee L, Feuerstein G. Acute and chronic effects of eicosapentaenoic acid (EPA) on the cardiovascular system. Res Comm Chem Path Pharm 1989; 66(3):355–374.
65. Head RJ, Mano MT, Bexis S, Howe PR, Smith RM. Dietary fish oil administration retards the development of hypertension and influences vascular neuroeffector function in the stroke prone spontaneously hypertensive rat (SHRSP). Prost Leuk Essent Fatty Acids 1991; 44(2):119–122.
66. Howe PR, Lungershausen YK, Rogers PF, Gerkens JF, Head RJ, Smith RM. Effects of dietary sodium and fish oil on blood pressure development in stroke-prone spontaneously hypertensive rats. J Hypertens 1991; 9(7):639–644.
67. Codde JP, Croft KD, Beilin LJ. The effect of salt loading on blood pressure and eicosanoid metabolism of spontaneously hypertensive rats fed a fish oil enriched diet. Clin Exp Pharmacol Physiol 1986;13:371–375.
68. Howe PR, Rogers PF, Lungershausen Y. Blood pressure reduction by fish oil in adult rats with established hypertension dependence on sodium intake. Prost Leuk Essent Fatty Acids 1991; 44(2):113–117.
69. Rayner TE, Howe PR. Purified omega-3 fatty acids retard the development of proteinuria in salt-loaded hypertensive rats. J Hypertens 1995; 13(7):771–780.
70. Mills DE, Ward RP, Mah M, DeVette L. Dietary N-6 and N-3 fatty acids and salt-induced hypertension in the borderline hypertensive rat. Lipids 1989; 24(1):17–24.
71. Codde JP, Beilin LJ. Dietary fish oil prevents dexamethasone induced hypertension in the rat. Clin Sci 1985; 69:691–699.
72. Yin K, Chu ZM, Beilin LJ. Study of mechanisms of glucocorticoid hypertension in rats: endothelial related changes and their amelioration by dietary fish oils. Brit J Pharmacol 1992; 106:435–442.
73. Codde JP, McGowan HM, Vandongen R, Beilin LJ. Changes to prostanoid synthesis in response to diet in the one-kidney, one-clip Goldblatt rat. Hypertension 1985; 7(6):886–892.
74. Hodge J, Sanders K, Sinclair AJ. Differential utilization of eicosapentaenoic acid and docosahexaenoic acid in human plasma. Lipids 1993; 28:525–531.
75. Mori TA, Codde JP, Vandongen R, Beilin LJ. New findings in the fatty acid composition of individual platelet phospholipids in man after dietary fish oil supplementation. Lipids 1987; 22:744–750.
76. Froyland L, Vaagenes H, Asiedu DK, Garras A, Lie O, Berge RK. Chronic administration of eicosapentaenoic and docosahexaenoic acid as ethyl esters reduced plasma cholesterol and changed the fatty acid composition in rat blood and organs. Lipids 1996; 31(2):169–178.

77. De Caterina R, Cybulsky MI, Clinton SK, Gimbrone MA Jr, Libby P. The omega-3 fatty acid docosahexaenoate reduces cytokine-induced expression of proatherogenic and proinflammatory proteins in human endothelial cells. Arterioscler Thromb 1994; 14:1829–1836.
78. Rambjor GS, Walen AI, Windsor SL, Harris WS. Eicosapentaenoic acid is primarily responsible for hypotriglyceridemic effect of fish oil in humans. Lipids 1996; 31:S45–S49.
79. Nelson GJ, Schmidt PS, Bartolini GL, Kelley DS, Kyle D. The effect of dietary docosahexaenoic acid on platelet function, platelet fatty acid composition, and blood coagulation in humans. Lipids 1997;32(11):1129–1136.
80. McLennan P, Howe P, Abeywardena M, Muggli R, Raederstorff D, Mano M, Rayner T, Head R. The cardiovascular protective role of docosahexaenoic acid. Eur J Pharmacol 1996; 300:83–89.
81. Kimura S, Minami M, Saito H, Kobayashi T, Okuyama H. Dietary docosahexaenoic acid (22:6 n-3) prevents the development of hypertension in SHRSP. Clin Exp Pharmacol Physiol 1995; (suppl. 1):S308–309.
82. Sasaki S, Nakamura K, Uchida A, Fujita H, Itoh H, Nakata T, Takeda K, Nakagawa M. Effects of gamma-linolenic and eicosapentaenoic acids on blood pressure in SHR. Clin Exp Pharmacol Physiol 1995;22(suppl. 1):S306–307.
83. Chu ZM, Yin K, Beilin LJ. Fish oil feeding selectively attenuates contractile responses to noradrenaline and electrical stimulation in the perfused mesenteric resistance vessels of spontaneously hypertensive rats. Clin Exp Pharmacol Physiol 1992; 19:177–181.
84. Lorenz R, Spengler U, Fischer S, Duhm J, Weber PC. Platelet function, thromboxane formation and blood pressure control during supplementation of the western diet with cod liver oil. Circulation 1983; 67:504–511.
85. Yoshimura T, Matsui K, Ito M, Yunohara T, Kawasaki N, Nakamura T, Okamura H. Effects of highly purified eicosapentaenoic acid on plasma beta thromboglobulin level and vascular reactivity to angiotensin II. Artery 1987; 14:295–303.
86. Chin JPF, Gust AP, Nestel PJ, Dart AM. Fish oils dose-dependently inhibit vasoconstriction of forearm resistance vessels in humans. Hypertension 1993; 21:22–28.
87. Chin JPF, Gust AP, Dart AM. Indomethacin inhibits the effects of dietary supplementation with fish oils on vasoconstriction of human forearm resistance vessels in vivo. J Hypertens 1993; 11:1229–1234.
88. Vekshtein VI, Yeung AC, Vita JA, et al. Fish oil improves endothelium-dependent relaxation in patients with coronary artery disease. Circulation 1989; 80(suppl. II):434.
89. Fleischhauer FJ, Yan W-D, Fischell TA. Fish oil improves endothelium-dependent coronary vasodilation in heart transplant recipients. J Amer Coll Cardiol 1993; 21:982–989.
90. Shimokawa H, Vanhoutte PM. Dietary cod-liver oil improves endothelium-dependent response in hypercholesterolaemic and atherosclerotic porcine arteries. Circulation 1988; 78:1421–1430.

91. Chin JPF, Dart AM. Therapeutic restoration of endothelial function in hypercholesterolaemic subjects: effect of fish oils. Clin Exp Pharmacol Physiol 1994; 21:749–755.
92. McVeigh GE, Brennan GM, Johnston GD, McDermott BJ, McGrath LT, Henry WR, Andrews JW, Hayes JR. Dietary fish oil augments nitric oxide production or release in patients with type 2 (non-insulin dependent) diabetes mellitus. Diabetologia 1993; 36:33–38.
93. Shimokawa H, Lam JYT, Chesebro JH, Bowie EJW, Vanhoutte PM. Effects of dietary supplementation with cod-liver oil on endothelium-dependent response in porcine coronary arteries. Circulation 1987; 76:898–905.
94. Schini VB, Durante W, Catovsky S, Vanhoutte PM. Eicosapentaenoic acid potentiates the production of nitric oxide evoked by interleukin-1β in cultured vascular smooth muscle cells. J Vasc Res 1993; 30:209–217.
95. Boulanger C, Schini VB, Hendrickson H, Vanhoutte PM. Chronic exposure of cultured endothelial cells to eicosapentaenoic acid potentiates the release of endothelium-derived relaxing factor(s). Br J Pharmacol 1990; 99:176–180.
96. Goodfellow J, Bellamy MF, Ramsey MW, Jones CJ, Lewis MJ. Dietary supplementation with marine omega-3 fatty acids improve systemic large artery endothelial function in subjects with hypercholesterolemia. J Am Coll Cardiol 2000; 35(2):265–270.
97. Engler MB, Engler MM, Ursell PC. Vasorelaxant properties of n-3 polyunsaturated fatty acids in aortas from spontaneously hypertensive and normotensive rats. J Cardiovasc Risk 1994; 1:75–80.
98. Harris WS, Rambjor GS, Windsor SL, Diederich D. n-3 Fatty acids and urinary excretion of nitric oxide metabolites in humans. Am J Clin Nutr 1997; 65:459–464.
99. Chin JP, Dart AM. How do fish oils affect vascular function? Clin Exper Pharm Physiol 1995; 22:71–81.
100. Fox PL, DiCorleto PE. Fish oils inhibit endothelial cell production of platelet-derived growth factor-like protein. Science 1988; 241:453–456.
101. Schini VB, Durante W, Elizondo E, Scott-Burden T, Junquero DC, Schafer AI, Vanhoutte PM. The induction of nitric oxide synthase activity is inhibited by TGF-β_1, $PDGF_{AB}$ and $PDGF_{BB}$ in vascular smooth muscle cells. Eur J Pharmacol 1992; 216:379–383.
102. McVeigh GE, Brennan GM, Cohn JN, Finkelstein SM, Hayes RJ, Johnston GD. Fish oil improves arterial compliance in non-insulin-dependent diabetes mellitus. Arterioscler Thromb 1994; 14(9):1425–1429.
103. Fischer S, Weber PC. Thromboxane A_3 (TXA_3) is formed in human platelets after dietary eicosapentaenoic acid (C20:5 ω3). Biochem Biophys Res Commun 1983; 116(3):1091–1099.
104. Knapp HR, Reilly IA, Alessandrini P, FitzGerald GA. In vivo indexes of platelet and vascular function during fish-oil administration in patients with atherosclerosis. N Engl J Med 1986; 314(15):937–942.
105. Fischer S, Weber PC. Prostaglandin I_3 is formed in vivo in man after dietary eicosapentaenoic acid. Nature 1984; 307(5947):165–168.

106. Needleman P, Raz A, Minkes MS, Ferrendelli JA, Sprecher H. Triene prostaglandins: prostacyclin and thromboxane biosynthesis and unique biological properties. Proc Natl Acad Sci USA 1979; 76(2):944–948.
107. Hashimoto M, Shinozuka K, Gamoh S, Tanabe Y, Hossain MS, Kwon YM, Hata N, Misawa Y, Kunitomo M, Masumura S. The hypotensive effect of docosahexaenoic acid is associated with the enhanced release of ATP from the caudal artery of aged rats. J Nutr 1999; 129:70–76.
108. De Mey JG, Vanhoutte PM. Role of the intima in cholinergic and purinergic relaxation of isolated canine femoral arteries. J Physiol 1981; 316:347–355.
109. Burnstock G. Local control of blood pressure by purines. Blood Vessels 1987; 24:156–160.
110. Nishiye E, Chen GF, Hirose T, Kuriyama H. Mechanical and electrical properties of smooth muscle cells and their regulations by endothelium-derived factors in the guinea pig coronary artery. Jpn J Pharmacol 1990; 54:391–405.
111. Hashimoto M, Hossain S, Yamasaki H, Yazawa K, Masumura S. Effects of eicosapentaenoic acid and docosahexaenoic acid on plasma membrane fluidity of aortic endothelial cells. Lipids 1999; 34(12):1297–1304.
112. Billman GE, Hallaq H, Leaf A. Prevention of ischemia-induced ventricular fibrillation by omega 3 fatty acids. Proc Natl Acad Sci USA 1994; 91(10): 4427–4430.
113. McLennan PL, Barnden LR, Bridle TM, Abeywardena MY, Charnock JS. Dietary fat modulation of left ventricular ejection fraction in the marmoset due to enhanced filling. Cardiovasc Res 1992; 26(9):871–877.
114. Grimsgaard S, Bonaa KH, Hansen JB, Myhre ESP. Effects of highly purified eicosapentaenoic acid and docosahexaenoic acid on hemodynamics in humans. Am J Clin Nutr 1998; 68(1):52–59.
115. Hartikainen JE, Malik M, Staunton A, Poloniecki J, Camm AJ. Distinction between arrhythmic and nonarrhythmic death after acute myocardial infarction based on heart rate variability, signal-averaged electrocardiogram, ventricular arrhythmias and left ventricular ejection fraction. J Am Coll Cardiol 1996; 28(2):296–304.
116. Christensen JH, Gustenhoff P, Korup E, Aaroe J, Toft E, Moller J, Rasmussen K, Dyerberg J, Schmidt EB. Effect of fish oil on heart rate variability in survivors of myocardial infarction: a double blind randomised controlled trial. BMJ 1996; 312(7032):677–678.
117. Christensen JH, Christensen MS, Dyerberg J, Schmidt EB. Heart rate variability and fatty acid content of blood cell membranes: a dose-response study with n-3 fatty acids. Am J Clin Nutr 1999; 70(3):331–337.
118. Leaf A, Kang JX. Dietary n-3 fatty acids in the prevention of lethal cardiac arrhythmias. Curr Opin Lipidol 1997; 8:4–6.
119. Hallaq H, Sellmayer A, Smith TW, Leaf A. Protective effect of eicosapentaenoic acid on ouabain toxicity in neonatal rat cardiac myocytes. Proc Natl Acad Sci. USA 1990; 87(20):7834–7838.
120. Abeywardena MY, McLennan PL, Charnock JS. Differential effects of dietary

fish oil on myocardial prostaglandin I_2 and thromboxane A_2 production. Am J Physiol 1991; 260(2 pt 2):H379–H385.
121. Pepe S, McLennan PL. A maintained afterload model of ischemia in erythrocyte-perfused isolated working hearts. J Pharmacol Toxicol Methods 1993; 29(4):203–210.
122. Kang JX, Leaf A. Protective effects of free polyunsaturated fatty acids on arrhythmias induced by lysophosphatidylcholine or palmitoylcarnitine in neonatal rat cardiac myocytes. Euro J Pharmacol 1996; 297(1–2):97–106.
123. Weylandt KH, Kang JX, Leaf A. Polyunsaturated fatty acids exert antiarrhythmic actions as free acids rather than in phospholipids. Lipids 1996; 31(9):977–982.
124. Krauss RM, Eckel RH, Howard B, Appel LJ, Daniels SR, Deckelbaum RJ, Erdman JW Jr, Kris-Etherton P, Goldberg IJ, Kotchen TA, Lichtenstein AH, Mitch WE, Mullis R, Robinson K, Wylie-Rosett J, St Jeor S, Suttie J, Tribble DL, Bazzarre TL. AHA Dietary Guidelines: revision 2000: a statement for healthcare professionals from the Nutrition Committee of the American Heart Association. Circulation 2000;102(18):2284–2299.
125. Kris-Etherton P, Daniels SR, Eckel RH, Engler M, Howard BV, Krauss RM, Lichtenstein AH, Sacks F, St Jeor S, Stampfer M, Eckel RH, Grundy SM, Appel LJ, Byers T, Campos H, Cooney G, Denke MA, Howard BV, Kennedy E, Krauss RM, Kris-Etherton P, Lichtenstein AH, Marckmann P, Pearson TA, Riccardi G, Rudel LL, Rudrum M, Sacks F, Stein DT, Tracy RP, Ursin V, Vogel RA, Zock PL, Bazzarre TL, Clark J. Summary of the scientific conference on dietary fatty acids and cardiovascular health: conference summary from the nutrition committee of the American Heart Association. Circulation 2001;103(7):1034–1039.
126. Sacks FM, Svetkey LP, Vollmer WM, Appel LJ, Bray GA, Harsha D, Obarzanek E, Conlin PR, Miller ER III, Simons-Morton DG, Karanja N, Lin PH. DASH-Sodium Collaborative Research Group. Effects on blood pressure of reduced dietary sodium and the Dietary Approaches to Stop Hypertension (DASH) diet. DASH-Sodium Collaborative Research Group. New Engl J Med 2001;344(1):3–10.

13

Biofeedback and Relaxation

Thomas Pickering and Mohammad Rafey
Mount Sinai Medical Center, New York, New York, U.S.A.

INTRODUCTION

Patients are always looking for a way of treating hypertension that does not sentence them to a lifetime of taking drugs, and since there is a common perception that hypertension is one of the results of the stressful lives we all lead these days, techniques that lead to stress reduction might be expected to lower blood pressure. Although procedures such as autogenic training and progressive muscular relaxation have been around for more than 50 years, the idea really took off in the early 1970s with the popularization of two forms of treatment, one ancient and the other novel—transcendental meditation and biofeedback. The former was championed by Dr. Herbert Benson in Boston, [1] and the latter by Dr. Chandra Patel in the United Kingdom [2,3]. Both groups published some quite dramatic results that indicated that these behavioral treatments could provide decreases of blood pressure of the same magnitude as drug treatment without the expense and side effects of drugs, and Benson reported a fall of 10.5/4.9 mmHg in patients on antihypertensive drugs who practiced the relaxation response regularly [4]. Thirty years later, neither procedure has established a place in the routine treatment of hypertension, although both are used for other purposes. Despite the lack of enthusiasm of the medical profession for this type of treatment, the public nevertheless is still interested. In a 1993 survey of the use of unconventional medicine in the United States [5], 11% of hypertensive patients reported using unconventional therapy in the past 12 months, mostly relaxation techniques and homeopathy.

BIOFEEDBACK

The idea of biofeedback originated with the work of Dr. Neal Miller, a renowned experimental psychologist, who first developed the concept of "visceral learning" [6]. It was based on a series of animal experiments that showed that rats could be trained to raise and lower their blood pressure using psychological conditioning techniques. This was translated into human studies, in which subjects were instructed to learn voluntary blood pressure control by attempting to keep a tone sounding, which was triggered by changes of blood pressure in the appropriate direction. Put another way, the rationale was that one reason why we cannot normally control our autonomic functions voluntarily is that we lack the conscious perception of them, and that if this is provided (by biofeedback) we can learn to "drive our own bodies," as one of the early enthusiasts put it. While the concept was attractive and supported by some positive early results, it has not stood the test of time.

A number of bodily functions have been used to provide biofeedback in addition to blood pressure. These include muscle tension (electromyography, or EMG), and skin temperature. In the former, case subjects are trained to reduce muscle tension and in the latter to warm their hands. There is no conclusive evidence that any one technique is superior to any other. While some studies have used pure biofeedback, most have combined it with relaxation training. While initially encouraging, studies using pure biofeedback were less likely to show significant effects on blood pressure when measurements made out of the office were included. An example is a study by Blanchard et al. [7], in which thermal biofeedback (training subjects to warm their hands and feet) was found to have no effect on home or ambulatory blood pressure. A meta-analysis reported by Eisenberg et al. [8] included six groups (n = 90) that underwent biofeedback without combination with other behavioral therapies. The blood pressure reduction was minimal (–2.6/0.2 mmHg) in comparison with patients who were wait-list controls or who underwent sham therapies (–2.9/–1.2 mmHg), and in whom the baseline blood pressure measurements had extended beyond 1 day. Even in the studies that show improvement in the blood pressure with direct biofeedback, long-term follow-up data beyond a 6-month period has been inconsistent or lacking.

TABLE 1 Meta-Analysis of Effects of Biofeedback (BFB) on Blood Pressure

Comparison	Mean change (mmHg)	95% CI	Number of studies
Systolic pressure			
BFB vs. active control	−2.1	−7.0, 2.9	6
BFB vs. inactive control	−6.7[a]	−10.2, −3.2	14
Diastolic pressure			
BFB vs. active control	−3.4	−7.4, 0.6	6
BFB vs. inactive control	−4.8[a]	−7.2, −2.3	13

[a] $p<0.05$
Source: Data from Yucha et al. [9].

A more recent meta-analysis by Yucha et al. [9] concluded that when biofeedback was compared against an active control group (such as relaxation training, cognitive behavioral therapy, or self-monitoring) the changes were insignificant, but when compared against an "inactive" control (wait-list control, or sham biofeedback), significant effects on clinic blood pressure were achieved. These changes are summarized in Table 1.

The same meta-analysis looked at the different types of biofeedback to see if any one appeared to be superior. The authors concluded that thermal and EDA (electrodermal activity) biofeedback were superior to combined EMG and blood pressure feedback (Table 2), but the numbers of studies are too small to allow any definitive conclusions.

TABLE 2 Meta-Analysis of Effects of Different Types of Biofeedback (BFB) on Blood Pressure

Comparison	Mean change (mmHg)	95% CI	Number of studies
Systolic pressure			
Thermal BFB vs. inactive control	−5.0	−9.1, −0.9	5
EDA BFB vs. inactive control	−7.1	−14.3, 0.2	3
EMG/BP BFB vs. inactive control	0.2	−5.6, 6.1	2
Diastolic pressure			
Thermal BFB vs. inactive control	−6.3	−9.9, −2.7	4
EDA BFB vs. inactive control	−3.8	−7.0, −0.6	3
EMG/BP BFB vs. inactive control	1.3	−1.6, 4.3	2

Note: EDA = electrodermal activity (skin resistance); EMG/BP = combined electromyogram and blood pressure feedback.
Source: Data of Yucha et al. [9].

A novel approach has been made by Hunyor, who has developed a blood pressure biofeedback technique using a device that monitors blood pressure continuously from a finger [10] using a method similar to the Finapres device. One of the attractive features of this is that it is possible to give false feedback, so that the placebo effect can be eliminated. Subjects in the true feedback condition can be trained to raise and lower their blood pressure by attempting to move a line on a computer screen, the position of which is determined by the blood pressure. Patients in the placebo group, however, were able to produce quite similar changes, and there were no significant effects on ambulatory pressure. A second study [11] extended the training period at home, and it was demonstrated that people can learn to improve their ability to lower blood pressure with practice. Despite this technical sophistication, the effectiveness of this procedure remains equivocal. Although clinic blood pressures fell more in the treatment group (154/98 to 144/91 mmHg, as compared to 152/96 to 147/93 mmHg in the control group), the differences between the two groups were not significant.

RELAXATION TECHNIQUES

In 1938 Edmund Jacobson proposed that patients with hypertension were hypermetabolic and had excessive muscle tension, and that a reduction in this muscle tension would lead to a corresponding decrease in blood pressure [12]. His technique, known as progressive muscle relaxation, has been used for many years, and is still used today, although its effects on blood pressure are questionable. Relaxation methods induce a state of physiologic hypometabolism described by Hess [13], which in cats is associated with decreased sympathetic activity. He concluded these were protective responses that countered overstress or flight or fright responses.

In practice, relaxation therapy may range from a physician's simple advice to his patient to "relax" to more formal structured techniques. These may include such meditative techniques as yoga and Zen, based on Eastern philosophy, progressive relaxation, developed by Jacobson, or autogenic training, as developed by Luthe [14]. The common denominator in all these techniques appears to be mental focusing, task awareness, quiet sitting, and relaxation of all muscle groups. Mental focusing involves directing attention to a constant or repetitive internal or external stimulus, such as the feeling accompanying relaxation or a silently repeated word or phrase.

The following relaxation methods have been identified by Shapiro for the treatment of hypertension [15]:

Progressive relaxation: a technique directed at relaxation of major skeletal muscle groups

Autogenic training: standard "autosuggestive" exercises for inducing altered physiologic and mental states
Hypnotic relaxation: hypnosis and posthypnotic suggestion to induce physiologic and mental relaxation
Zen meditation: methods of meditation involving passive concentration on respiration and an exercise to elicit a relaxation response
Hatha yoga: relaxation elicited through bodily postures and exercises, breath control, and meditation
Transcendental meditation: a cognitive technique derived from Vedic practices in which individuals assume a comfortable position, breathe peacefully, close their eyes, and repeat a "mantra" as each breath is exhaled

Since the early 1970s several studies have shown a significant reduction in both systolic and diastolic blood pressures with relaxation therapy as the sole intervention [1,4]. Benson's group [16] showed that practicing a standardized meditation technique for 1 month resulted in reduction in blood pressure in 22 untreated borderline hypertensives (average reduction of 7 mmHg systolic and 4 mmHg diastolic) and 14 treated hypertensive patients (average blood pressure reduction of 11 mmHg systolic and 5 mmHg diastolic) that persisted for a 5-month period. Brady et al. used a metronome-conditioned relaxation therapy that achieved a significant reduction of up to 10 mmHg diastolic blood pressure in four hypertensive patients [17].

Most of the early studies were limited by weaknesses in methodology, including small sample size, absence of control groups, confounding factors such as pharmacological treatment or placebo response, statistical artifacts, including regression to the mean, and reliance on clinic or laboratory blood pressure measurements [18]. Later studies that used ambulatory blood pressure as the measure of success have provided mixed results. Two have reported positive findings. Southam et al. [19] studied the effects of relaxation therapy on 42 patients with diastolic pressures of greater than 90 mmHg who were randomized to either relaxation training or no intervention. At 6 months there was a significant reduction in the daytime ambulatory blood pressure in the treatment group (mean change of −6.0/−12.1 as compared to +1.3/−2.2 mmHg in the control group). The changes in the clinic pressure were somewhat larger than the ambulatory pressures. In a study of 39 subjects randomized to either a meditation group or a cognitive stress education control group Wenneberg et al. reported a net reduction of 9 mmHg in ambulatory diastolic pressure in the meditation group [20].

Others have found no effect on ambulatory blood pressure. A study by Jacob et al. [21] on the effect of relaxation therapy as compared with antihypertensive medications (atenolol and chlorthalidone) showed a modest but marginally significant reduction in clinic blood pressure (2 to 3 mmHg decrease in systolic and diastolic blood pressures), but no effect on ambulatory blood pressure. In contrast, the effects of the drugs were substantial and significant for both measures of blood pressure. A later one by van Montfrans et al. found a modest reduction in clinic pressure (2 mmHg), but no change in intra-arterial 24-hr pressure [22]. This issue is thus still unresolved.

As with biofeedback studies, one of the problems with relaxation studies has been that similar falls of blood pressure are often seen in both the active treatment and control groups. A good example of this is a study conducted by Irvine and Logan [23] in 100 untreated hypertensives, who were randomized to either a 12-week course of relaxation training (with a little biofeedback included in some sessions) or a nonspecific support group. Both groups received weekly sessions with the same therapists. Blood pressure fell by the same amount (5/5 mmHg) in both groups. The same thing occurred in an industry-based study by Chesney et al. [24], who found a marked reduction of clinic blood pressure of 7.4/4.5 mmHg in the treatment group (relaxation plus biofeedback), but this was also observed in the control (blood pressure monitoring) group, in which the fall was 9.0/5.9 mmHg. This study measured blood pressure not only in the clinic, but also at the worksite, where the changes were less pronounced but again virtually identical for the two groups (Fig. 1).

One factor that appears to be very important in determining the magnitude of the effects of any of these techniques on blood pressure is the pretreatment level of pressure, as shown by a meta-analysis conducted by Jacob et al. [18]. Many of the negative studies have, thus included subjects whose initial pressures were essentially normal. One example is the Trial of Hypertension Prevention, phase I (TOHP-I) [25], in which 562 healthy participants (diastolic blood pressures of 80 to 89 mm Hg) were randomized to either stress management intervention or an assessment-only (control) group. The interventions included training in relaxation techniques in addition to cognitive techniques, anger management, and improvement of communication skills and time management. Intention to treat analysis showed an absence of blood pressure-lowering efficacy in the intervention group. A second example is a study by Fiedler et al. [26], who investigated the effects of a stress management program in 66 hazardous waste workers that utilized a combination of progressive muscular relaxation and meditation techniques, and found no change in ambulatory blood pressure in either the experimental or control group. This is hardly surprising since the pretreatment work blood pressures were 124/80 mmHg and 124/79 mmHg in the experimental and control groups. The Jacob

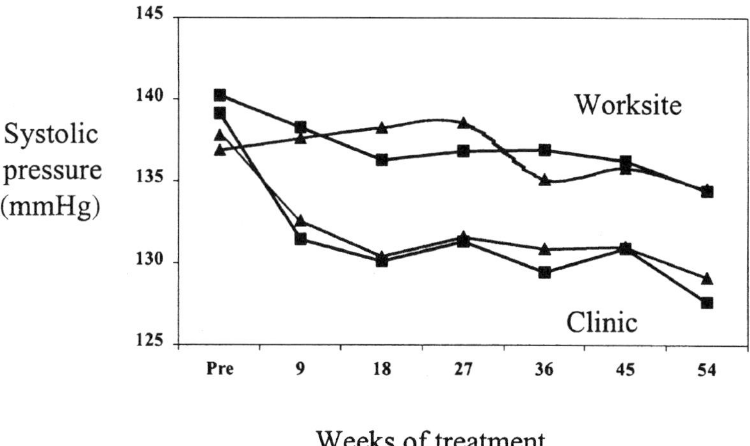

FIGURE 1 Decline of blood pressure measured both at the worksite and in the clinic during a controlled trial of relaxation therapy. Solid lines show changes in the active treatment group, and hatched lines the control group. *Source*: Data of Chesney et al. [24].

meta-analysis included 75 treatment groups and 41 control groups [18], and showed that the reduction of blood pressure after treatment was directly related to the height of the pressure before treatment. The analysis also established that the treatment effect was related to the number of pretreatment baseline readings. The expected decrease of systolic pressure with a pretreatment pressure of 140 mmHg and one baseline session thus was 9.4 mmHg, whereas if there were four baseline visits the expected decrease would be only 3.3 mmHg. This analysis suggests that regression to the mean could explain much of the treatment effects in such studies, but of course one would expect the same decrease of pressure to be seen in both the treatment and control groups (as was observed, e.g., in the Irvine and Logan study).

Several studies have compared different varieties of biofeedback and relaxation techniques, but with the exception of the controlled breathing device described below, none have shown any consistent superiority over the others [27]. Linden et al. [28] reported substantial reductions of ambulatory blood pressure (6/4 mmHg) as a result of a stress management program that utilized a variety of interventions that included autogenic training, biofeedback, cognitive therapy, and anxiety management. The exact mode of treatment was individualized, which makes it very difficult to generalize these results.

CAN THE EFFECTS OF BIOFEEDBACK AND RELAXATION BE ATTRIBUTED TO PLACEBO EFFECTS?

One of the issues has to do with the measurements of blood pressure by which the effects of the interventions were judged. The early trials used clinic measurements [2,4,29], which are known to be very susceptible to the placebo effect. It is thus now clearly recognized that blood pressure tends to increase just before a clinic visit, a phenomenon commonly called the white coat effect, which has been attributed to the anxiety associated with the visit. Any intervention that reduces anxiety thus may lower the clinic blood pressure without necessarily affecting the pressure at other times. As shown in Fig. 2, a reduction in the clinic pressure could reflect a similar reduction in the pressure measured outside the clinic, or it could simply be the result of a reduction of the white coat effect (the difference between the clinic and ambulatory pressure) without any change in the pressure outside the clinic. The former would be regarded as a therapeutic effect, while the latter may be a placebo effect. Antihypertensive drugs lower both the clinic and the ambulatory pressure, but the reduction of clinic pressure is typically greater, so that the white coat effect is diminished, but not eliminated.

One of the most dramatic demonstrations of the powers of the placebo and the effectiveness of reassurance was provided by an ingenious experiment designed by Dr. William Goldring and his colleagues, the

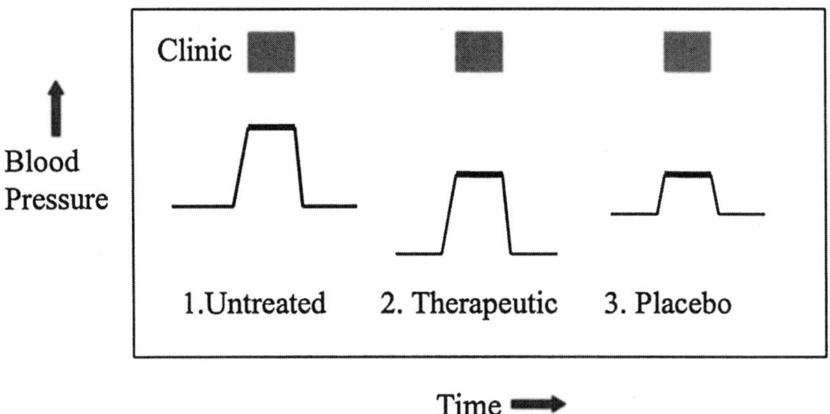

FIGURE 2 Shows how the white coat effect (the increase of blood pressure at the time of a clinic visit) may confuse the response to treatment, which lowers the clinic pressure. Panel 1 shows pattern before treatment; panel 2 a sustained reduction of blood pressure (a therapeutic response); and panel 3 a reduction of the clinic pressure without a change of the pressure outside the clinic (a placebo response).

results of which were published in 1956 [30]. They made an impressive-looking device that they called the "electron gun," which consisted of a large metal coil surmounted by a conical "gun," and an oscilloscope. The patient was seated in a darkened room with the gun pointing at his or her chest. When it was turned on the nozzle of the gun began to glow as if it was red hot, and to emit sparks and crackling sounds. At the same time a series of sinusoidal waves was displayed on the oscilloscope. The treatment was carried out by a sympathetic nurse twice a week for several months, and then discontinued. In about half of the patients the blood pressure decreased during the treatment period, with an average drop of 36/27 mmHg—a very impressive change. In addition, the patients all reported an improvement in their symptoms, and several were able to return to work. Once the treatment was discontinued, however, the pressure gradually climbed back to pretreatment levels.

One critical aspect of the placebo effect on blood pressure is the expectations of the patients, and it has been suggested that an expectation of positive results is a necessary if not sufficient condition for placebo effects [31]. Two lines of evidence support the notion that at least some of the benefits of behavioral forms of treating hypertension derive from placebo effects. First, Agras et al. studied the effects of relaxation training on blood pressure, and divided patients into two groups [32]. One was informed that the relaxation would not have an immediate effect on blood pressure, while the other was told that it would. The group with the more positive expectations showed the biggest fall in pressure. The second line of evidence comes from the control groups of these studies. In general, it has been found that the more closely the control procedure resembles the "active" treatment the more likely it is to show a fall of blood pressure [33].

Another problem with the meditation and biofeedback studies was that other investigators were unable to replicate the dramatic early results. Some of the individual studies were quite small, which limits their generalizability, and this led the National Heart, Lung, and Blood Institute to form the Hypertension Intervention Pooling Project [34], which collected data from 733 patients in nine randomized studies, all of which used various types of biofeedback or relaxation training. The results, published in 1988, were disappointing; there was no effect of the interventions in treated patients, and in untreated patients there was a modest reduction of diastolic pressure but no change in systolic. A few years later (1993) another wound to these behavioral forms of treatment was inflicted by a meta-analysis by Eisenberg et al. [8]. The authors reviewed studies using a variety of behavioral techniques, which included biofeedback, relaxation, and stress management, and identified only 26 that satisfied the selection criteria for scientific rigor. The results, while generally negative, were of interest; studies that used only a single day's readings to measure the baseline pressure and then compared the effects of the intervention with wait-list controls achieved an average reduction of 13.4/9.0 mmHg more than the controls, while those that used a longer baseline period achieved a smaller reduction (4.1/4.0 mmHg), and those that used a placebo-treated control group did not achieve any net reduction of blood pressure. One interpretation of this analysis is that the positive reports of the behavioral interventions may have been attributable to regression to the mean and the placebo effect. Most of the studies had sample sizes that may have been too small to be able to demonstrate a significant difference among the groups, however.

It could be argued that it does not matter whether the reduction of blood pressure is specific to the type of treatment or to a placebo effect, since any reduction is therapeutic. The important thing is whether the reduction is sustained over 24 hr as opposed to merely lowering the clinic pressure (a diminution of the white coat effect; see below). The solution to the placebo question is to use 24-hr ambulatory monitoring, which is the ultimate determinant of therapeutic efficacy. Any intervention that lowers blood pressure throughout the day and night can be regarded as therapeutically effective, while one that merely lowers the clinic pressure is ineffective. In general, placebos have been found to lower clinic pressure but not 24-hr pressure. Most of the studies of biofeedback and relaxation used clinic pressure, but there were some early ones that claimed a reduction of ambulatory pressure [19].

TREATMENT OF WHITE COAT HYPERTENSION

White coat hypertension is defined as a persistently elevated clinic blood pressure combined with a normal pressure outside the clinic. It is generally accepted to have a relatively benign prognosis, as shown by several prospective studies. Treatment with antihypertensive drugs tends to lower the clinic pressure, but has little effect on the ambulatory blood pressure, which by definition is normal to begin with. What little evidence there is suggests that drug treatment does not reduce the risk of cardiovascular morbidity, which is also low in the untreated condition [35]. White coat hypertension must be distinguished from the white coat effect, which is usually defined as the difference between the clinic and daytime ambulatory pressure. This is present to a greater or lesser degree in most hypertensives, but in patients with sustained hypertension the ambulatory pressures, while often markedly lower than the clinic pressures, are still elevated. The white coat effect is thus a measure of change, whereas white coat hypertension is a measure of levels.

A possibility that has to date received little attention is whether or not behavioral forms of treatment might have a beneficial effect in patients with white coat hypertension. Some years ago we attempted to treat it using systematic desensitization, which has been used with some success to treat specific phobias, such as fear of flying. The rationale for this was that white coat hypertension also appears to be characterized by an increase in blood pressure that is relatively specific to the clinic setting, as opposed to a more generalized increase in reactivity to any type of pressor stimulus. Unfortunately, the treatment was unsuccessful. Two studies, however, suggest that behavioral techniques such as biofeedback and relaxation may selectively lower clinic blood pressure. In the first, Jacob et al. [18] randomized hypertensive patients whose pressure was uncontrolled by medication to treatment with temperature biofeedback-assisted relaxation or a control (stress education) group. Blood pressure was assessed in four ways: by the therapist in the office, by a nurse in the clinic, by a physician, and by 24-hr ambulatory monitoring. No significant changes were seen in any of the measures in the control group, but in the experimental group the most striking change was in the physician pressures. These were expressed as the difference between the physician and the nurse-measured pressures (roughly equivalent to the white coat effect), and were reduced

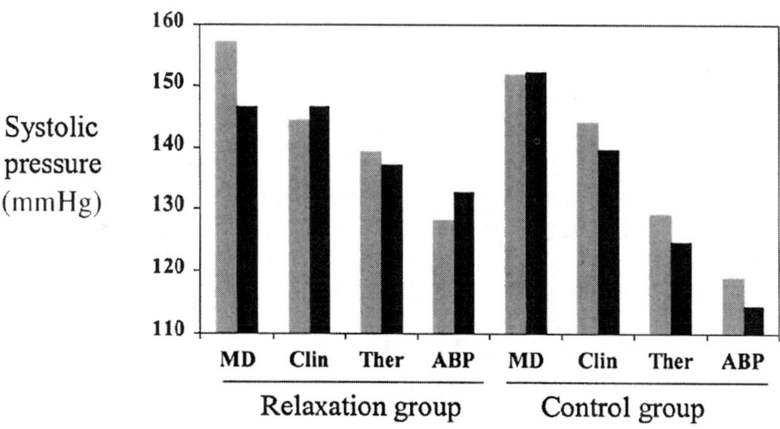

FIGURE 3 Systolic pressure before (pale bars) and after (dark bars) treatment by biofeedback-assisted relaxation or stress education (control group): MD = physician measurement; Clin = clinic measurement by a nurse; Ther = therapist measurement; ABP = ambulatory blood pressure. Note that the most marked change was the decrease in the MD pressures in the relaxation group. *Source*: Plotted from data of Jacob et al. [18].

by 14.6/5.8 mmHg in the relaxation treatment group, whereas in the control group the white coat effect was unchanged (+0.4/−1.0 mmHg). The daytime ambulatory pressure actually increased slightly in the treatment group (4.8/5.5mmHg) and decreased slightly in the control group (−4.6/3.5 mmHg). These changes are shown in Fig. 3.

The second study to show a reduction of the white coat effect was performed by Nakao et al. [36], using biofeedback from blood pressure measured continually (beat-to-beat) by a Finapres device. All the patients were hypertensive in the clinic, but were classified as sustained or white coat hypertensive according to whether their home pressures were elevated (>135/85 mmHg) or normal. Patients were randomized to a treatment group or a wait-list control group. The treatment lowered the clinic pressures by 22/11mmHg in the white coat hypertensives, but the home pressures were lowered by only 4/2 mmHg. In the sustained hypertensives the reduction of clinic pressures was a little smaller (14/8 mmHg), but the effects on home pressures were similar (4/3 mmHg). The blood pressure reactivity to mental arithmetic was also reduced in both hypertensive groups. In contrast, none of the blood pressure measures were affected in the control group. When, however, these were given the active biofeedback treatment at the end of the study, they also responded to the treatment.

CONTROLLED BREATHING TECHNIQUE—A REAL BREAKTHROUGH

The most exciting technique in this area is one that combines features of both biofeedback and relaxation training using a novel device that trains patients to lower their breathing rate to about 6 breaths per min. The device, which is marketed as the RespeRate, comprises a belt that goes round the chest to record breathing movements. The RespeRate is linked to a battery-operated monitor that detects the movements and emits a series of musical tones that have a different pitch for expiration and inspiration. The patients are instructed to synchronize their breathing to the music, and after a few breaths the device gradually begins to prolong the expiratory phase notes so that the patient gradually slows the breathing rate to a minimum of about 6/min. The device also has a data log that records the duration of use on a daily basis, and also the breathing rates achieved. Patients are encouraged to practice this for about 15 min per day. Several studies based on the use of the device have been published, and suggest that the effects are both sustained and substantial. It takes about 4 weeks for the full effects on blood pressure to be realized (Fig. 4). One study has used 24-hr blood pressure monitoring [37] and reported that in 13 hypertensive patients the average reduction was 7.2/2.3 mmHg during the day, but less at night.

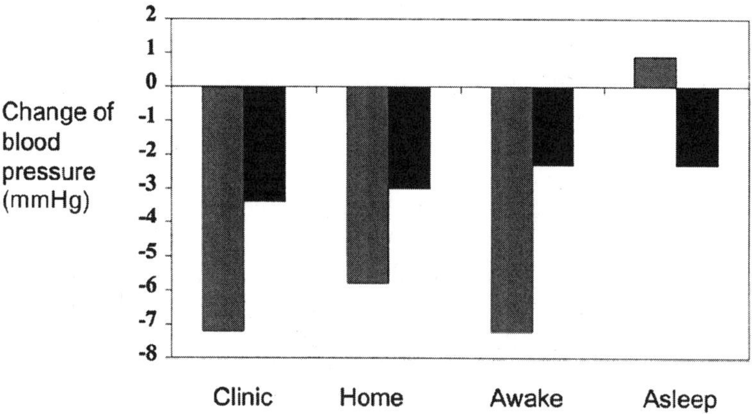

FIGURE 4 Blood pressure response to treatment with RespeRate, measured in the clinic, at home (self-monitoring), and by ambulatory monitoring (awake and asleep). *Source*: Data of Rosenthal et al. [37].

Similar changes were seen in both home and clinic pressures. The effects were greatest in older patients. Another study used a randomized controlled study design [38], with a Walkman tape player that played relaxing music as the control condition. At the end of 8 weeks there was a bigger reduction in clinic pressure in the treated group (15.2/11.3 mmHg) than in the Walkman control group (11.3/5.6 mmHg), but it should be noted that the reduction was still substantial in the latter, underscoring the need for placebo controls in studies of this nature.

MECHANISMS OF BLOOD PRESSURE REDUCTION WITH BEHAVIORAL TECHNIQUES

On the assumption that behavioral interventions can have a sustained and beneficial effect on blood pressure, it is germane to ask what mechanisms might be involved. Short-term changes of blood pressure occurring at the time of a biofeedback or relaxation training session are not hard to explain, since it has been known for years that psychological factors that lead to arousal or relaxation can have a profound acute effect on blood pressure. Since there is obviously a huge overlap between the various techniques described here, it is likely that a common set of mechanisms are involved.

Such mechanisms could be direct (i.e., operating through a primary effect on blood pressure) or indirect (i.e., operating through some other mechanism that affects blood pressure, such as increased compliance with medication). Direct mechanisms must involve either some resetting of the blood pressure-regulating processes at a lower level or a reduction of reactivity to stimuli that normally raise pressure. The two could be distinguished by the changes on nocturnal blood pressure. Antihypertensive medications generally work by the first of these, since blood pressure is usually lowered similarly throughout the day and night, but short-term variability is little changed. A study by Wenneberg et al. [20] reported that transcendental meditation (TM) resulted in a significant reduction of ambulatory pressure of 9 mmHg, but resulted in no change in the cardiovascular response to acute stressors. Other studies have also found no effect on reactivity [18]. This would suggest that a suppression of stress reactivity is not the primary mechanism of sustained blood pressure reduction. There have also been studies however, in which the reactivity to stress has been reduced [36], and in which the principal effect has been to reduce the white coat effect with little influence on ambulatory or home pressures.

A study by Barnes et al. looked at the acute hemodynamic changes in subjects who were skilled practitioners of TM, and compared them with a control group of naive subjects. The main finding was that TM resulted in a reduction of systolic pressure that was not seen in the control group when they were asked to relax with their eyes closed for 20 min. This reduction was associated with a reduction of total peripheral resistance (measured by impedance cardiography). Other studies [39] have reported that TM is associated with a decreased respiration rate, and that the mediating mechanisms linking the central nervous system and peripheral circulation might include reduced activity of the sympathetic nervous system and the hypothalamic-pituitary-adrenal axis. Patel et al. [3] reported that blood pressure reductions that resulted from a biofeedback trial were associated with a reduction of both plasma renin activity and aldosterone.

Bernardi et al. [40] trained healthy normotensive subjects to breathe at 6 breaths per min, which did not significantly change blood pressure or heart rate levels, although the variability of both was increased. More interestingly, baroreflex sensitivity was markedly increased, and the chemoreflexive responses to hypoxia and hypercapnia were both reduced. A breathing rate of 6/min may be of particular physiological significance, since it coincides with the frequency of the naturally occurring Mayer waves. Interestingly, it has also been recently pointed out [41] that this frequency is the same as the frequency of the repetitive recitation of the Ave Maria prayer used by Catholics, as well as of yoga mantras. Both of these, of course, induce a sense of calmness and well-being. Recitation of the Ave Maria induces not only a cyclical fluctuation of respiration at 6/min, but also of systolic and diastolic pressure, although the levels are not acutely changed.

It might be anticipated that the treatment effects would be greatest in those patients who have the greatest stress component to their high blood pressure. While some studies have reported that higher pretreatment levels of anxiety are associated with a more favorable blood pressure response, others did not. An example of the former was a study by Cottier et al. (see the Jacob meta-analysis [18]), who found that patients responding best to progressive muscle relaxation had higher anxiety scores, higher heart rates, and higher plasma norepinephrine levels than nonresponders. Irvine and Logan found that pretreatment stress levels did not predict the blood pressure response to treatment, and some studies even found that lower stress levels predicted a more favorable response [18].

Indirect mechanisms could also be effective, thus in the study of Irvine and Logan quoted above, alcohol consumption decreased in both the experimental and control groups (which showed similar blood pressure decreases), and this decrease of alcohol consumption appeared to correlate across groups with the fall in blood pressure.

CAN BEHAVIORAL FORMS OF TREATMENT BE COST-EFFECTIVE?

A general problem facing any type of behavioral or lifestyle intervention is that it typically involves a series of training sessions between the patient and the therapist. A typical example would be 12 weekly sessions of 45 min each [18]. This means that such interventions are not cheap. A major determinant of the cost-effectiveness of such interventions would be the duration of the effects. Most studies have not included long-term follow-up, but one that did was conducted by Agras et al. in a worksite setting [42]. The patients all had uncontrolled hypertension at entry (diastolic pressures above 90 mmHg despite taking antihypertensive therapy), and the treatment consisted of eight relaxation training sessions over 8 weeks, done either individually or in small groups. After that there were monthly follow-up sessions. As shown in Fig. 5, both groups showed a marked improvement in the rate of blood pressure control, but immediately posttreatment the rate of control was much higher in the treatment group than in the control group (69.4% vs. 41.5%). Over the next 2½ years, however, the difference between the two groups was gradually eroded, probably because the physicians changed the patients' medications. This would indicate that the cost-effectiveness of the relaxation training was low.

An exception to the necessity for intensive and prolonged personal contacts may be provided by the RespeRate device. This sells for about $400, and requires virtually no personal training by a skilled therapist. In addition, it can be used for an indefinite period. If the encouraging early work is

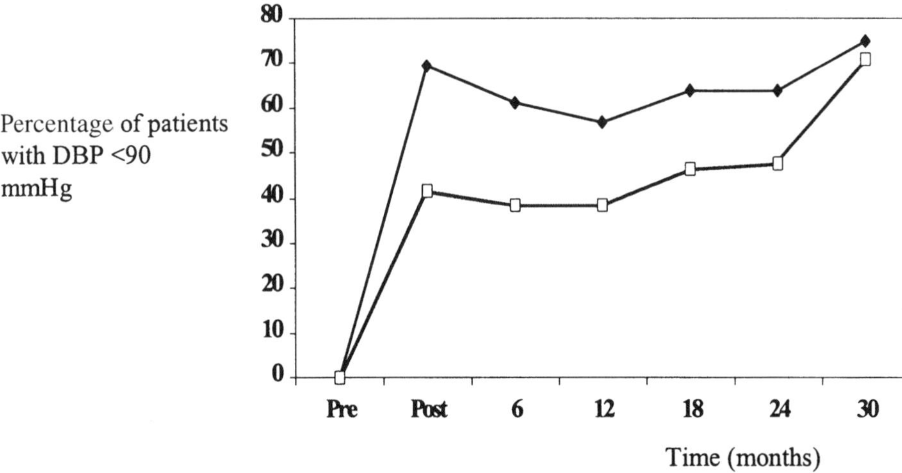

FIGURE 5 The rates of blood pressure control in patients with initially uncontrolled hypertension who were in the active treatment (relaxation) group (solid lines) or control group (hatched lines). Immediately after the treatment the control was better in the treated group (59 vs. 41%), but these differences gradually disappeared. Medications were changed during the follow-up period. *Source*: Data of Agras et al. [42].

confirmed, it thus has the capability of proving to be the first really cost-effective modality for the behavioral treatment of hypertension.

CURRENT GUIDELINES ON BEHAVIORAL TECHNIQUES

These changing fortunes of behavioral forms of treatment have been reflected in the Joint National Committee (JNC) recommendations over the years. In 1980 the committee concluded that "these methods are still experimental and cannot yet be recommended for sustained control of hypertension" [43]. The 1984 report [44] was more optimistic: "various relaxation and biofeedback therapies may consistently produce modest but significant blood pressure reduction" and they "should be considered in the context of a comprehensive treatment program that may include both pharmacologic and non-pharmacologic therapeutic approaches". In 1988 the pendulum had begun to swing the other way: "these promising methods have yet to be subjected to rigorous clinical trial evaluation and should not be considered as definitive treatment for patients with high blood pressure" [45]. The latest report (the sixth, published in 1997) [46] stated: "Relaxation therapies and biofeedback have been studied in multiple controlled trials with little effect beyond that seen in control groups... the available literature does not support the use of relaxation therapies for definitive therapy or prevention of hypertension."

CONCLUSION

Although behavioral forms of treatment are currently out of fashion for the treatment of hypertension, it is facile to dismiss the many positive results of individual studies as merely placebo effects, and probably overly simplistic. There are encouraging preliminary reports indicating that controlled breathing using a biofeedback device may lower ambulatory blood pressure. Another promising area is the treatment of white coat hypertension, in which the use of antihypertensive drugs is controversial, but in which the behavioral techniques appear to be particularly effective. The last word has not yet been said in this area.

REFERENCES

1. Benson H. The relaxation response: history, physiological basis and clinical usefulness. Acta Med Scand Suppl 1982; 660:231–237.
2. Patel C, Marmot MG, Terry DJ, Carruthers M, Hunt B, Patel M. Trial of relaxation in reducing coronary risk: four year follow up. Br Med J (Clin Res Ed) 1985; 290:1103–1106.
3. Patel C, Marmot MG, Terry DJ. Controlled trial of biofeedback-aided behavioural methods in reducing mild hypertension. Br Med J (Clin Res Ed) 1981; 282:2005–2008.
4. Benson H, Rosner BA, Marzetta BR, Klemchuk HM. Decreased blood-pressure in pharmacologically treated hypertensive patients who regularly elicited the relaxation response. Lancet 1974; 1:289–291.
5. Eisenberg DM, Kessler RC, Foster C, Norlock FE, Calkins DR, Delbanco TL. Unconventional medicine in the United States: prevalence, costs, and patterns of use. N Engl J Med 1993; 328:246–252.
6. Miller NE. Editorial: Biofeedback: evaluation of a new technic. N Engl J Med 1974; 290:684–685.
7. Blanchard EB, Eisele G, Vollmer A, Payne A, Gordon M, Cornish P, et al. Controlled evaluation of thermal biofeedback in treatment of elevated blood pressure in unmedicated mild hypertension. Biofeedback Self Reg 1996; 21: 167–190.
8. Eisenberg DM, Delbanco TL, Berkey CS, Kaptchuk TJ, Kupelnick B, Kuhl J, et al. Cognitive behavioral techniques for hypertension: are they effective? [see comments.] Ann Int Med 1993; 118:964–972.

9. Yucha CB, Clark L, Smith M, Uris P, LaFleur B, Duval S. The effect of biofeedback in hypertension. Appl Nurs Res 2001; 14(1):29–35.
10. Hunyor SN, Henderson RJ, Lal SK, Carter NL, Kobler H, Jones M, et al. Placebo-controlled biofeedback blood pressure effect in hypertensive humans. Hypertension 1997; 29:1225–1231.
11. Henderson RJ, Hart MG, Saroj KL, Hunyor SN. The effect of home training with direct blood pressure biofeedback of hypertensives: a placebo-controlled study. J Hypertens 1998; 16:771–778.
12. Jacobson E. Progressive Muscular Relaxation. Chicago: University of Chicago Press, 1938.
13. Hess WR. The Functional Organization of the Diencephalon. New York: Grune & Stratton, 1957.
14. Luthe W. Autogenic Therapy. New York: Grune and Stratton, 1969.
15. Shapiro AP, Schwartz GE, Redmond DP, Ferguson DC, Weiss SM. Non-pharmacologic treatment of hypertension. Ann NY Acad Sci 1978; 304:222–35.
16. Caudill MA, Friedman R, Benson H. Relaxation therapy in the control of blood pressure. Bibl Cardiol 1987; 106–119.
17. Brady JP, Luborski L, Kron RE. Blood pressure reduction in patients with essential hypertension through metronome-conditioned relaxation: a preliminary report. Behav Ther 1974; 5:203–209.
18. Jacob RG, Chesney MA, Williams DM, Ding Y, Shapiro AP. Relaxation therapy for hypertension: design effects and treatment effects. Ann Behav Med 1991; 13:5–17.
19. Southam MA, Agras WS, Taylor CB, Kraemer HC. Relaxation training: blood pressure lowering during the working day. Arch Gen Psych 1982; 39: 715–717.
20. Wenneberg SR, Schneider RH, Walton KG, Maclean CR, Levitsky DK, Salerno JW, et al. A controlled study of the effects of the Transcendental Meditation program on cardiovascular reactivity and ambulatory blood pressure. Int J Neurosci 1997; 89:15–28.
21. Jacob RG, Shapiro AP, Reeves RA, Johnsen AM, McDonald RH, Coburn PC. Relaxation therapy for hypertension: comparison of effects with concomitant placebo, diuretic, and beta-blocker. Arch Int Med 1986; 146:2335–2340.
22. van Montfrans GA, Karemaker JM, Wieling W, Dunning AJ. Relaxation therapy and continuous ambulatory blood pressure in mild hypertension: a controlled study. BMJ 1990; 300:1368–1372.
23. Irvine MJ, Logan AG. Relaxation behavior therapy as sole treatment for mild hypertension. Psychosom Med 1991; 53:587–597.
24. Chesney MA, Black GW, Swan GE, Ward MM. Relaxation training for essential hypertension at the worksite. I. the untreated mild hypertensive. Psychosom Med 1987; 49:250–263.
25. Batey DM, Kaufmann PG, Raczynski JM, Hollis JF, Murphy JK, Rosner B, et al. Stress management intervention for primary prevention of hypertension: detailed results from phase I of Trials of Hypertension Prevention (TOHP-I). Ann Epidemiol 2000; 10(1):45–58.

26. Fiedler N, Vivona-Vaughan E, Gochfeld M. Evaluation of a work site relaxation training program using ambulatory blood pressure monitoring. J Oc Med 1989; 31:595–602.
27. McCaffrey RJ, Blanchard EB. Stress management approaches to the treatment of essential hypertension. Ann Behav Med 1985; 7:5–12.
28. Linden W, Lenz JW, Con AH. Individualized stress management for primary hypertension: a randomized trial. Arch Int Med 2001; 161(8):1071–1080.
29. Patel C, Marmot M. Can general practitioners use training in relaxation and management of stress to reduce mild hypertension? Br Med J (Clin Res Ed) 1988; 296:21–24.
30. Goldring W, Chasis H, Schreiner GE, Smith HW. Reassurance in the management of benign hypertensive disease. Circ 1956; 14:260–264.
31. Chesney MA, Black GW. Behavioral treatment of borderline hypertension: an overview of results. J Cardiovasc Pharmacol 1986; 8(suppl. 5)S57–S63.
32. Agras S, Horne M, Taylor CB. Expectation and the blood pressure lowering effects of relaxation. Psychom Med 1982; 44:389–395.
33. Wadden T, Luborski L, Greer S, Crits-Christoph P. The behavioral treatment of essential hypertension: an update and comparison with pharmacological treatment. Clin Psych Rev 1984; 4:403–429.
34. Kaufmann PG, Jacob RG, Ewart CK, Chesney MA, Muenz LR, Doub N, et al. Hypertension Intervention Pooling Project. Health Psychol 1988; 7(suppl.): 209–224.
35. Fagard RH, Staessen JA. Treatment of isolated systolic hypertension in the elderly: the Syst-Eur trial. Systolic Hypertension in Europe (Syst-Eur) Trial Investigators. Clin Exp Hypertens 1999; 21:491–497.
36. Nakao M, Nomura S, Shimosawa T, Fujita T, Kuboki T. Blood pressure biofeedback treatment of white-coat hypertension. J Psychosom Res 2000; 48(2):161–169.
37. Rosenthal T, Alter A, Peleg E, Gavish B. Device-guided breathing exercises reduce blood pressure: ambulatory and home measurements. Am J Hypertens 2001; 14(1):74–76.
38. Schein MH, Gavish B, Herz M, Rosner-Kahana D, Naveh P, Knishkowy B, et al. Treating hypertension with a device that slows and regularises breathing: a randomised, double-blind controlled study. J Human Hypertens 2001; 15(4):271–278.
39. Barnes VA, Treiber FA, Turner JR, Davis H, Strong WB. Acute effects of transcendental meditation on hemodynamic functioning in middle-aged adults. Psychosom Med 1999; 61:525–531.
40. Bernardi L, Gabutti A, Porta C, Spicuzza L. Slow breathing reduces chemoreflex response to hypoxia and hypercapnia, and increases baroreflex sensitivity. J Hypertens 2001; 19(12):2221–2229.
41. Bernardi L, Sleight P, Bandinelli G, Cencetti S, Fattorini L, Wdowyczyc-Szulc J, et al. Effect of rosary prayer and yoga mantras on autonomic cardiovascular rhythms: comparative study. BMJ 2001; 323:1446–1449.
42. Agras WS, Taylor CB, Kraemer HC, Southam MA, Schneider JA. Relaxation

training for essential hypertension at the worksite. II. the poorly controlled hypertensive. Psychosom Med 1987; 49:264–273.
43. The 1980 report of the Joint National Committee on prevention, detection, evaluation, and treatment of high blood pressure. Arch Int Med 1980; 140: 1280–1285.
44. The 1984 report of the Joint National Committee on prevention, detection, evaluation, and treatment of high blood pressure. Arch Int Med 1984; 144: 1045–1057.
45. The 1988 report of the Joint National Committee on detection, evaluation, and treatment of high blood pressure. Arch Int Med 1988; 148:1023–1038.
46. The sixth report of the Joint National Committee on prevention,detection, evaluation,and treatment of high blood pressure. Arch Intern Med 1997; 157: 2413–2446.

14

Intervention in Children

Elaine Urbina
Tulane University School of Medicine, New Orleans, Louisiana, U.S.A.

Sathanur R. Srinivasan and Gerald S. Berenson
Tulane University School of Public Health and Tropical Medicine
New Orleans, Louisiana, U.S.A.

INTRODUCTION

Essential hypertension and hypertensive cardiovascular-renal disease are leading causes of morbidity and mortality worldwide. Hypertension is an underlying basis for strokes and heart failure, and is a major contributor to the development of atherosclerosis and complications of diabetes mellitus. Observations on cultural and ethnic differences in the prevalence of hypertension provide insights into understanding mechanisms in the development of hypertension and also approaches to interrupt the natural course of the disease. Importantly, from observations in adults, understanding the early natural history of essential hypertension can provide rational approaches to its prevention much earlier in life.

In 1973 we began research on the early natural history of cardiovascular diseases in a semirural, biracial (black–white) community of Bogalusa, Louisiana [1,2]. We recognized that precursors of essential hypertension begin very early in life and that intrinsic physiologic and genetic factors as well as environmental factors play roles in the early development of underlying "silent" hypertensive disease. Further, the observations about a black–white population living in a similar environment have contributed to appreciating the complexity of hypertension.

Major advances are yet to be made in the prevention of early hypertension. Its early detection and appreciation of the early subtle effects are challenges, in contrast to the vast studies of clinical hypertension in adults. The question remains whether or not the early natural history underlying pathophysiologic mechanisms producing the disease can be altered. Intervention beginning very early has the potential to reduce the burden of hypertensive disease in a large part of the population. The following material focuses on (1) measurement of blood pressure and definitions of abnormal levels, (2) anatomic evidence of early hypertensive changes in the cardiovascular–renal system, (3) ethnic (black–white) contrasts as clues to different mechanisms of the disease, and (4) strategies for prevention.

MEASURING BLOOD PRESSURE IN CHILDHOOD

Evidence has been accumulated over the past three decades from studies of children and young adults, and suggests that risk factors and lifestyles related to hypertensive cardiovascular disease are preventable [3–7]. The importance of recognizing of hypertension and its pathobiologic consequences beginning in childhood is based on how it is defined. However, it is important to measure blood pressures regularly in children and observe levels over time. There is considerable controversy regarding methods of measurement, the choice of Korotkoff fourth or fifth phase for diastolic pressure, and levels that are appropriate for intervention [8,9]. Reasonable measurements can be obtained by indirect methods starting around age 5 years, and since blood pressure levels reflect beat-to-beat and moment-to-moment variations, serial measurements are needed. Recording fourth and fifth diastolic phases are recommended since controversy still remains on which is more important [10]. Studies from 1139 children, ages 4 to 17 years and representing 68,000 measurements, showed K–4 to be a more reliable measure of diastolic blood pressure and a better predictor of adult hypertension than K–5 [10]. The percentile distributions of blood pressure levels have been reported from population studies in several task force reports [11]. Comparison of a given individual to these distributions requires a similar methodology of recording blood pressure, however. Levels of growing children are considerably lower than reported in adults. The adult task force reports, such as Joint National Commission VI, begin at 19 years of age and at an age much later than the onset of underlying hypertensive target organ changes. Both systolic and diastolic blood pressures increase as the child grows. Systolic levels increase approximately 1.5 mmHg per year, while diastolic blood pressure increases approximately 0.7 mmHg per year [12]. Studies of growing children indicate that weight, height, body mass, and skinfolds account for approximately 40% of the variability [13], thus levels should not be related to age alone but more to the body mass or height.

Observations on the Bogalusa population further suggest that obesity in white children has a much stronger relationship to higher blood pressure levels than in black children, especially black males. Although obesity has been found to be a strong determinant of high blood pressure [14,15], young black males are thin and yet have high blood pressure and high peripheral resistance. Since levels of obesity vary considerably, height appears to be a better reference point for determining abnormal blood pressure levels. It has therefore been recommended that blood pressure levels should be adjusted for the height of the child [13]. After serial observations, individuals tracking consistently at or above the ninetieth percentile for height should be considered for intensive prevention. This level is chosen arbitrarily because at this level structure–function changes of the cardiovascular system are noted (discussed below). To obtain a representative level, a series of four to six serial measurements are needed [16]. A precise definition of hypertension, however, that produces underlying tissue damage still remains difficult because clinical methodology, like electrocardiography and echocardiography of a single individual, is technically limited.

CHARACTERISTICS OF BLOOD PRESSURE IN CHILDREN

Twenty-Four-Hour Blood Pressure Measurements

Because blood pressure varies from moment to moment and varies with physiologic stress a representative level is difficult to obtain in childhood by a single casual measurement. Although serial measurements can obtain a representative level, ambulatory blood pressure measurements are of an additional value to identify risk. In studies of children, 2 days of measurements accounted for approximately 90% of the variability [17]. It is of interest that nighttime blood pressures are exceptionally low and an early morning rise tends to occur, as in adults. The drop of blood pressure during the nighttime is less apparent in black children, especially those with high levels [18]. Since there are multiple measurements during the 24 hr, various criteria have been used to evaluate high levels as abnormal. As suggested by White [19] a percent occurring above a specific cut point, like the ninetieth percentile related to height, seems to be appropriate. Children with levels more consistently above the ninetieth percentile should be diagnosed as hypertensive, and should be targeted for treatment. Since the methodology of 24-hr ambulatory blood pressures may not be feasible, the multiple series of casual observations are practical for identifying hypertensive individuals.

Evidence of Tracking and Prediction of Adult Hypertension

The recommendation of repeated readings of blood pressure at multiple visits over time assists in the prediction of future hypertension as adults. Tracking of blood pressure refers to the tendency for levels of an individual to remain, in relationship to their peers, in a respective rank over time. Voors et al. [16] demonstrated that tracking of blood pressure begins in childhood. Correlation coefficients for systolic and diastolic blood pressure measured 9 years apart were approximately 0.55 and 0.30, respectively. Serial blood pressure measurements increased the percentage remaining in the upper quartile to 68% for systolic blood pressure and 62% for diastolic blood pressure. Observations over a 15-year follow-up demonstrated that childhood blood

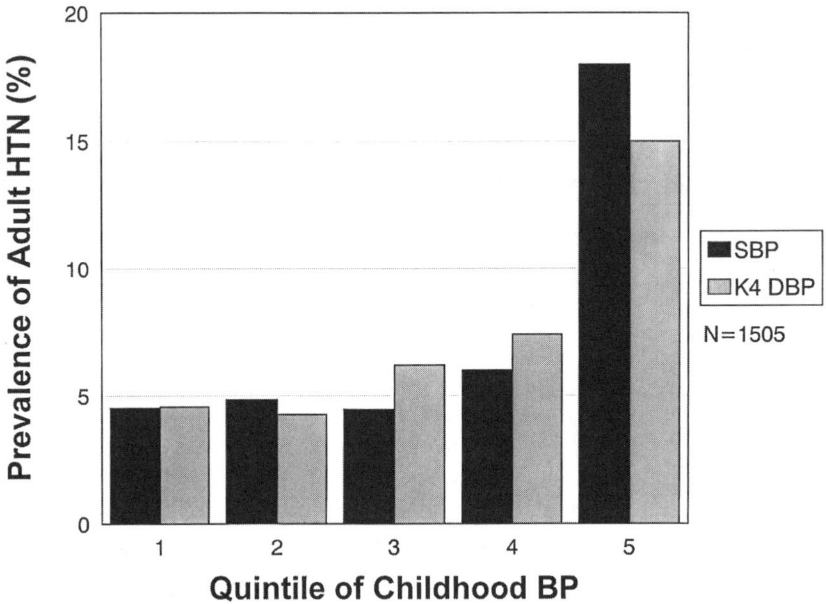

FIGURE 1 Prevalence of adult hypertension by childhood blood pressure quintiles. Childhood blood pressure in the top quintile is associated with a greater prevalence of hypertension in adulthood some 15 years later. *Source*: From Ref. 20.

pressure levels were predictive of adult hypertension and that those in the highest quintile during childhood were 3.6 times more likely to remain in the highest quintiles as young adults (Fig. 1) [20].

Association of Family History and Hypertension in Youth

An underlying genetic basis is supported by familial associations. Parental history of hypertension was found to be significantly associated with higher blood pressure levels in offspring [21]. Furthermore, children from hypertensive parents were found to have higher blood pressure levels after 10 years of age along with dyslipidemia, irrespective of weight. Black children with parental hypertension also had higher insulin levels than white offspring. Generally, those children selected with higher casual levels were more likely to have a higher percentage of high readings in the 24-hr period, with less of the nighttime dip. The evidence of tracking and the relationship with a family history therefore contribute to understanding that hypertension exists in childhood.

Since hypertension is familial, the diagnosis of hypertension in parents gives added credence to more aggressive management of children tracking at the higher percentile levels. In addition, the presence of high levels with other risk factors, such as in insulin resistance (syndrome X) and a strong family history, emphasizes the need of beginning prevention early in life.

HIGH BLOOD PRESSURE AND THE CARDIOVASCULAR SYSTEM IN EARLY LIFE

Autopsy Studies

The strongest evidence that hypertensive disease occurs in childhood was found by autopsies of young subjects, mostly with accidental deaths, conducted as part of the Bogalusa Heart Study [22]. Of 190 cases, ages 3 to 31 years, 85 had antemortem cardiovascular risk factor data, including blood pressure levels. Aortas and coronary arteries were stained with sudan 4, and gross evaluation of fatty streaks and fibrous plaques were performed according to the protocol developed by the International Atherosclerosis Project [23]. Significant associations were demonstrated between fatty streak involvement in the coronary arteries with systolic blood pressure, even after adjustment for age. Additionally, fibrous plaques in the coronary arteries correlated with age-adjusted antemortem systolic and diastolic blood pressure levels. Histologic evaluation revealed a relationship between the extent of foam cell infiltration and intensive lipid staining in the aorta with antemortem levels of blood pressure, adjusted for age and especially for black males. Some intimal thickening of the coronary arteries were noted with a weak correlation with blood pressure levels. In addition, studies were conducted on vascular structures of the kidney [24]. A thickening of coronary intima was found to be strongly related to hyalinization of renal arterioles. Also, a relationship between blood pressure and renal vascular abnormalities was noted by studying the medial thickness of renal arteries (50 to 400 uM) [25]. The severity of vascular involvement correlated with antemortem levels of blood pressure and other cardiovascular risk factors. These findings, obtained in a population with a mean age of less than 20 years, confirms that the atherosclerotic-hypertensive process begins in youth.

Cardiovascular–Renal Structure and Function Changes and Early Onset of Hypertension

Cardiac changes have been demonstrated both by electrocardiography (ECG) and echocardiography. Aristimuno et al. [26] demonstrated subtle ECG changes occurred in children at the highest decile of blood pressure. These changes were consistent with left ventricular hypertrophy and cardiac structural effects associated with relatively high blood pressure in childhood. Burke et al. [27] correlated echocardiographic measures of left ventricular wall thickness and systolic blood pressure in the top quintile of young subjects, even after adjusting for body size, race, and sex. Similarly, findings relating blood pressure levels to increased left ventricular mass, especially in males, have been reported by Scheiken et al. [28] and others [29]. Longitudinal echocardiographic studies of left ventricular mass relate linear growth of height as a major determinant of increasing heart size in children. In addition, excess weight gain and obesity was also shown to relate to increased left ventricular mass in children, while a relationship between fasting insulin and left ventricular mass, implicating metabolic factors, was also noted [30].

Evidence that cardiovascular function is associated with blood pressure levels has been shown in children and young adults [31]. Left ventricular stroke volume and cardiac output were positively correlated with both systolic and diastolic blood pressure in white males more than in black males. In contrast, black males were found to have higher peripheral resistance than whites (Fig. 2). Racial differences in hemodynamic mechanisms are suggested to occur and operate in the early phase of hypertension. Studies employing microneurography to measure muscle sympathetic nerve activity have confirmed an increased musculosympathetic nerve activity in blacks related to higher blood pressure levels as compared with whites, suggesting an enhanced α-adrenergic sensitivity in blacks [32,33]. In contrast, the early natural history of hypertension in whites may involve an initial increase in cardiac output

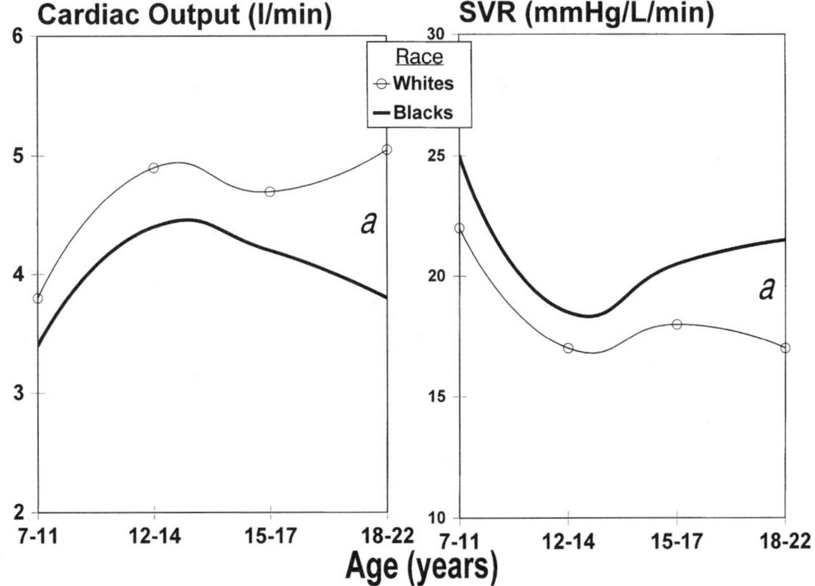

FIGURE 2 Echocardiographic examinations showing a greater cardiac output in white males vs. black males and a higher peripheral resistance in black males vs. white males. Race difference, a:p < 0.01. *Source*: From Ref. 31.

followed by down regulation of β-adrenergic receptors, ultimately progressing to an increase in systemic vascular resistance. Taken together, these observations show that early hemodynamic factors have a potential effect on cardiac size and function as well as on other target organ sites.

Noninvasive ultrasonic examination of carotid arteries have provided further evidence of vascular function and a relationship to cardiovascular risk factors in early life [34]. The pressure-strain elastic modulus (Ep), a measure of wall stiffness, was calculated from ultrasonic measurements of the carotid arteries. Increased Ep values in young subjects were found to relate to a positive parental history of hypertension and diabetes. While parental history could be used as a surrogate measure of future heart disease, functional differences were already detectable in carotid arteries of children and adolescents. Carotid artery studies on young adults have also shown intima media thickness of the far wall of the common carotid and bifurcation with a strong relationship to blood pressure levels [35]. Clearly cardiac and vascular structural and functional changes related to blood pressure levels occur in youth.

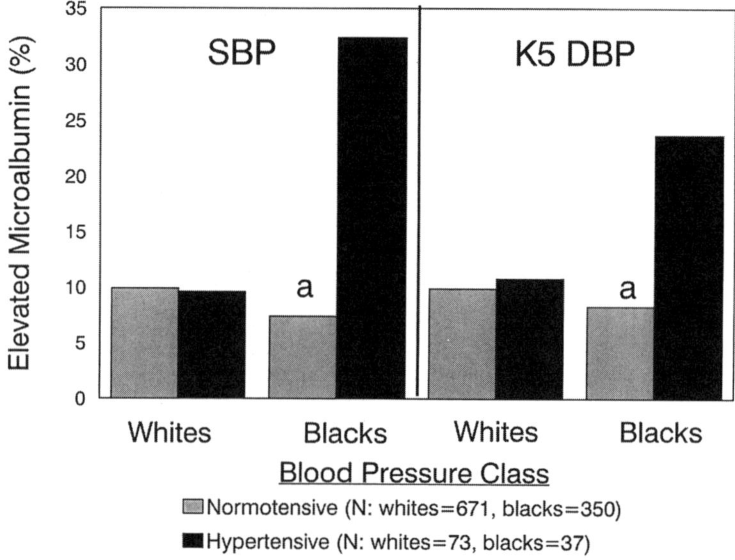

FIGURE 3 Association between albumin excretion and blood pressure levels in blacks. Normotensive denotes blood pressure <90th percentile; hypertensive ≥90th percentile. Higher percentage of blacks, but not whites, show microalbuminuria at this age, a: $p < 0.01$. *p value for race difference ≤0.0001. *Source*: From Ref. 36.

Evidence of the impact of early hypertension on renal function can be seen by the presence of microalbuminuria [36]. Microalbuminuria is associated with the development of hypertensive and/or diabetic nephropathy in young adults. A significant and positive correlation has been found between urine micro amounts of albumin excretion and higher levels of systolic and diastolic blood pressure as well as a greater prevalence of hypertension in "healthy" blacks (Fig. 3). Such associations were not found in young white subjects. This finding, along with observations of cardiovascular structure and function changes, indicate that even at a young age elevated blood pressure levels are detrimental to the cardiovascular–renal system.

RACE (BLACK–WHITE) AND GENDER CONTRASTS

Hemodynamic and Metabolic Factors

Finding differences in biologic variables based on race and gender are valuable in providing clues or questions regarding mechanisms contributing to the disease. In the routine screening of young children using an automatic

TABLE 1 Black–White Characteristics Related to Blood Pressure Levels of Children

All blood pressure strata	
Whites	Blacks
Percentage body fat[a]	
Plasma renin activity[a]	
Serum dopamine β–hydroxylase[a]	Blood pressure
24-hr urine potassium[a]	Peripheral resistance[b]
Fasting serum glucose[c]	
High blood pressure strata	
Resting heart rate[b]	Positive association of 24-hr urine sodium with resting blood pressure[c]
Cardiac output[c]	Negative association of plasma renin with systolic blood pressure in boys[d]
Renin activity and serum dopamine β -hydroxylase[d]	
1-hr postglucose load plasma glucose[d]	

Note: p values: [a]≤0.0001; [b]≤0.001; [c]≤0.01; [d]≤0.05. Variables listed for all blood pressure groups and those in high blood pressure groups are greater than for all other subjects. Higher values are shown.

instrument, higher values of blood pressure were detected in blacks at an early age (5 to 14 years) than in whites. This racial difference becomes evident using the mercury sphygmomanometer for indirect blood pressure measurements beginning at the adolescent age. Based on this racial contrast, extensive studies were performed on children selected with low, middle, and high levels of blood pressure [37,38]. Several metabolic and hemodynamic contrasts emerged, especially in the high blood pressure strata (Table 1). At higher blood pressure levels, white children, unlike black children, tended to be more obese, have higher insulin and glucose levels, and have faster heart rates. Plasma renin activity was higher in white children, and in the high blood pressure strata, dopamine β-hydroxylase (DBH) levels were also found to be lower in blacks. Based on these findings, it is postulated that racial differences in sympathomimetic-hormonal influences occur as part of the divergent mechanisms contributing to development of early essential hypertension.

Role of Sodium and Potassium

In studies of children with high and low blood pressure levels blacks displayed considerably lower urinary potassium excretion (Fig. 4), and somewhat lower creatinine clearance [37,38]. In addition, a positive relationship between 24-hr sodium excretion was suggested in blacks, but very clearly in blacks the 24-hr

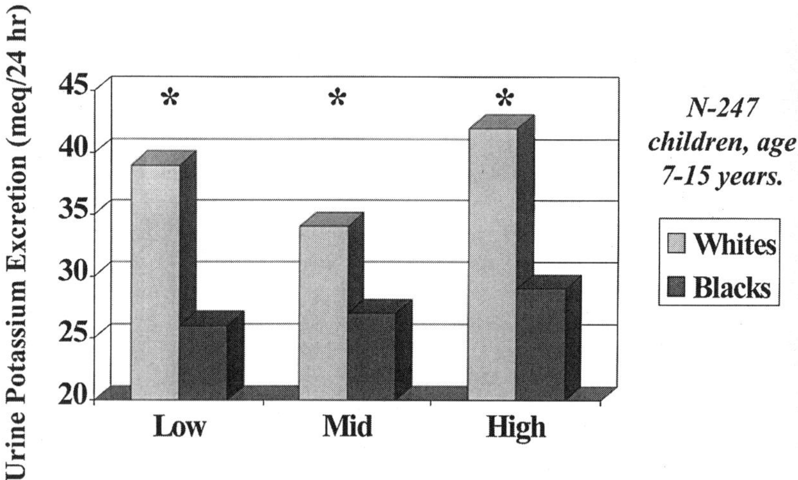

FIGURE 4 Twenty-four-hr urinary potassium excretion in black and white children by blood pressure strata. Blacks vs. whites excreted considerably lower potassium. *p value for race influence ≤ 0.0001. *Source*: From Ref. 38.

urine sodium-to-potassium clearance ratio and blood pressure levels were significantly different, implicating difference in renal handling of electrolytes. Further studies on young subjects indicate racial differences in the handling of electrolytes after administration. Voors et al. [39] and Weinberger et al. [40] illustrated differences in the response to electrolytes in blacks compared to whites with hypertension. Falkner et al. [41] have shown that blacks with higher blood pressure also have greater hyperinsulinemia/insulin resistance and salt sensitivity. These findings complement the hormonal and metabolic contrasts interacting with hemodynamic factors noted above.

In a study supplementing 80 mEq of potassium chloride with the usual diet, young black adults had a greater natruresis and a negative urine sodium balance with a greater cumulative potassium balance than whites [39]. Potassium administration resulted in a lowering of blood pressure levels—more so in blacks than in whites, with a delayed excretion of potassium in blacks. Such differences were found despite an overall similar sodium-potassium dietary intake between the races. Dietary intake studies of children in general indicated an excessively high intake of sodium, exceeding the recommended range of 2 g/day by two- to three fold. A considerable number had potassium intakes below half of the recommended dietary allowance (2 mEq/kg/day). These observations indicate that dietary modifications of reducing sodium and increasing potassium consumption are critically important in preventing early essential hypertension, especially in blacks and genetically salt-sensitive individuals. Because of the interaction of sodium and potassium as well as such other electrolytes as calcium and magnesium with metabolic and hemodynamic factors, it is crucial to focus on changing the environmental conditions contributing to the early natural history of hypertension.

Strategies to Prevent Hypertension

Controversy exists on whether or not to examine children for risk factors and at what ages screening should begin. Guidelines have been suggested incorporating a high-risk approach directed toward families with evidence of cardiovascular disease. Studies, including those from the Bogalusa Heart Study, have shown that parental history is a surrogate measure of future cardiovascular disease risk in "healthy" young offspring. A positive parental history links cardiovascular risk factors, including high blood pressure, in their offspring. With regard to coronary artery disease and stroke, however, a parental history for children is limited because parents are too young. The lack of recognition of hypertension even in adults indicates a further limitation of parental history to detect children at risk [21]. A history of heart attack appears more prevalent in white males, and as expected, increases as children age, along with their parents age. Similarly,

TABLE 2 General Guidelines for Examination of Children for Cardiovascular Risk

Family history
Premature heart disease; i.e., myocardial infarction in males <55 years and females <65 years
Hypertension
Hyperlipidemia: high-LDL cholesterol
Low-HDL cholesterol
Diabetes mellitus
Cerebrovascular accident
Routine examination by physician
Blood pressure, height, weight, skinfolds, waist measurement
Venipuncture for determination of cholesterol, triglycerides, and lipoproteins: as a minimum serum total cholesterol and HDL cholesterol
Examination of all school-age children; preschool examination
Evaluation of
Type A–B behavior
Cigarette smoking
Exercise

Note: LDL = low-density lipoprotein; HDL = high-density lipoprotein.

the prevalence of hypertension increases with age. Further, parental diabetes and hypertension show strong relationships in black children that increase with age. Table 2 provides general guidelines for screening, including the use of a family history. Since blood pressure is readily measured beginning around 5 to 7 years of age by indirect auscultation techniques, measurements should be incorporated in routine examinations. As discussed above, population percentile grids related to height can be used to evaluate significance of levels [2].

Change of Lifestyles to Prevent Hypertension in Early Life

Lifestyle modifications have been useful to bring hypertension under control in adults, especially as an adjunct to drug treatment. Incorporating increased fruit and vegetables in the DASH diet has resulted in slight reductions of blood pressure, as has reducing weight [42]. Based on those observations in adults, indoctrination of children in healthy lifestyles should alter the natural history of essential hypertension beginning in early life. Individuals with an increased genetic susceptibility to development of hypertension, particularly blacks, however, will require more intensive intervention. Since criteria for adult hypertension are inappropriate for young individuals, we suggested above that tracking at a level of ninetieth percentile be used as a guide for intervention. As pointed out, at this level subtle end organ changes occur. Since body mass and obesity relate strongly with the development of higher percentiles of blood pressure, control of obesity is important (Fig. 5). Along with the high sodium and low potassium found in diets in the United States, obesity is a fundamental contributor to the development of hypertension. Additionally, parental hypertension implies the need for intervention involving the family, which would also include the offspring. Additional consideration should be given offspring of parents with a history of diabetes, since diabetes is a major contributor to renal disease and coronary heart disease morbidity and mortality. Since diabetes is two- to three fold greater in blacks than in whites and hypertension much more common in blacks, a family history of the two diseases should raise more concern for the health of the offspring. In the context of preventing early essential hypertension there are compelling observations that hypertension is a rather complex, inherited syndrome. As discussed above, hypertension is a syndrome that involves multiple abnormalities, such as insulin resistance, alterations of renal function, hormonal changes, dyslipidemia, and even abnormalities of coagulation. Consequently, prevention strategies should focus on controlling multiple risk factors.

Central to prevention are a prudent diet, weight control, and exercise. An intensive exercise program is known to reduce heart rate and blood pressure, but alterations of the usual dietary intake of the U.S. population is

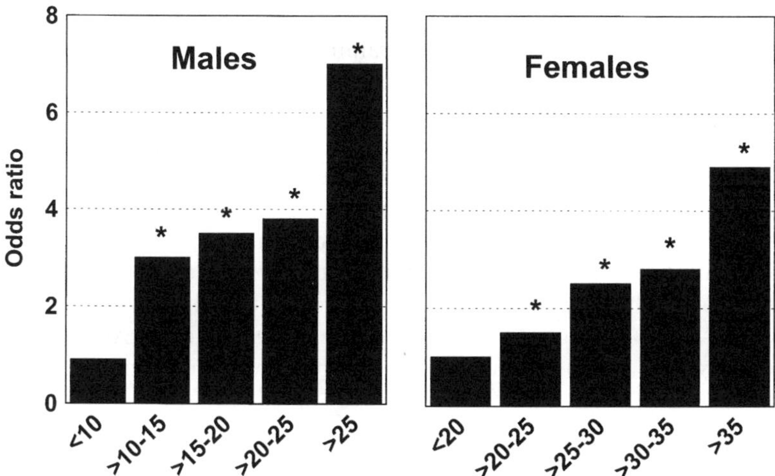

FIGURE 5 Odds for having elevated (top quintile) blood pressure by percentage body fat in children ages 5 to 18 years. *Note*: N = 3320 children, ages 5 to 18 years. *95% CI does not include 1.00. *Source*: From Ref. 15.

also needed. In addition to a balanced caloric intake and energy expenditure, a reduction of sodium and an increase of potassium, magnesium, and calcium are important. A reduction of saturated fat to control excess caloric intake has also aided blood pressure control. The above observations about young subjects have shown the importance of increasing potassium intake, especially in blacks, and may be crucial to management of salt-sensitive individuals.

Efforts to get young individuals to adopt healthy lifestyles face challenges. Apathy, a sense of immortality, resistance against changing diets, poor exercise habits, smoking, and alcohol consumption are part of childhood and adolescence. Support is therefore needed from education and the health care systems. Although prevention is cost beneficial, the medical profession is becoming more and more concerned with the need for prevention because of high health care costs. Lifestyles are adopted in childhood; therefore it would be prudent to begin to encourage healthy lifestyles early by various approaches [43].

High-Risk Approach

There are two general approaches to intervention, the high-risk and the population or public health approach. Both strategies are needed and complement each other. The high-risk approach addresses individuals or families found to be at risk based on the presence of cardiovascular disease, stated above. Implementation of this strategy requires a multidisciplinary approach, integrating educational and training programs by primary care physicians, nutritionists, exercise physiologists, and behavioral trained personnel [44]. A medical team of this nature provides an optimum opportunity for changing lifestyles. For children detected with hypertension, more aggressive management and medication may be required.

In an effort to thwart the early natural history of hypertension, clinical trials using low-dose medication along with education, nutrition, and exercise programs have been implemented successfully to lower blood pressure levels [3,6,7]. An algorithm for diagnosis and control of high blood pressure in children is shown in Fig. 6 [45]. Efforts are being made to expand this methodology of coupling medication with education, diet, and exercise.

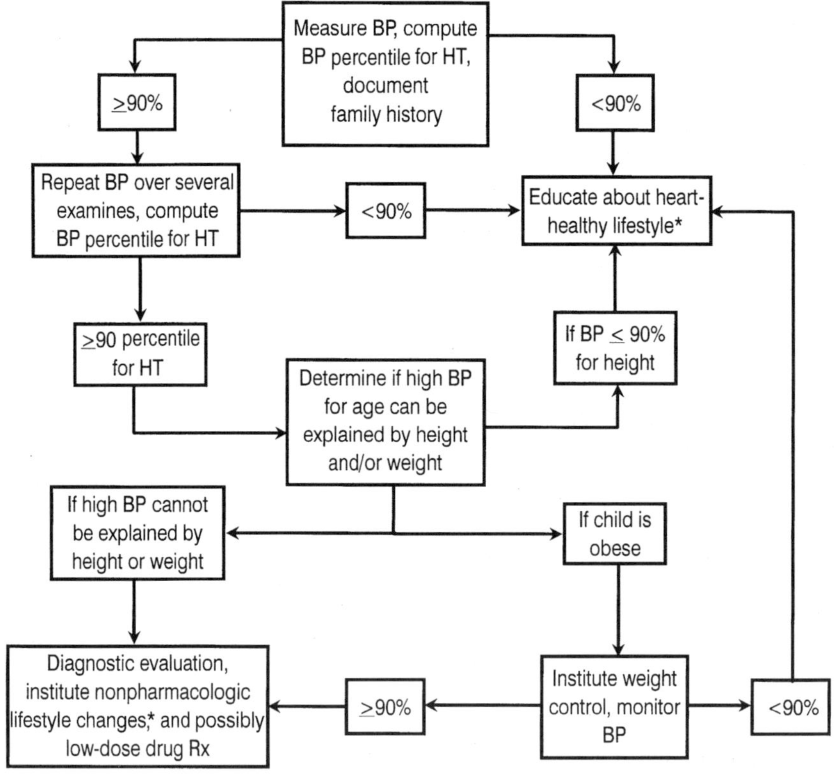

FIGURE 6 An algorithm for detection and treatment of children with elevated (≥90th percentile) blood pressure. *Prevent obesity, encourage physical activity. *Source*: From Ref. 45.

Children tracking at the ninetieth percentile or greater, especially when found with a positive parental history of hypertension, should be targeted for treatment with low-dose antihypertensive medication. Primary care physicians can play a role in encouraging prevention of hypertension in the general population by identifying of young individuals, especially in families with hypertension. Recognition of hypertension beginning in early life should be at a high priority in preventive cardiology.

Population Approach

Since hypertension is so prevalent in the adult society, prevention by the population approach in early life is advocated. Such comprehensive educational programs for young children like Health Ahead/Heart Smart, the Know Your Body program, and Growing Healthy are now available, and introduction into the school system beginning in elementary school is the most practical and long term method to prevent cardiovascular diseases, such as hypertension, obesity, and poor lifestyles. Comprehensive or coordinated health promotion programs dealing with all aspects of the school environment must become an integral component and a priority of the educational system for young children. A program of health education for elementary school age, Health Ahead/Heart Smart, was developed based on findings in the Bogalusa Heart Study [46]. This program addresses the entire school environment, including the classroom, the cafeteria, physical education, and programs for teachers and parents, and encourages physicians and cardiologists to become involved [47].

CONCLUSION

Beginning prevention in early life should be a focus in addressing hypertension as a disease. Epidemiologic studies of cardiovascular risk factors in children prove that hypertensive disease as well as atherosclerosis begin at a young age. Consequently, prevention efforts should begin early in life to obtain maximum benefit, particularly primary intervention. If pharmacotherapeutics is needed, dietary alterations and increased physical activity should be incorporated as adjunctive therapy. Prevention of obesity, along with attention to diet and physical activity, remains the cornerstone to overall health and the prevention of hypertension.

ACKNOWLEDGMENTS

This research was supported by funds from the National Heart, Lung and Blood Institute (HL38844) and the National Institute on Aging (AG16592).

The Bogalusa Heart Study is a joint effort of many individuals whose cooperation is gratefully acknowledged. We are especially grateful to the study participants.

REFERENCES

1. Berenson GS, McMahan CA, Voors AW, Webber LS, Srinivasan SR, Frank GC, Foster TA, Blonde CV. Cardiovascular Risk Factors in Children—The Early Natural History of Atherosclerosis and Essential Hypertension. New York: Oxford University Press, 1980: 450.
2. Berenson GS, ed. Causation of Cardiovascular Risk Factors in Children: Perspectives on Cardiovascular Risk in Early Life. New York: Raven, 1986: 408.
3. Frank GC, Farris RP, Ditmarsen P, Voors AW, Berenson GS. An approach to primary preventive treatment for children with high blood pressure. J Am Coll Nutr 1982; 1:357–374.
4. Arbeit ML, Johnson CC, Mott DS, Harsha DW, Nicklas TA, Webber LS, Berenson GS. The Heart Smart cardiovascular school health promotion: behavior correlates of risk factor change. Prev Med 1992; 21:18–32.
5. Hetzel BS, Coonan WE, Maynard EJ, Dwyer T. Perspectives on implementation of intervention programs. In Hetzel BS, Berenson GS, eds. Cardiovascular Risk Factors in Childhood: Epidemiology and Prevention, Amsterdam: Elsevier, 1987: 263–279.
6. Berenson GS, Voors AW, Webber LS, Frank GC, Farris RP, Tobian L, Aristimuno GG. A model of intervention for prevention of early essential hypertension in the 1980's. Hypertension 1983; 5:41–55.
7. Berenson GS, Shear SL, Chiang YK, Webber LS, Voors AW. Combined low-dose medication and primary intervention over a 30-month period for sustained high blood pressure in childhood. Am J Med Sci 1990; 299:79–86.
8. Update on the 1987 Task Force Report on high blood pressure in children and adolescents: a working group report from the National High Blood Pressure Education Program, National Heart, Lung and Blood Institute. Pediatrics 1996; 98:649–658.
9. Hammond IW, Urbina EM, Wattigney WA, Bao W, Steinmann WC, Berenson GS. Comparison of fourth and fifth Korotkoff diastolic blood pressure in 5- to 30-year old individuals: the Bogalusa Heart Study. Am J Hypertens 1995; 8:1083–1089.
10. Elkasabany AM, Urbina EM, Daniels SR, Berenson GS. Prediction of adult hypertension by K4 and K5 diastolic blood pressure in children: the Bogalusa Heart Study. J Ped 1998; 132:687–692.
11. Report of the Second Task Force on Blood Pressure Control in Children. Pediatrics 1987; 79:1–25.
12. Voors AW, Webber LS, Berenson GS. Time course studies of blood pressure in children: the Bogalusa Heart Study. Am J Epidem 1978; 109:320–334.

13. Voors AW, Webber LS, Berenson GS. Relationship of blood pressure levels to height and weight in children. J Cardiovasc Med 1978; 3:911–918.
14. Lauer RM, Clark WR. Childhood risk factors for high adult blood pressure: the Muscatine Study. Pediatrics 1984; 84:633–641.
15. Williams DP, Going SB, Lohman TG, Harsha DW, Srinivasan SR, Webber LS, Berenson GS. Body fatness and risk for elevated blood pressure, total cholesterol, and serum lipoprotein ratios in children and adolescents. Am J Pub Health 1992; 82:358–363.
16. Voors AW, Webber LS, Berenson GS. Time course study of blood pressure in children over a three-year period: the Bogalusa Heart Study. Hypertension 1980; 2 (suppl. 1):I-102–108.
17. Berenson GS, Dalferes ER Jr, Savage D, Webber LS, Bao W. Ambulatory blood pressure measurements in children and young adults selected by high and low casual blood pressure levels and parental history of hypertension: the Bogalusa Heart Study. Am J Med Sci 1993; 305:374–382.
18. Vaughn CJ, Murphy MB. The use of ambulatory blood pressure monitoring in the evaluation of racial differences in blood pressure. J Cardiovasc Risk 1994; 1:132–135.
19. White WB. Assessment of patients with office hypertension by 24 hour noninvasive ambulatory blood pressure monitoring. Arch Int Med 1986; 146:2194–2199.
20. Bao W, Threefoot SA, Srinivasan SR, Berenson GS. Essential hypertension predicted by tracking of elevated blood pressure from childhood to adulthood: the Bogalusa Heart Study. Am J Hypertens 1995; 8:657–665.
21. Bao W, Srinivasan SR, Wattigney WA, Berenson GS. The relation of parental cardiovascular disease to risk factors in children and young adults: the Bogalusa Heart Study. Circulation 1995; 91:365–371.
22. Berenson GS, Srinivasan SR, Bao W, Newman WP III, Tracy RE, Wattigney WA. Association between multiple cardiovascular risk factors and atherosclerosis in children and young adults. N Engl J Med 1998; 338(23): 1650–1656.
23. McGill HC, ed. The Geographic Pathology of Atherosclerosis. Baltimore: Williams & Wilkins, 1968.
24. Tracy RE, Newman WP III, Wattigney WA, Srinivasan SR, Strong JP, Berenson GS. Histologic features of atherosclerosis and hypertension from autopsies of young individuals in a defined geographic population: the Bogalusa Heart Study. Atherosclerosis 1995; 116:163–179.
25. Newman WP III, Freedman DS, Voors AW, Gard PD, Srinivasan SR, Crescendo JL, Williamson GD, Webber LS, Berenson GS. Relation of serum lipoprotein levels and systolic blood pressure to early atherosclerosis: the Bogalusa Heart Study. N Engl J Med 1986; 314:138–144.
26. Aristimuno GG, Foster TA, Berenson GS, Akman D. Subtle electrocardiographic changes in children with high levels of blood pressure. Am J Cardiol 1984; 54:1272–1276.
27. Burke GL, Arcilla RA, Culpepper WS, Webber LS, Chiang RA, Berenson GS.

Blood pressure and echocardiographic measures in children: the Bogalusa Heart Study. Circulation 1987; 75:106–114.

28. Schieken RM, Clarke WR, Mahoney LT, Lauer RM. Measurement criteria for group echocardiographic studies. Am J Epidemiol 1979; 110:504–514.
29. Laird WP, Fixler DE. Left ventricular hypertrophy in adolescents with elevated blood pressure: assessment by chest roentgenography, electrocardiography, and echocardiography. Pediatrics 1981; 67:255.
30. Urbina EM, Gidding SS, Bao W, Elkasabany A, Berenson GS. Association of fasting blood sugar level, insulin level, and obesity with left ventricular mass in healthy children and adolescents: the Bogalusa Heart Study. Am Heart J 1999; 138:122–127.
31. Soto LF, Kikuchi DA, Arcilla RA, Berenson GS. Echocardiographic functions and blood pressure levels in children and young adults from a biracial population: the Bogalusa Heart Study. Am J Med Sci 1989; 296: 271–279.
32. Urbina EM, Bao W, Pickoff AS, Berenson GS. Ethnic (black–white) differences in heart rate variability during cardiovascular reactivity testing in male adolescents with high and low blood pressure: the Bogalusa Heart Study. Am J Hyper 1998; 11:,196–202.
33. Guzzetti S, Dassi S, Pecis M, Casati R, Masu AM, Longoni P, Tinelli M, Cerutti S, Pagani M, Milani A. Altered pattern of circadian neural control of heart period in mild hypertension. J Hypertens 1991; 9:831–838.
34. Riley WA, Freedman DS, Higgs NA, Barnes RW, Zinkgraf SA, Berenson GS. Decreased arterial elasticity associated with cardiovascular disease risk factors in the young: the Bogalusa Heart Study. Arteriosclerosis 1986; 6: 378–386.
35. Urbina EM, Srinivasan SR, Tang R, Bond MG, Kieltyka RL, Berenson GS. The impact of multiple coronary risk factors on the intima-media thickness of different segments of carotid artery in healthy young adults: the Bogalusa Heart Study. Am J Cardiol 2002; 90:953–958.
36. Jiang X, Srinivasan SR, Radhakrishnamurthy B, Dalferes ER Jr, Bao W, Berenson GS. Microalbuminuria in young adults related to blood pressure in a biracial (black–white) population: the Bogalusa Heart Study. Am J Hypertens 1995; 7:794–800.
37. Voors AW, Berenson GS, Dalferes ER, Webber LS, Shuler SE. Racial differences in blood pressure control. Science 1979; 204:1091–1094.
38. Berenson GS, Voors AW, Webber LS, Dalferes ER Jr, Harsha DW. Racial differences of parameters associated with blood pressure levels in children: the Bogalusa Heart Study. Metabolism 1979; 28:1218–1228.
39. Voors AW, Dalferes ER, Frank GC, Aristimuno GG, Berenson GS. Relation between ingested potassium and sodium balance in young blacks and whites. Am J Clin Nutr 1983; 37:583–594.
40. Weinberger MH. Racial differences in renal sodium excretion: relationship to hypertension. Am J Kidney Dis 1993; 21:41–45.
41. Falkner B, Hulman S, Kushner H. Hyperinsulinemia and blood pressure sensitivity to sodium in young blacks. J Am Soc Nephrol 1992; 3:940–946.

42. Sacks FM, Svetkey LP, Vollmer WM, Appel LJ, Bray GA, Harsha D, Obarzanek E, Conlin PR, Miller ER III, Simons-Morton DG, Karanja N, Lin P-H. Effects on blood pressure of reduced dietary sodium and the dietary approaches to stop hypertension (DASH) diet. N Engl J Med 2001; 344: 3–10.
43. Berenson GS, Pickoff AS. Preventive cardiology and its potential influence on the early natural history of adult heart diseases: the Bogalusa Heart Study and the Heart Smart Program. Am J Med Sci 1995; (suppl.):S133–S138.
44. Johnson CC, Nicklas TA, Arbeit ML, Harsha DW, Mott DS, Hunter SM, Wattigney W. Cardiovascular intervention for high-risk families: the Heart Smart Program. So Med J 1991; 84:1305–1312.
45. Bronfin DR, Urbina EM. The role of the pediatrician in the promotion of cardiovascular health. Am J Med Sci 1995; suppl.:542–547.
46. Downey AM, Frank GC, Webber LS, Harsha DW, Virgillio SJ, Franklin FA, Berenson GS. Implementation of "Heart Smart": a cardiovascular school health promotion program. J Sch Health 1987; 57:98–104.
47. Downey AM, Cresanta JL, Berenson GS. Cardiovascular health promotion: "Heart Smart" and the changing role of the physician. Am J Prev Med 1989; 5:279–295.

15

Intervention in the Elderly

Jeff D. Williamson and William B. Applegate
Wake Forest University School of Medicine, Winston-Salem, North Carolina, U.S.A.

INTERVENTION IN THE ELDERLY

Introduction

Elevations of either systolic blood pressure (SBP) or diastolic blood pressure (DBP) are prevalent problems with major health implications in older patients [1–7]. A number of lifestyle modifications are effective at reducing abnormal elevations in blood pressure and their associated adverse outcomes in the elderly. These modifications include dietary changes, regular aerobic physical activity, smoking cessation, appropriate alcohol consumption, and weight reduction for obese individuals. This chapter will review the epidemiology of hypertension and its special impact on older people, the approach to diagnosing hypertension in the elderly, and specific nonpharmacologic approaches to the initial management of high blood pressure in this growing population.

Epidemiology

In all industrialized countries, average SBP rises throughout the life span, whereas average DBP rises until age 55 to 60 years and then levels off or even declines [8]. These changes are important because epidemiologic data indicate that in the elderly, SBP but not DBP is a strong predictor of both total and cardiovascular mortality [9], and thus most of the increase in the prevalence of hypertension-related disease in older persons is due to an increase in isolated systolic hypertension (SBP > 140 to 160 mmHg, DBP >90 mmHg) [10]. For instance, population-based studies from East Boston indicate that as persons approach advanced old age (ages 80 and older), elevations of SBP are the single strongest cardiovascular risk factor, while elevations of DBP are associated with only a relatively small cardiovascular disease (CVD) risk. Therefore, because systolic blood pressure plays a major role in determining cardiovascular events, the benefits of therapy aimed at SBP should be stressed more than DBP in discussing treatment with older people [10]. Estimates of the prevalence of hypertension (both systolic and diastolic hypertension; SDH) and isolated systolic hypertension (ISH) in people older than 65 years vary greatly, depending on the age and race of the group studied, the blood pressure cutoff point used for the definition of hypertension, and the number of measurements made. Because levels of DBP tend to stabilize at about age 55, the prevalence of SDH tends to be constant at age 55 and older. Based on estimates from the Hypertension Detection and Follow-up Program (HDFP), the prevalence of SDH in people older than age 65 is about 15% in whites and 25% in African Americans. In screening for the pilot study of the Systolic Hypertension in the Elderly (SHEP), ISH was found in about 10% of people age 70 to 80 and in 20% of people older than age 80 (in both blacks and whites). Not simply the prevalence but also the importance of ISH as a risk factor grows with each decade after age 65. Hypertension remains a powerful risk factor for CVD in both the old and very old, and while the risk of CVD for each incremental increase in blood pressure diminishes with age beyond the age of 65, the attributable risk remains unchanged [11]. This is because the prevalence of hypertension and the absolute risk of CVD are substantially greater in older people. For men, the absolute risk of CVD due to hypertension levels off beyond the age of 75. For women, however, the absolute risk continues to rise through age 94 and may continue to rise beyond the age of 94, but data are lacking in this age group. In addition to the importance of hypertension in incident CVD-related mortality and morbidity, hypertension is also an important contributor to the onset of disability and loss of independence in older people. This outcome, which often results in institutionalization, is perhaps a more feared outcome than mortality for many elderly persons. Figure 1 shows the results of a recent analysis of longitudinal data from the Women's Health and Aging Study demonstrating that SBP elevations above 140 mmHg are associated with a significantly higher probability of incident loss of ability to walk across a small room.

Recent analyses of epidemiologic data indicate that in older persons an increased pulse pressure (which is generally a result of the combined decrease

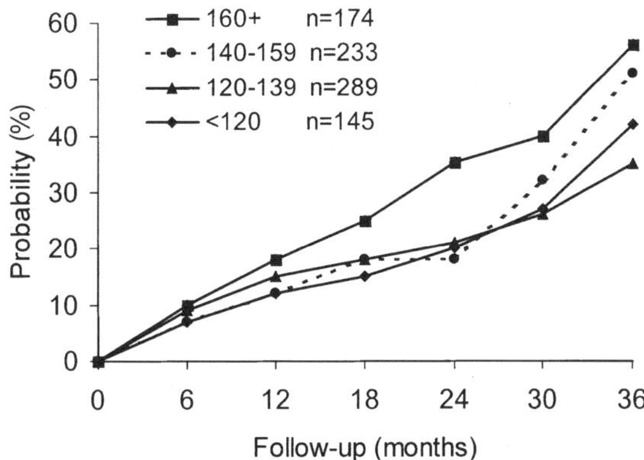

FIGURE 1 Baseline blood pressure and 3-year incidence of inability to walk across a small room.

in DBP and elevation in SBP) is an even better predictor of CVD risk than SBP alone [12]. Figure 2 clearly shows the importance of pulse pressure as a risk factor for mortality relative to SBP and DBP [13]. These data show that for equivalent levels of SBP, persons with isolated systolic hypertension are actually at greater risk for CVD than those with combined SDH. The risk increases as the separation between the SBD and DBP increases. This finding has important therapeutic implications; while lowering SBP in elderly

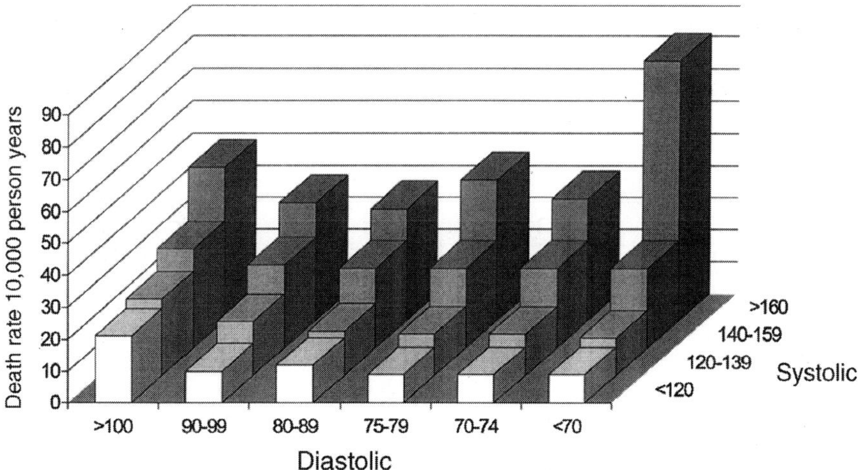

FIGURE 2 Blood pressure and age-adjusted coronary heart disease (CHD) death rate per 10,000 person-years (men).

patients with ISH is clearly beneficial, lowering DBP to below 70 mmHg with active treatment has been associated with an increased risk of stroke, coronary heart disease, and CVD [14]. This relationship between DBP and cardiovascular events is more marked at diastolic pressures below 60 mmHg, in which case it is thought to reflect underlying subclinical CVD. Low blood pressure in older adults, especially the very old, may thus be a consequence of disease and not a cause of it. This creates the false impression that excess mortality observed in individuals with low blood pressures is a consequence of reduced blood pressure. Data from Framingham, however, have shown that this excess mortality is observed only in the subset of older people with known coronary heart disease [11]. For example, persistent reductions in blood pressure, especially DBP, are often observed in older adults after experiencing a myocardial infarction [15]. Most important, however, epidemiologic data clearly show that high SBP is related to excess mortality and CVD for adults over the age of 80 who are free of existing, observed CVD [11].

Presentation and Evaluation of the Older Hypertensive Patient

High blood pressure is usually detected in an asymptomatic older person at a routine office visit or through various programs that offer blood pressure screening examinations to older individuals. In about 10% of older persons, however, high blood pressure is first diagnosed on presentation of a clinical event probably triggered by long-standing high blood pressure such as a stroke, congestive heart failure, or myocardial infarction (Table 1). At times, older patients will complain of dizziness or headaches that they believe may be associated with elevations of blood pressure, but studies have consistently shown that unless the blood pressure is either extremely high or extremely low, symptoms are usually absent unless the patient

TABLE 1 Symptoms Related to High Blood Pressure

Symptoms related to pressure rise	Symptoms related to chronic effects of high blood pressure	Symptoms/conditions related to cardiovascular morbidity
Headache	Postprandial syncope	Low energy
Clouded sensorium	Postural syncope	Symptoms of multi-infarct dementia
Syncope	Edema	Stroke
Seizure	Dyspnea	Myocardial infarction
Tachycardia		Congestive heart failure
Dysnea		Renal failure

presents with a cardiovascular clinical event (and, as in younger patients, high blood pressure is an uncommon cause of headache). As blood pressure increases with age, however, the baroreceptor reflex is diminished and hypertensive patients may present with either postural hypotension or postprandial hypotension.

Based on epidemiologic data, the Sixth Report from the Joint National Commission on Detection, Evaluation and Treatment of High Blood Pressure recommends that the upper limit of normal systolic pressure for elderly persons should also be 140 mmHg [26]. Despite this widely published recommendation, there remains a commonly held erroneous opinion that SBP elevations above 140 mmHg are physiologically appropriate in older people.

Physical Examination

The physical exam of the hypertensive older adult is important because of the high probability of encountering advanced atherosclerosis, therefore although hypertension is usually asymptomatic, it is important to question the older patient about potential symptoms related to acute rises in blood pressure as well as symptoms related to the vascular complications of high blood pressure (Table 1). For instance, questions regarding syncope, tachycardia, flushing, headaches, chest pain, nocturnal dyspnea, and numbness or trends in paralysis of a focal part of the body are all appropriate. Of course, it is important to question the patient about previous times when blood pressure may have been measured, and if possible, it is important to document the duration that the blood pressure has been elevated. Often, older persons who present with elevations of blood pressure will report having been treated previously with nonpharmacologic therapy or antihypertensive agents. It is important to document the type of therapy used, its effectiveness, and any reason for discontinuation. Finally, older patients frequently take multiple prescription or over-the-counter medicines, some of which can cause an elevation of blood pressure. These include sympathomimetics, nonsteroidal anti-inflammatory drugs (NSAIDS), alcohol, caffeine (acutely only), postmenopausal hormone replacement therapy (rarely), and corticosteroids (including heavy topical use).

The physical examination should focus on examining the patient for potential signs of organ damage from high blood pressure and for any potential underlying physical abnormalities that might contribute to the rise in blood pressure. Evaluate for bradycardia in the presence of hypertension, as this may guide the use of specific behavioral therapy such as exercise and will factor into potential medication usage for future therapy. Examination of the retina for signs of arteriolar damage and other funduscopic changes, of the heart (particularly heart size), and of the peripheral blood vessels is critical. Many older persons with long-standing untreated high blood pressure will present with a combination of high blood pressure-related funduscopic changes, a diffuse lateral point of maximal impulse (PMI), and diminished peripheral pulses. Auscultation of the major vessels for bruits is important to help assess the degree of atherosclerosis. Of particular importance are the carotid arteries and abdominal aorta. Carotid bruits may influence a decision on how rapidly the target blood pressure is to be achieved. In addition, auscultation should be done over the kidneys (in the midepigastrium), because renal artery stenosis is the most common secondary cause of hypertension in older adults. Upper abdominal bruits radiating laterally are indicative of possible renal artery stenosis and should raise awareness as to the risk of producing acute renal failure should angiotensin-converting enzyme inhibitors be chosen as a blood pressure agent in a patient with bilateral renal artery stenosis [16].

Meticulous and accurate measurement of the blood pressure itself is the most critical component of the physical examination in an elderly person with high blood pressure. This is also the part of the physical examination that may be the most poorly performed in terms of reliability and accuracy. First, blood pressure should only be measured in an older person who is seated, with his or her back supported, and after 5 min of rest. The blood pressure cuff should be placed just above the elbow and the arm should be resting so that the cuff is at the same level as the heart in the chest cavity. Blood pressure should never be taken over clothing, and use of an appropriate cuff size is critical. The width of the cuff should be about 80% of the circumference of the patient's arm. If the clinician is in doubt about the size cuff to use, using an oversized cuff introduces very little measurement error, whereas using an undersized cuff can induce a great deal of measurement error. While the sphygmomanometer cuff is being inflated, the clinician should palpate the radial artery and continue to inflate the cuff until the pulse at the radius is obliterated. (This will avoid mismeasurement caused by to an auscultatory gap.) A standard mercury sphygmomanometer is the instrument of choice, although aneroid sphygmomanometers are reasonably accurate if standardized every few months against a mercury sphygmomanometer. A common source of measurement error is too rapid deflation of the cuff. The cuff should be deflated at the rate of 2 mm per sec. Measure blood pressure in both arms and use the arm with the highest blood pressure for all subsequent determinations. It can be readily appreciated that obtaining an accurate blood pressure measurement can be time consuming. It is consequently often performed by nonphysician personnel. Their training and the periodic reinforcement of that training and standardization of techniques are important in proper management of hypertension, however, especially in the older person. The diagnosis of high blood pressure should be based on the average of three measures over two or three visits. This process is critical in accounting for the variations in blood pressure commonly seen in older people. Once the average of three to six measures over

TABLE 2 Classification of Blood Pressure for Adults

Category	Systolic (mmHg)		Diastolic (mmHg)
Optimal[a]	<120	and	<80
Normal	<130	and	<85
High-normal	130–139	or	85–89
Hypertension[b]			
Stage 1	140–159	or	90–99
Stage 2	160–179	or	100–109
Stage 3	>180	or	>110

Note: Not taking antihypertensive drugs and not acutely ill. When systolic and diastolic blood pressures fall into dierent categories, the high category should be selected to classify the individual's blood pressure state.
[a] Optimal blood pressure with respect to cardiovascular risk is below 120/80 mmHg. Unusually low readings should be evaluated for clinical significance, however.
[b] Based on the average of two or more readings taken at each of two or more visits after an initial screening. *Source*: Ref. 26, p. 2413.

three separate visits is obtained, the patient can be classified according to the potential severity of high blood pressure. The most recent classification system for older adults is shown in Table 2. It is important to note that ISH is covered by this classification system because the stage for a given patient is determined by the component of blood pressure (SBP or DBP), whichever is higher. Other concerns in regard to accuracy of office blood pressure measurements, namely "white coat hypertension" and ambulatory blood pressure monitoring (ABPM), are beyond the scope of this chapter. Because the prevalence of postural hypotension increases as the blood pressure increases, older persons with elevations of blood pressure should regularly have their blood pressure also measured both supine and after standing for 1 to 3 min. As many as 10–15% of untreated elderly persons with high blood pressure will have a decrease in standing SBP of 20 mmHg or more.

Laboratory Evaluation

The laboratory evaluation of older adults can provide important clues as to the severity of complications from hypertension and also the appropriate treatment regimen for specific individuals. Current national guidelines for laboratory tests include a urinalysis, complete blood count, fasting serum glucose and cholesterol [with high-density lipoprotein (HDL), triglycerides and estimation of low-density lipoprotein (LDL)], serum potassium, creatinine, uric acid, and a 12-lead electrocardiogram. Although older persons with high blood pressure have a higher prevalence of cardiac enlargement than younger persons, routine echocardiographic screening is not recommended.

While these recommendations do not differ across all ages, the prevalence of comorbid disease and subclinical CVD is much higher with advancing age, and so the likelihood of laboratory evaluation providing assistance and guiding therapy is greater. The following areas of laboratory evaluation can be of benefit:

1. *BUN-to-creatinine ratio.* A ratio greater than 20 is an indicator of possible dehydration or poor cardiac function [17]. Patients with this finding should be approached cautiously when beginning therapy or when adding a diuretic to behavioral therapies for hypertension.
2. *Serum potassium.* The high prevalence of ventricular arrhythmia and the frequent use of digoxin in older people demands a careful evaluation of potassium status with a special focus on hypokalemia (serum potassium below 3.5 mmol/liter).
3. *Serum sodium.* Reduced ability of the kidney to concentrate or dilute urine is a common phenomenon in aging. Hyponatremia can also be a clue indicating high renin levels in a patient with congestive heart failure. Such patients may experience significant hypotension with exercise therapy or on initiation of therapy with an ACE inhibitor [18].
4. *Proteinuria.* Dipstick valves of 2+ or more indicate the need for an evaluation for possible diabetic nephropathy.

Differential Diagnosis

The diagnosis of high blood pressure in older people is relatively straightforward except for the issues of measurement, misclassification, and stress responses. Measurement problems have been discussed above. There is one major type of misclassification that is limited to the older adult population, specifically pseudohypertension. Pseudohypertension is thought to occur in elderly persons who have very rigid arteries. It is known that the rigidity of arteries on average increases with age. The indirect sphygmomanometer can overestimate the true intra-arterial pressure because increased pressure is required for the blood pressure cuff to compress a stiff artery. Unfortunately, the studies of this phenomenon do not contain representative samples of older persons, so it is difficult to assess the potential prevalence of this condition in the general population. In addition, prior investigations indicate that while there may be some increased estimate of blood pressure by indirect sphygmomanometry in older persons, the actual magnitude of misclassification in most patients is not that high and often does not alter whether or not an older person would be classified as having hypertension. Ancillary studies associated with SHEP indicated that the prevalence of pseudohypertension is low in an aging cohort. Also, other recent studies indicate that Osler's maneuver is neither sensitive nor specific for a true diagnosis of pseudohypertension.

A diagnosis of pseudohypertension should be suspected in older persons who either have relatively high blood pressures but no evidence of end-organ damage or who have symptoms of excessive low blood pressure on antihypertensive therapy even though their measured blood pressures appear to be in the normal range. In other words, pseudohypertension is really only diagnosed based on clinical presentation and is not a common disorder.

The other aspect of differential diagnosis of primary (essential) systolic or diastolic hypertension in older persons is whether or not there may be underlying secondary causes that could be treated so that the blood pressure would return to the normal range. Probably less than 1% of older persons have a secondary cause of hypertension amenable to targeted therapy. The most common cause of secondary hypertension in older people is atherosclerotic renal artery stenosis. The risk of renal artery stenosis increases progressively with advancing age. This diagnosis (renal vascular hypertension) is difficult to make, and surgical treatment is often less than curative. Renovascular high blood pressure or hypertension is associated with an increase in both systolic and diastolic pressure. It is rarely, if ever, associated with ISH with normal levels of DBP, therefore further evaluation is not indicated in an older person who has a treated blood pressure that remains elevated in the systolic range with a normal diastolic pressure. While renal artery atherosclerosis may be present it is unlikely to contribute to isolated elevation of the SBP. In contrast, a new finding of DBP elevation (especially greater than 110 mmHg) in a previously well-controlled patient is reason to pursue the diagnosis of renal artery stenosis if invasive therapy would be recommended should the diagnosis ultimately be made. Other commonly thought of secondary causes of hypertension are rare with advancing age. Primary aldosteronism is relatively rare after age 50. While pheochromocytoma is possible beyond age 65, its incidence is dramatically reduced and there is only one reported case of a pheochromocytoma presenting in a person above the age of 80.

BEHAVIORAL APPROACHES TO MANAGEMENT OF HYPERTENSION IN OLDER PATIENTS

Overview

Nonpharmacologic (i.e., behavioral or lifestyle) modifications are a cornerstone of therapy for high blood pressure in older people, as has been published in the National High Blood Pressure Program Guidelines [26]. Evidence for the efficacy of specific lifestyle interventions is strong for all but the oldest old (age > 85). Nonpharmacological interventions help reduce blood pressure and thus the associated risk of stroke, myocardial infarction, and heart failure. These interventions are valuable in initial therapy or as adjuncts to pharmacologic therapy for older people with high blood pressure. The advantages of nonpharmacologic therapies are magnified in older people and include their low rate of adverse side effects, the active involvement of patients in the treatment process, and collateral benefits on other disease processes, such as obesity, arthritis, and depression. There are also disadvantages for behavioral interventions. These include the possibility of lower levels of compliance common to all ages plus poor compliance due to comorbid disease. Other disadvantages include slower progress toward achievement of treatment goals, and in some cases their potential cost.

Once the diagnosis of high blood pressure is firmly established in an older person, the first step in managing the patient is to assess his or her nutritional status, dietary intake patterns, activity levels, and tobacco and alcohol use. The central components of a good behavioral program for reducing the risk associated with high blood pressure include decreasing dietary sodium, increasing dietary potassium intake, reducing body weight, especially in those who have abdominal obesity, moderating any alcohol intake, increasing physical activity, and controlling stress. Cessation of smoking and reduction of excess alcohol intake is also critical and non-negotiable. While this chapter does not focus on drug therapy for hypertension, part of a health care provider-directed nonpharmacologic approach to hypertension therapy also involves evaluation of the use of certain drugs, such as oral sympathomimetics or non-steroidal anti-inflammatory drug (NSAIDs) (alone or in combination), which may actually cause high blood pressure. It is therefore prudent to review all over-the-counter and prescription medications for all older persons prior to drug treatment for high blood pressure.

For all patients with hypertension and for older patients in particular, combining nonpharmacologic strategies at modest levels is very important. A good approach is to initiate one or two of these strategies monthly with frequent follow-up. This avoids frustration and initial noncompliance and reduces the number of perceived "adverse side effects" from intensive behavioral interventions. A more global strategy of nonpharmacologic intervention therefore should be ultimately implemented in this older population.

SPECIFIC NONPHARMACOLOGIC ANTIHYPERTENSIVE INTERVENTIONS IN OLDER PATIENTS

Salt Restriction

In the area of salt intake, increasing age is generally associated with increasing salt sensitivity, which means that blood pressure increases with a salt load and blood pressure decreases with salt restriction [20]. The Trial of Nonpharmacologic Intervention in the Elderly (TONE) included more than 900 older people age 60 to 80 years and clearly documented the efficacy of salt restriction and weight reduction, alone and in combination, in reducing the need to begin medication therapy for hypertension [21]. While the clinical trial evidence base for recommendations for salt restriction in those persons over age 85 is lacking, the limited evidence indicates an equal if not greater benefit in this growing population. Only small studies have been done in persons beyond this age. These studies involving the oldest old, however, found that blood pressure response to sodium restriction was substantial and indicated that sodium restriction is likely to be effective at all ages. In fact, blood pressure response to sodium restriction may be greater at the highest ages relative to the youngest ages [22,23], thus sodium restriction may be as important and effective as medication therapy for reducing blood pressure in the very old hypertensive. Sodium restriction is also safe at any age, and because of the important goal of limiting polypharmacy, it should be strongly supported in older populations with hypertension. Finally, dietary sodium restriction is inexpensive and therefore may contribute to reduced drug costs, an especially important consideration for most elderly persons with mild to moderate elevations in blood pressure. Clinicians treating older hypertensives should therefore advise all of these patients to maintain as high a degree of dietary sodium restriction as possible.

There are a number of factors associated with salt sensitivity (see Table 3), and age alone identifies an important subpopulation of individuals with hypertension or at risk for incident hypertension who benefit from

TABLE 3 Factors Associated with Salt Sensitivity in Adults

Age
Female gender
Abdominal obesity
Alcoholism
African-American origin
Degree of blood pressure elevation in hypertension
Isolated systolic hypertension (ISH)
Hypertension with low plasma renin
Impaired glucose tolerance
Diabetes
Renal insufficiency
Strong family history of salt-sensitive hypertension
Higher amounts of microalbuminuria

carefully monitored intake of salt. With age, the blood pressure–naturesis curve is shifted to the right (toward higher blood pressure values) for a specified salt load. A higher filtration pressure is therefore needed. This shift is the result of a number of hormonal changes, in particular alterations in the renin-aldosterone system. Because age is probably the most important nonmodifiable factor affecting salt sensitivity, reduction of salt intake is a very important dietary modification in older people.

Table 3 also illustrates that clinicians should make special note of patients with combinations of factors indicative of salt sensitivity. For example, older adults who have obesity and are also African American are particularly important to target for reductions in dietary salt intake. In older adult African Americans, as many as three out of every four individuals with hypertension will be salt-sensitive, and the higher the blood pressure, the greater the likelihood of salt sensitivity and therefore the greater the potential benefit of restricted salt intake. Type 2 diabetes, which increases in prevalence with age, is also associated with salt sensitivity. In general, combinations of risk factors drawn from Table 3 should prompt intensive discussions regarding salt restriction with patients who are either hypertensive or whose borderline blood pressure indicates the potential risk of developing hypertension.

In the United States, the Third National Health and Nutrition Evaluation Survey (NHANES III) has shown that current sodium intake for the U.S. population corresponds to about 8.3 g of salt per day, with 1 g of salt (sodium chloride) containing 393 mg of sodium. Nearly half of all salt in foods is discretionary; in other words, salt that is added either during the cooking process or at the table. Dietary strategies as outlined in the DASH (Dietary Approaches to Stop Hypertension) diet and by the American Heart Association (see below) provide effective guidelines for reducing salt in the diet and optimizing salt-related decreases in blood pressure.

While current guidelines recommend that such nonpharmacologic strategies as salt reduction be attempted for a 3-to-6-month period, in older patients an initial 2-to 3-week trial of total compliance with aggressive salt restriction is a practical approach. Using the 3-week trial as a test, patients should be restricted to no more than 2.4 g of sodium or 6 g of sodium chloride per day. At 3 weeks, a follow-up blood pressure measurement can often be effective in impressing upon salt-sensitive hypertension patients and borderline hypertensives the efficacy of long-term salt restriction. Significant falls in blood pressure after even this short period of sodium restriction suggest the presence of salt sensitivity and the need for lifelong salt intake control in these older patients. The DASH diet, described in Chap. 11, is an excellent long-term strategy for maintaining a low-sodium diet in older people [24,28]. Diets with additional, more aggressive reduction in sodium intake have also clearly demonstrated the efficacy of incorporating the largest possible reductions in sodium intake into the diet, but are particularly difficult to implement in older people. One important obstacle to effective and adequate salt restriction in elderly persons with hypertension is that they may already have a reduced appetite and be at risk for protein calorie malnutrition. For example, taste perception declines for many older adults, and the desire for salt actually may increase in order to make food more palatable. Extreme sodium restriction (reducing salt to less than 6 g/day) may therefore be counterproductive for total reduction in protein–calorie intake in terms of its effect on skeletal muscle mass, but sizeable studies in this population are lacking.

Dietary Potassium and Calcium Intake

Increasing potassium intake in some older hypertensives can be as important as restricting sodium intake [19,27]. Both epidemiologic and interventional studies have shown that enhanced dietary potassium can produce blood pressure lowering in salt-sensitive subjects, and it appears that potassium lowers the blood pressure by limiting the effects of sodium. Potassium also has a substantial natriuretic effect and reduces the release of renin into the systemic circulation. For older patients who have successfully reduced their sodium intake to very low levels, however, dietary potassium has minimal effects on blood pressure. In addition, before enhancing dietary potassium, an assessment of current medication use and also the serum potassium should be completed. (See discussion above.)

Clinical trials have clearly shown a substantial reduction in SBP through the use of diets with enhanced potassium content. The DASH study tested a diet (see Chap. 11) incorporating the concept of effective combinations of salt reduction and potassium maintenance as one strategy for reducing hypertension. The initial DASH study (DASH I) tested the effect of a combination diet rich in fruits and vegetables and low-fat dairy products relative to a typical U.S. diet. This combination diet demonstrated a significant reduction of blood pressure in hypertensive subjects, and in some people eliminated the need for medication to treat hypertension [24].

Calcium is an example of another mineral that has been shown to reduce blood pressure in both clinical and observational trials. Calcium supplements are safe, and many older adults take them, especially older women at risk for the complications of osteoporosis. Compared to interventions involving sodium and potassium intake, however, the blood pressure-lowering effects of calcium are very modest and the consistency of the effect is limited. The DASH study does include calcium-containing milk products such as low-fat milk, yogurt, and cottage cheese as part of its successful, more global, approach to nutritional reductions in blood pressure. These foods are also especially well tolerated in older adults. Here, calcium in combination with potassium, magnesium, and moderate sodium restriction may have the greatest effect. It is important to emphasize that in persons with normal potassium, dietary potassium maintenance should be accomplished through specific foods that are rich in potassium and not by potassium supplements. Potassium supplements for the purpose of blood pressure reduction are ineffective and should be avoided because they have the potential to result in dangerous levels of hyperkalemia. This is a particular concern in hypertensive individuals with undetected degrees of renal insufficiency and in those patients taking a potassium-sparing diuretic. An additional problem with salt substitutes containing potassium is that they often do not enhance food taste, and but for many patients leave a bitter aftertaste, leading to ever-increasing amounts of the potassium supplement.

In summary, for older adults who have responded well to a 3-week trial of dietary sodium restriction, continuing maintainence therapy with the DASH diet is a good strategy and one that is relatively well tolerated. If sufficient gains in blood pressure reduction cannot be achieved with DASH then further sodium restrictions as outlined in a follow-up DASH study [29] would be warranted, although the difficulty of following this diet with increasing age should be noted. The DASH diet was most effective in persons with SBP in the 140-to-160 mmHg range. In these individuals, SBP declined an average of 11.4 mmHg. For the remaining hypertensive older patients who are unable to effectively limit their sodium intake due to adverse effects on protein-calorie intake or other reasons, continued emphasis on moderate sodium restriction in conjunction with an increase intake of potassium through higher levels of fruit and vegetables would be the appropriate recommendation. Furthermore, virtually all unprocessed potassium-containing foods are low in sodium. In addition, the American Heart Association has recently published revised dietary guidelines for sodium intake, maintenance of body weight, and alcohol intake for both middle- and older-age adults. As with the DASH diets, these recommendations emphasize a dietary pattern that maintains a high intake of fruits, vegetables, and low-fat dairy products, and is also low in fat [30].

Alcohol and Caffeine Intake

In terms of alcohol use and hypertension in older adults (age 60 to 80 years), data from the NHANES show a strong relationship between SBP and alcohol consumption of more than 2 oz a day [25]. Excessive alcohol intake by older adults is a growing problem and is very often missed by health care providers [31]. For practitioners treating many patients with high blood pressure, intervening on the degree of alcohol intake is probably one of the more important strategies that can be incorporated. Alcohol is one of the most commonly used pressor agents in society and many difficult-to-treat hypertensive patients are those who are experiencing excessive alcohol intake. The blood pressure-elevating effect of alcohol has been reported in many studies. Alcohol acts through a number of mechanisms, including adversely impacting baroreceptor function, alterations in angiotensin, renin, and insulin metabolism, alterations in electrolyte metabolism, and alterations in the secretion and efficacy of adrenal hormones. As with many conditions and substances, there is a dose–effect relationship; low to moderate alcohol intake (up to two drinks a day) is not associated with increased blood pressure, but higher amounts are.

There are factors in all alcohol users, but especially older adults with excessive alcohol intake, that promote difficult-to-control blood pressure. For example, compliance with therapy is often worse in persons who use alcohol. For those patients who also require antihypertensive medication, metabolism of antihypertensive drugs may be adversely impacted through the systemic effects of alcohol. In addition, a heightened degree of potential side effects for behavioral interventions such as exercise and interactions with the many medications used by older adults (both prescribed and over-the-counter) may occur. Older women are especially susceptible to the effects of alcohol on blood pressure because of gender differences in absorption in combination with age. There is both a lower "first pass" metabolism of alcohol in the stomach, and the volume of distribution for alcohol is lower in women, leading to higher blood alcohol levels for a given dose of intake. As the levels of intake increase, gender differences disappear, but for persons with marginal elevations in blood pressure, it may be that strategies for reducing blood pressure in women may be more effective than men at similar levels of blood pressure and moderate alcohol intake. For any individual that a practitioner suspects is consuming too much alcohol and thus hampering efforts to control blood pressure, a strategy similar to that recommended above for initial dietary salt restriction should be adopted. Specifically, the practitioner should recommend to the patient a 3-week reduction in the frequency of alcohol consumption. For example, patients may be encouraged to limit alcohol to one drink or two drinks every other day but to eliminate the daily dose of alcohol.

Caffeine is another dietary substance that has been linked to blood pressure, but its effect on elevations in blood pressure is generally seen with individuals who are caffeine-naïve. For regular consumers of caffeine products, the risk of blood pressure elevations appears to be less. This is based on data from the studies in which regular caffeine and coffee consumers experienced no adverse impact on blood pressure compared to placebo challenged nonconsumers, even in borderline hypertension [32,33].

Smoking Cessation

Discontinuing tobacco smoking has an immediate effect on reducing high blood pressure and smoking cessation remains a powerful tool for reducing high blood pressure and preventing coronary heart disease death even at advanced ages [34]. Nevertheless, the Cardiovascular Health Study data have shown an adjusted relative risk (RR) of mortality of 1.58 (95% confidence interval 1.25 to 2.0) for adults 65 years and older who have more than a 50 pack-year history of tobacco smoking [7]. Tobacco use is lowest in those age 65 years and older (10.9%); however, risk reduction remains high for cessation of tobacco smoking at any age. During the first 2 years of cigarette smoking cessation, the approximate 50% risk reduction in CVD ages holds true for even the oldest subgroups of adults. Physicians should therefore continue to counsel older smokers about the health benefits of quitting tobacco smoking just as vigorously as they counsel younger smokers. As with all ages, a reasonable approach with older patients is to provide a steady encouragement at each office visit to reduce smoking as much as possible, with the ultimate goal being smoking cessation.

Weight Loss and Exercise

Weight loss is also a highly effective strategy in reducing blood pressure in older people. A 10% reduction in body weight for individuals with mild to moderate obesity can have a considerable impact on reduction in blood pressure and other CVD risk factors. Obviously, for patients who are morbidly obese, nutritional measures are often inadequate in the short term to reduce blood pressure. Long-term strategies to reduce weight, however, can over time reduce or completely eliminate the need for pharmacologic interventions for hypertension. For many older adults (age 60 to 80 years), an important weight and blood pressure control strategy is simply maintaining and not adding body weight. As with all other interventions, weight loss does not automatically produce a reduction in blood pressure, and the response is variable. While the effects of weight reduction on blood pressure may vary, however, the associated improved cardiovascular and overall health risk profile is generalizable across all individuals.

Sedentary lifestyle and hypertension are highly prevalent in the older adult population in the United States, and together present tremendous opportunities for the prevention of CVD-related disability and death. According to the 1996 surgeon general's report on physical activity and health, the elderly are one of the demographic groups at highest risk for inactivity. Nearly one-third of adults over the age of 65 can be classified as sedentary [35]. This same report concluded that regular, sustained physical activity can substantially reduce the risk of developing or dying from high blood pressure. Improving health fitness and quality of life through the adoption and maintenance of regular daily physical exercise is therefore now a stated public health goal.

Cardiovascular disease is strongly associated with functional dependency in older people [4], and physical activity lowers the risk of developing CVD. In 1996, the Committee on Exercise and Cardiac Rehabilitation of the American Heart Association issued a statement outlining the CVD-related benefits of exercise and emphasizing that these benefits extend over the entire life span. These recommendations are based upon a large body of scientific data providing reassurance as to the efficacy and safety of exercise even in the oldest old [36]. Older men and women who engage in regular physical activity experience significant benefit in terms of cardiovascular risk profiles, regardless of their blood pressure status. In particular, endurance exercise in older adults both with and without hypertension have shown decreases in SBP. While the mechanisms of exercise for the reduction of the risk of death and disability in CVD remain unclear, they are no doubt related to a combination of positive effects on blood pressure, body weight, and metabolism.

The power of exercise as a prevention tool in elderly hypertensives relative to other behavioral interventions is illustrated by the fact that while only 10% of adults over the age of 65 smoke tobacco, between 70–80% of the adult population of the United States is less than optimally physically active. Even obesity, which has approximately half the prevalence of physical inactivity, has a lower potential for overall public health impact relative to improvements in physical activity. Increases in physical activity thus provide more opportunity to benefit the health of the population, including elderly hypertensives, than any other behavioral change. Elderly women are at particularly high risk for sedentary behavior relative to men, and so this subpopulation of older adults is an especially important group for physicians and other providers to focus upon in terms of activity-related reductions in high blood pressure.

There is a great deal of misunderstanding in older populations about the benefits of moderate as compared to vigorous exercise and also the benefits of the periodic as opposed to continuous exercise during a daily period. It is most important to note that a structured, vigorous exercise program is not necessary to experience benefit in terms of a reduction in hypertension-related CVD complications. It is critical that physical activity be performed regularly in order to maintain these benefits, however. The Institute of Medicine recently doubled its recommendation for exercise from 30 min to 1 hr of exercise on a daily basis. Health providers should emphasize to older adults with hypertension that intermittent and shorter periods of activity spanning at least 10 min are adequate if accumulated over a day's period and total up to 30 to 60 min. These activities can occur during both occupational and non-occupational settings and range from the traditional forms of exercise, such as brisk walking, cycling, and swimming, to doing yard work and home repair, walking the dog, and strolling young children. All of these activities contribute to cardiovascular fitness and reductions in blood pressure-associated risk. Older adults frequently fail to appreciate the importance of simple walking as exercise.

Sedentary individuals who are older can usually safely begin exercise programs without extensive testing from their physician, and simply need to discuss briefly with their physician their plans before beginning an exercise program [37]. The contraindications for exercise do not differ between young and very old populations, although specific modalities for exercise often need to be altered to accommodate individual disability. A general physical exam to assess and treat any acute medical condition is necessary, but this recommendation consists of no more than what is currently recommended for all older people, regardless of plans to exercise on a periodic basis. The presence of CVD, diabetes, stroke, osteoporosis, depression, dementia or chronic pulmonary disease, chronic renal failure, peripheral vascular disease, or arthritis is not a contraindication to exercise. A small number of untreatable or serious conditions are in fact exclusions for vigorous exercise, and these include such conditions as an enlarging aortic aneurysm, a known cerebral hemorrhage or aneurysm, a history of malignant ventricular arrhythmia, critical aortic stenosis, and end-stage congestive heart failure. Even for the oldest old (>age 80) there is a large amount of literature on exercise training, and to date this literature does not include any reports of increases in serious cardiovascular incidents, sudden death, myocardial infarction, or other serious adverse events.

Table 4 lists some of the recent studies that have demonstrated the cardiovascular benefits of a moderate exercise regimen (and also diet studies) in older persons. Simple changes in behavior can result in important gains in improving cardiovascular fitness. For example, increased walking during daily life, using of stairs, and shifting toward more active recreational pursuits and less reliance on automated devices decreases a sedentary life and confers benefits. Studies have shown that it is possible to change habitual physical activity levels even in older sedentary adults for up to 2 years using both supervised and home-based settings [38]. As noted, walking regimens are one of the most widely studied, feasible, safe, accessible, and economic approaches to cardiovascular training and can be used by adults at almost any age and state of health as long as they can walk. Exercise to reduce the

TABLE 4 Cardiovascular Benefits of Exercise and Diet in Older Adults

Study	Population	Intervention	Endpoint	Reduction
Exercise studies				
Honolulu heart	Men 71 to 93 years old	Walking 1.5 miles/day	CHD	51%
		Walking > 2 miles/day, walking/cycling 20 min tiw	Mortality	41%
Zutphen	Men 64 to 84 years old		CV mortality	31%
Cardiovascular health	Men and women 65 to 101 years old	Moderate exercise	Mortality	22%
Wannamethee et al.	Men, mean age 63 years	At least light activity	Mortality	45%
Diet Studies				
TONE	Men and women 60 to 80 years old, mild HTN	Reduced salt with and without weight loss	Decreased BP; decreased need for medication	31%
DASH	Men 64 to 84 years old with HTN	High in fruits/vegetables; low in meat, fowl, fish, high-fat dairy	Decreased BP to < 140/90 mmHg	70%
Health professional	Men, 40 to 75 years old	Observed on high fiber, potassium, and magnesium	Reduced stroke risk	38%

Note: CHD, coronary heart disease; CV, cardiovascular.

complications of hypertension and improve cardiovascular fitness is probably the easiest recommendation to integrate into daily practice and activities. It simply requires a few behavioral choices to be made and adhered to for reasonable success. Such decisions include the following:

1. Never use an escalator or elevator when stairs are available.
2. Never take the car for errands that can be accomplished by a walk of 10 minutes or less.
3. Avoid using remote control/lower exercise-associated devices as a substitute for manual devices (lawnmowers, mixers, brooms, etc).
4. Park further from a store entrance in the parking lot whenever shopping.

In summary, targeting sedentary older adults with hypertension should be a common approach for clinicians concerned with preventing coronary heart disease complications in this population. More research is needed on the effects of increased physical activity on sedentary older adults with hypertension. Ultimately, increasing physical activity may hold the greatest potential for reducing mortality from hypertension-related coronary heart disease and other CVDs.

Pitfalls and Complications

Once a plan for management with nondrug therapy is devised for an older patient with high blood pressure, the issue of adherence becomes critical. Unfortunately, self-report of adherence has proven to be less than totally accurate. Laboratory testing, such as urine screening for sodium levels for those on dietary interventions, have also proven to be inadequate. Nevertheless, it is important to assess adherence as best as one can (getting a self-report, taking a pill count, or talking with the spouse or significant other). If the physician or other health care provider does this on a routine basis, compliance will probably increase or be maintained even though the physician will never have a precise estimate of the actual level of patient adherence.

Complications or problems in the behavioral management of high blood pressure in older persons are rare. Most involve combinations of behavioral and pharmacologic therapies and include postural hypotension, falls, depression, and reduced protein-calorie intake. On every visit, the clinician should include a formal evaluation of mental status and mood and should directly measure postural changes in blood pressure as well as question the patient about symptoms of dizziness. It is also crucial to obtain a history from family members with regard to the patient's relative vitality, cognition, and overall state of health. Elderly patients should be encouraged to utilize various compliance aids, and older persons' families and caregivers should be enlisted in the effort to maintain adherence to the therapeutic regimen. On the other hand, if older persons adhere rigidly to a nonpharmacologic regimen, they may encounter problems from the side effects of medications. Frequently, older persons who experience side effects from these interventions (musculoskeletal discomfort, loss of taste) are more likely to attribute the cause of the side effect to the aging process than the intervention itself. Both patients and their families must therefore be cautioned with regard to potential problems and their solutions.

REFERENCES

1. Kaplan RC, Psaty BM, Heckbert SR, Smith NL, Lemaitre RN. Blood pressure level and incidence of myocardial infarction among patients treated for hypertension. Am J Pub Health 1999; 89(9):1414–1417.
2. Psaty BM, Furberg CD, Kuller LH, Cushman M, Savage PJ, Levine D, et al. Association between blood pressure level and the risk of myocardial infarction, stroke, and total mortality: the cardiovascular health study. Arch Int Med 2001; 161(9):1183–1192.
3. Prevention of stroke by antihypertensive drug treatment in older persons with isolated systolic hypertension. Final results of the Systolic Hypertension in the Elderly Program (SHEP). SHEP Cooperative Research Group. JAMA 1991; 265(24):3255–3264.
4. Ettinger WH Jr, Fried LP, Harris T, Shemanski L, Schulz R, Robbins J. Self-reported causes of physical disability in older people: the Cardiovascular Health Study. CHS Collaborative Research Group. J Am Geriatr Soc 1994; 42(10):1035–1044.
5. Kannel WB. Rational for treatment of hypertension in the elderly. Am J Geriatr Cardiol 1994; 3(3):33–45.
6. Applegate WB. Hypertension in elderly patients. Ann Int Med 1989; 110(11): 901–915.
7. Fried LP, Kronmal RA, Newman AB, Bild DE, Mittelmark MB, Polak JF, Robbins JA, Gardin JM. Risk factors for 5-year mortality in older adults: the Cardiovascular Health Study. JAMA 1998; 279(8):585–592.
8. Franklin SS. Ageing and hypertension: the assessment of blood pressure indices in predicting coronary heart disease. J Hypertens 1999; 17 (suppl. 5): S29–S36.
9. Alli C, Avanzini F, Bettelli G, Colombo F, Torri V, Tognoni G. The long-term prognostic significance of repeated blood pressure measurements in the elderly: SPAA (Studio sulla Pressione Arteriosa nell'Anziano) 10-year follow-up. Arch Int Med 1999; 159(11):1205–1212.
10. Lloyd-Jones DM, Evans JC, Larson MG, O'Donnell CJ, Levy D. Differential impact of systolic and diastolic blood pressure level on JNC-VI staging. Joint National Committee on Prevention, Detection, Evaluation, and Treatment of High Blood Pressure. Hypertension 1999; 34(3):381–385.

11. Kannel WB, D'Agostino RB, Silbershatz H. Blood pressure and cardiovascular morbidity and mortality rates in the elderly. Am Heart J 1997; 134(4): 758–763.
12. Franklin SS, Khan SA, Wong ND, Larson MG, Levy D. Is pulse pressure useful in predicting risk for coronary heart disease? The Framingham heart study. Circulation 1999; 100(4):354–360.
13. Izzo JL Jr, Black HR. The hypertension primer project: an educational experiment. Hypertension 1999; 33(1):167–168.
14. Somes GW, Pahor M, Shorr RI, Cushman WC, Applegate WB. The role of diastolic blood pressure when treating isolated systolic hypertension. Arch Int Med 1999; 159(17):2004–2009.
15. Langer RD, Criqui MH, Barrett-Connor EL, Klauber MR, Ganiats TG. Blood pressure change and survival after age 75. Hypertension 1993; 22(4): 551–559.
16. Hricik DE, Browning PJ, Kopelman R, Goorno WE, Madias NE, Dzau VJ. Captopril-induced functional renal insufficiency in patients with bilateral renal-artery stenoses or renal-artery stenosis in a solitary kidney. N Engl J Med 1983; 308(7):373–376.
17. Badr KF, Ichikawa I. Prerenal failure: a deleterious shift from renal compensation to decompensation. N Engl J Med 1988; 319(10):623–629.
18. Packer M, Medina N, Yushak M. Relation between serum sodium concentration and the hemodynamic and clinical responses to converting enzyme inhibition with captopril in severe heart failure. J Am Coll Cardiol 1984; 3(4):1035–1043.
19. Suter PM. Potassium and hypertension. Nutr Rev 1998; 56(5 pt. 1):151–153
20. Luft FC, Weinberger MH, Fineberg NS, Miller JZ, Grim CE. Effects of age on renal sodium homeostasis and its relevance to sodium sensitivity. Am J Med 1987; 82(1B):9–15.
21. Whelton PK, Appel LJ, Espeland MA, Applegate WB, Ettinger WH Jr, Kostis JB, et al. Sodium reduction and weight loss in the treatment of hypertension in older persons: a randomized controlled trial of nonpharmacologic interventions in the elderly (TONE). TONE Collaborative Research Group. JAMA 1998; 279(11):839–846.
22. Palmer RM, Osterweil D, Loon-Lustig G, Stern N. The effect of dietary salt ingestion on blood pressure of old-old subjects: a double-blind, placebo-controlled, crossover trial. J Am Geriatr Soc 1989; 37(10):931–936.
23. Cutler JA, Follmann D, Allender PS. Randomized trials of sodium reduction: an overview. Am J Clin Nutr 1997; 65(2 suppl.):643S–651S.
24. Appel LJ, Moore TJ, Obarzanek E, Vollmer WM, Svetkey LP, Sacks FM, et al. A clinical trial of the effects of dietary patterns on blood pressure. DASH Collaborative Research Group. N Engl J Med 1997; 336(16):1117–1124.
25. Welte JW, Greizerstein HB. Alcohol consumption and systolic blood pressure in the general population. Subst Alcohol Actions Misuse 1984; 5(6):299–306.
26. The Sixth Report of the Joint National Committee on Prevention, Detection, Evaluation, and Treatment of High Blood Pressure. Arch Int Med 1997; 157(21):2413–2446.

27. Whelton PK, He J, Appel LJ, Cutler JA, Havas S, Kotchen TA, Roccella EJ, Stout R, Vallbona C, Winston MC, Karimbakas J, the National High Blood Pressure Education Program Coordinating Committee. Primary prevention of hypertension: clinical and public health advisory from the National High Blood Pressure Education Program. JAMA 2002; 288(15):1882–1888.
28. Vollmer WM, Sacks FM, Ard J, Appel LJ, Bray GA, Simons-Morton DG, Conlin PR, Svetkey LP, Erlinger TP, Moore TJ, Karanja N, DASH–Sodium Trial Collaborative Research Group. Effects of diet and sodium intake on blood pressure: subgroup analysis of the DASH-sodium trial. Ann Int Med 2001; 135(12):1019–1028
29. Sacks FM, Svetkey LP, Vollmer WM, Appel LJ, Bray GA, Harsha D, Obarzanek E, Conlin PR, Miller ER 3rd, Simons-Morton DG, Karanja N, Lin PH, DASH–Sodium Collaborative Research Group. Effects on blood pressure of reduced dietary sodium and the Dietary Approaches to Stop Hypertension (DASH) diet. N Engl J Med 2001; 344(1):3–10
30. Krauss RM, Eckel RH, Howard B, Appel LJ, Daniels SR, Deckelbaum RJ, Erdman JW Jr, Kris-Etherton P, Goldberg IJ, Kotchen TA, Lichtenstein AH, Mitch WE, Mullis R, Robinson K, Wylie-Rosett J, St Jeor S, Suttie J, Tribble DL, Bazzarre TL. Revision 2000: a statement for healthcare professionals from the Nutrition Committee of the American Heart Association. J Nutr 2001; 131(1):132–146
31. Conigliaro J, Kraemer K, McNeil M. Screening and identification of older adults with alcohol problems in primary care. J Geriatr Psychiatry Neurol 2000; 13(3):106–114
32. MacDonald TM, Sharpe K, Fowler G, Lyons D, Freestone S, Lovell HG, Webster J, Petrie JC. Caffeine restriction: effect on mild hypertension. BMJ 1991; 303(6812):1235–1238.
33. Robertson D, Hollister AS, Kincaid D, Workman R, Goldberg MR, Tung CS, Smith B.Caffeine and hypertension. Am J Med 1984; 77(1):54–60.
34. Cigarette smoking among adults—United States 1999. Morbid Mortal Wkly Rep 2001; 50(40):869–873.
35. U.S. Dept. of Health and Human Services. Physical activity and health: a report of the surgeon general. Atlanta: U.S. Dept. of Health and Human Services, Centers for Disease Control and Prevention, National Center for Chronic Disease Prevention and Health Promotion, 1996.
36. Fries JF. Exercise and the health of the elderly. Am J Geriatr Cardiol 1997; 6(3):24–32
37. Gill TM, DiPietro L, Krumholz HM. Role of exercise stress testing and safety monitoring for older persons starting an exercise program. JAMA 2000; 284(3):342–349.
38. Campbell AJ, Robertson MC, Gardner MM, Norton RN, Buchner DM. Falls prevention over 2 years: a randomized controlled trial in women 80 years and older. Age Ageing 1999; 28(6):513–518.

16

Intervention in Minorities

Daniel W. Jones and Marion R. Wofford
University of Mississippi Medical Center, Jackson, Mississippi, U.S.A.

INTRODUCTION

The principles of prevention and treatment of hypertension in majority populations hold true in general in minority populations. There are differences, however, in prevalence of hypertension, age of onset, prevalence of target organ damage, associated risks, lifestyle habits, and lifestyle management that are of practical significance to consider. African Americans, in particular, have notable differences to consider. This chapter will focus primarily on intervention in the African-American population.

African Americans have a higher prevalence [1] and incidence [2,3] of hypertension at a given age. African-American men and women have a hypertension prevalence 33% and 50% higher than their European-American counterparts. Mean blood pressures in African Americans are higher than European-Americans' blood pressures at any age, and the age of onset of essential hypertension is usually earlier as well. The higher blood pressure readings begin in childhood and adolescence. Lifestyle factors, particularly factors leading to obesity and dietary choices, play a major role in these early differences [4].

The Coronary Artery Risk Development in Young Adults (CARDIA) study examined a biracial cohort of 5116 persons aged 18 to 30. African Americans had higher mean systolic and diastolic blood pressures at baseline compared to European Americans. Over a 7-year follow-up period, these differences increased. Adjustments for several lifestyle factors including body mass index, physical activity, and alcohol intake, reduced the differences [3]. In the past, there have been large racial disparities in hypertension awareness, treatment, and control rates, but these differences have narrowed in recent surveys, especially among women [5].

Not only does hypertension occur at a younger age, but death and disability related to hypertension complications often occur at a younger age in African Americans [6,7]. While Americans in general have had improving death rates for coronary heart disease and stroke over the last few years, the improvements have been less impressive in African Americans, especially in those living in the southeastern United States [8].

Apparently the excess cardiovascular morbidity and mortality seen in African Americans is primarily due to higher blood pressures with less adequate control as opposed to more disease at a given blood pressure level. At a given blood pressure, African Americans and European Americans seem to have equal risk [9].

Additionally, much of the racial difference in morbidity and mortality in the United States can be attributed to socioeconomic differences. African Americans are more likely to be poor and attain a lower education level. Adjusting for socioeconomic status accounts for much of the racial difference in hypertension and cardiovascular disease outcomes. These effects are more than economic [6], however. There appear to be affects that are not eradicated by one generation of higher income and some that are related to neighborhood of residence [10]. African Americans at any income level have higher rates for hypertension and cardiovascular disease than European Americans [11,12].

There is evidence that racial disparities in target organ damage can be overcome with treatment. In the Hypertension and Detection Program (HDFP), African Americans had similar cardiovascular disease outcomes to non-African Americans [13]. The approach to therapy in HDFP overcame many social issues that make access to care more difficult. Although this was a drug treatment study, there is every reason to believe that equally fair access to lifestyle therapy would lead to similar improvements in outcome.

It is tempting to consider most racial differences in hypertension and other disease states accountable to genetic differences. This is far too simplistic, however, and as it turns out, not accurate. There are compelling data that demand environmental influences be considered a major part of the explanation of racial differences.

First, migration studies of the African diaspora reveal a graded level of blood pressure and hypertension prevalence, with the lowest rates occurring in rural Africa and the highest rates occurring in the southeastern United States [14]. As Africans move toward more "Western" lifestyles, mean blood pressure and hypertension prevalence increase. Factors associated with changes in blood pressure include high caloric, fat, and sodium content in the diet and a more sedentary lifestyle [15,16]. African Americans are substantially more obese than Africans. Persons of African descent living in the Caribbean have intermediate findings in all these areas.

Within the United States, there are also substantial geographic differences in hypertension, other cardiovascular risk factors, and cardiovascular disease rates. This is true of African Americans as well as European Americans [8,14]. Most of the geographic disparity in hypertension and cardiovascular disease is likely related to differences in lifestyles, including diet and physical activity. Residents of the southeastern United States tend to be more obese, tend to have lower intakes of potassium and calcium, and perhaps higher intakes of sodium, and are more sedentary than residents of other regions [14].

The baseline data from the Dietary Approaches to Stop Hypertension (DASH) study provide evidence of the difference in nutrient intake in African Americans compared to European Americans [17]. Data for diets taken prior to the study (usual diets) demonstrated lower intakes of dairy products, calcium, and magnesium for African Americans. African-American women were heavier than European-American women. Heavier women reported lower intakes of protein and potassium and higher intake of fat. Overall, young, overweight African-American women had the least favorable diets among the DASH participants. African-American women had a more atherogenic diet than did white women. Although African-American men did not have higher obesity rates than European-American men, the intake of dairy products and potassium were lower. Data from the National Health and Nutrition Examination Survey (NHANES) confirms significant racial differences in nutrient intake [18].

Other data comparing body mass index for African Americans and European Americans are seen in the Atherosclerosis Risk in Communities Study (ARIC). Obesity rates are substantially higher in African-American women [19,20]. Obesity rates for African-American children are higher than for European-American children as well [21].

Obesity is not only associated with higher blood pressures [22], but also accounts for other cardiovascular renal risk [23]. Obesity is associated with left ventricular hypertrophy [24] and albuminuria [25,26]. Some believe it is the most likely explanation for increasing prevalence rates of hypertension and end stage renal disease in this country [23].

Though genetic influences are almost certainly a part of the reason for racial differences in hypertension prevalence and associated risk, it is clear that environmental influences (lifestyle) must play a major role. The good news that derives from this fact is that modification of lifestyle habits in minority populations should be useful in the prevention and treatment of hypertension.

There is evidence that supports aggressive intervention in lifestyle management in minority groups. We will first examine the evidence in detail for African Americans. Lifestyle topics addressed in other chapters will be considered, including a comprehensive dietary approach (DASH), dietary sodium, potassium, weight, physical activity, and stress.

COMPREHENSIVE DIETARY APPROACH

The evidence regarding the use of diet as a successful intervention for prevention and treatment of hypertension was dramatically changed with the presentation and publication of the DASH study [27]. This study was designed to address several frustrating issues in dietary intervention research.

First, the study was designed as a feeding study to address the effects of change in nutritional intake without having to deal with issues of food selection in an environment in which selection is so challenging. Participants were provided with food prepared by study personnel. Participants in the study included a broad age range of adults, both hypertensive and normotensive. Because of the hypertension challenge in African Americans, this group was oversampled to allow for subgroup analysis by race [27].

Another important design issue was the decision to test blood pressure response to a comprehensive diet approach, rather than to test one element of diet, such as sodium or potassium. In the initial study, participants were given a control diet (similar to the typical American diet), a diet high in fruits and vegetables, or the fruit and vegetable diet plus low-fat diary products. In all three diets, calories and sodium intake were held equal. The diets were designed to maintain weight at baseline.

The diet high in fruits, vegetables, and low-fat dairy products proved to be the best of the three for blood pressure reduction. This diet reduced systolic blood pressure 11.4 mmHg ($p < 0.001$) and diastolic blood pressure 2.8mmHg ($P = 0.013$) in the entire group [27]. There are several reasons to predict a good response in African Americans to this diet: (1) the higher stage of hypertension in African Americans; (2) knowledge that dietary intake of African Americans was not as healthy as European Americans at baseline in this study, and (3) the strength of the evidence that lifestyle has a significant effect on hypertension risk. Rarely have study results confirmed as nicely what one would predict and hope [28]. African Americans, both hypertensive and normotensive, had better responses to the diet than European Americans [27].

Among African Americans with hypertension, the DASH diet reduced blood pressure by 13.2/6.1 mmHg (95% confidence interval −18.2 to −8.1/ −9.1 to −0.8) Among white hypertensives blood pressure decreased 6.3/4.4 mmHg (95% confidence interval −12.9 to 0.4/−9.4 to 0.6). Among normotensive African Americans, blood pressure was reduced by 4.3/2.6 (95% confidence interval −6.5 to −2.2/−4.4 to −0.8). The diet reduced blood pressure in normotensive whites by 2.0/1.2 mmHg (95% confidence interval −4.3 to 0.3/−3.2 to 0.8) [29].

This study demonstrated the clear utility of dietary intervention for both treatment and prevention of hypertension. Just as important, it demonstrated the most benefit in those at highest risk; African Americans had a better response than European Americans.

DIETARY SODIUM

Because sodium was held constant in the initial study, it needed to be determined whether or not a reduction in sodium content in the diet would improve on the response of the DASH diet. The DASH-sodium study was designed to answer this important question [30]. Participants were provided with either the DASH diet or a control diet (typical American diet), with sodium controlled in both at three levels: 3300 mg/day (the average consumed by most Americans), 2400 mg/day (the upper limit of current recommendations), and a lower intake of 1500 mg/day. Again, both hypertensive and normotensive persons participated (African Americans as well as European Americans).

Once again, the results were impressive. Those eating the DASH diet had better blood pressures than those eating the control diet at all three sodium intakes. Also, the lower the sodium intake, the lower the blood pressure, regardless of whether participants were on the DASH or control diet. The lowest blood pressures were in those on the DASH low-sodium diet. The highest blood pressures were in those on the control diet at the highest sodium level. Again, African Americans had a larger reduction in blood pressure in all the diet subgroups compared to their European-American counterparts [30].

The effects of sodium reduction were greater in African-American participants than in others. Compared to the combination of the control diet and high sodium intake, the lowest-sodium DASH diet decreased systolic blood pressure by 12.6 mmHg in African-American hypertensives compared to 9.5 mmHg in non-African-American hypertensives. In normotensives, the difference was 7.2 mmHg for African Americans and 6.9 mmHg for others ($P < 0.001$ for all subgroups). These data confirm that both the DASH diet and sodium reduction (with or without the DASH diet) are powerful tools for lowering blood pressure in African Americans. Dietary intervention is effective to treat those with hypertension and to prevent hypertension in the normotensive [30,31].

It is a common misconception that sodium intake is higher in African Americans than other ethnic groups in this country. This may have been true in the distant past, but recent data suggest similar intakes of dietary sodium in African Americans and European Americans [32]. African Americans do tend to have more sensitivity to sodium, however (more rise in blood pressure for a given exposure to dietary sodium). Both short-term [33] and chronic exposure to sodium [34] raises blood pressure in a high percentage of African Americans, both normotensive and hypertensive. Demographic characteristics associated with more sodium sensitivity are African-American race, older age, female gender, and high body weight [35,36]. The failure to appropriately excrete a sodium load leads to short-term and long-term elevation of blood pressure.

Though African Americans do not have higher sodium intakes in general, they do have lower intakes of dietary potassium [37] and higher body weights [20] than European Americans do. Both of these have been demonstrated to increase sodium sensitivity, producing higher blood pressures at a given dietary sodium intake than those without risks [35,36]. Physical inactivity also affects sodium sensitivity [38]. African Americans are more sedentary than other groups, and this may contribute to the adverse affects of dietary sodium [6].

Prior to the publication of the DASH-sodium study results, there has been considerable controversy regarding the benefits of restricting dietary sodium. Some have even suggested that restriction of dietary sodium might have harmful affects [39]. Data regarding the association between dietary sodium and blood pressure has been confusing [40].

The majority of the world's populations eat much more sodium than is physiologically necessary and within a fairly narrow range. In designing studies, this has made inclusion of populations with a diverse intake of sodium difficult, leading to results in some studies suggesting little or no relationship [41]. Intervention studies have been difficult because of challenging compliance to a low-sodium diet over prolonged periods. Participants in studies eating foods that they buy and prepare themselves have great challenges in this country in maintaining low sodium intakes. The DASH-sodium diet overcame these challenges with the feeding study methodology [30].

DIETARY POTASSIUM

Just as there has been confusion regarding the benefits of restricting dietary sodium, confusion exists regarding the benefit of increased potassium intake. This is partly because of the complex interaction between sodium and potassium [42]. Some believe much of the benefit of reduced sodium intake may actually be due to an increase in the intake of potassium. In a low-sodium diet, high-sodium, low-potassium foods are usually replaced by low-sodium, high-potassium foods. Some studies have reported an inverse relationship between dietary potassium and blood pressure [42,43], especially in African Americans [44]. Many studies, however, have failed to demonstrate a benefit to blood pressure with increased potassium intake.

A meta-analysis by Whelton of 33 randomized trials provides clarity regarding dietary potassium [45]. This analysis demonstrated that the greatest reduction in blood pressure related to potassium supplementation was seen in subjects with the lowest baseline potassium intakes. This included those with hypertension, African Americans, and those with high dietary sodium intakes.

Aside from its benefit on blood pressure, higher potassium intake appears to have cardiovascular-protective effects. In stroke-prone rats, very high potassium supplementation essentially eliminates stroke risk [46]. In human observational studies, those with the highest intake of fruits and vegetables that are high in potassium had the lowest stroke rates [47]. African Americans have lower potassium intake than European Americans [37]. Increasing dietary potassium in African Americans likely improves not only blood pressure, but may have a direct effect on the reduction of cardiovascular disease risk.

WEIGHT

In this country, obesity is epidemic in all groups, but especially among African-American women. More than 75% of the African-American women in the ARIC cohort (age 45 to 64) were obese [19,20]. Obesity rates are high and increasing in this country. The increasing levels of obesity are a major part of the increase in hypertension and type II diabetes mellitus rates [24]. In African Americans in ARIC, 23% of the women and 19% of the men have diabetes [6]. Childhood overweight is also epidemic in the United States, with the greatest prevalence seen in African-American and Hispanic children [21].

Blood pressure and body weight are strongly associated across a wide range of body weights [22]. At any given weight, a decrease of a few pounds will improve blood pressure, make antihypertensive medications more effective, and reduce the number of antihypertensive medications needed for control [48].

Though the evidence for the benefit of weight loss is clear, challenges remain. Weight loss is difficult to achieve and much more difficult to maintain [48]. In African Americans, there are many cultural and socioeconomic factors to consider in designing treatment programs regarding weight control. Issues of body image, access to healthy foods, education, and literacy are all issues that must be addressed [49–56].

PHYSICAL ACTIVITY

The evidence that regular physical activity improves cardiovascular outcomes is strong, yet each year Americans become more sedentary. Among all race and gender groups in this country, the prevalence of physical inactivity is highest in African-American women [6]. Many studies in normotensive and hypertensive persons have demonstrated a benefit to aerobic exercise. In a group of black men with severe hypertension requiring multiple medications, 16 weeks of regular aerobic exercise improved blood pressure, reduced medication use, and reduced left ventricular mass [57].

STRESS

Nothing in lifestyle influences in minority populations is more controversial or confusing than stress. There are many potential contributors to stress that are unique to African Americans [58]. Racism and discrimination are social realities in many societies. Many consider racism and the individual response to racism (John Henryism) as a factor in the disparity in blood pressure and cardiovascular disease [59].

Stress and its effects are difficult to measure, therefore quantification of this problem has been challenging [60]. Newer studies focusing on African-American issues are addressing this difficult issue [6]. Some existing data shed some light. African-American children have a greater pressor response to stress than European-American children [61]. African-American adults have enhanced peripheral sympathetic nerve activity with exposure to stress [62].

OTHER MINORITY GROUPS

Many of the challenges seen in the African-American community are experienced in other minority groups in this country. Obesity is a major problem in Hispanics [63]. Obesity is associated with high rates of type II diabetes mellitus, but hypertension rates are somewhat lower in Hispanics than in other ethnic groups. Hispanic Americans do experience high rates of cardiovascular disease [64].

CHALLENGES OF INTERVENTION

Now that we know certain lifestyle interventions are useful in improving blood pressure in minority populations, it would seem that implementation would be simple and automatic. This is far from reality. The DASH and DASH-sodium studies provided the best support to date for lifestyle intervention in African Americans. A strong study design was achieved, contributing to the success of the studies. The feeding study approach necessary to prove benefit is impossible to implement on a populationwide basis, however. Short-term and long-term compliance to lifestyle interventions have been and remain a major challenge [65].

Current strategies call for interventions of education and behavior modification that depend on individual choice. The results of the education and behavior interventions are highly dependent on educational level, motivation, and access to appropriate foods and exercise opportunities.

Even the best educated and motivated have difficulties maintaining healthy dietary choices in our general culture. Our lifestyles dictate little time for food preparation. Most Americans consume a diet high in processed foods purchased in grocery stores, restaurants, and fast food chains. African-American neighborhoods tend to have fewer healthy choices for both food and exercise. Despite one's personal education or income, our health is connected to the neighborhoods in which we live [10]. African Americans are much more likely to live in low-income neighborhoods, regardless of personal income. Further influence of culture includes body image in African-American women and certain ethnic food patterns adverse to health.

An important next step in research is to determine if the highly effective DASH-sodium study can be replicated in a study design more suited to everyday life [65]. It will not be surprising if it is challenging for individuals to adhere to the DASH-sodium diet through an educational and behavioral intervention and without protocol-provided foods. The problem is food choice. Currently, we are faced with easy access to less healthy foods and difficult access to healthier foods.

If we are to successfully implement the use of diets similar to DASH-sodium in the prevention and treatment of hypertension, we must have access to better food choices. At the least, this will require cooperation of the food and restaurant industries in this country. Persons of all races will have better opportunities for prevention and treatment of hypertension through lifestyle management if this is accomplished.

REFERENCES

1. Burt VL, Whelton P, Roccella EJ, Brown C, Cutler JA, Higgins M, Horan MJ, Labarthe D. Prevelance of hypertension in the US adult population: results from the Third National and Nutrition Examination Survey, 1988–1991. Hypertension 1995;25: 305–313.
2. Dyer AR, Liu K, Walsh M, Kiefe C, Jacobs DR Jr, Bild DE. Ten-year incidence of elevated blood pressure and its predictors: the CARDIA study. Coronary Artery Risk in Young Adults. J Hum Hypertens 1999;13: 12–21.
3. Liu K, Ballew C, Jacobs DR Jr. Ethnic Differences in BP, pulse rate, and related characteristics in young adults: the CARDIA study. Hypertension 1989; 14: 218–226.
4. Berenson GS, Wattigney WA, Webber LS. Epidemiology of hypertension from childhood to young adulthood in black, white, and Hispanic population samples. Pub Health Rep 1996;111: 3–6.
5. Burt VL, Cutler JA, Higgins M, Horan MJ, Labarthe D, Whelton P, Brown C, Roccella EJ. Trends in the prevalence, awareness, treatment, and control of hypertension in the adult US population: data from the health examination surveys, 1960 to 1991. Hypertension 1995; 26: 60–69.
6. Jones DW, Sempos CT, Thom TJ, Harrington AM, Taylor HA, Fletcher BW, et al. Rising levels of cardiovascular mortality in Mississippi, 1979–95. Am J Med Sci 2000; 319: 131–137.
7. Sempos CT, Bild DE, Manolio TA. Overview of the Jackson Heart Study: a study of cardiovascular diseases in African American men and women. Am J Med Sci 1999; 317: 142–146.
8. Jones DW, Basile J, Cushman W, Egan B, Ferrario C, Hill M, et al. Consortium for southeastern hypertension control. managing hypertension in the southeastern United States: applying the guidelines from the Sixth Report of the Joint National Committee on Prevention, Detection, Evaluation, and Treatment of High Blood Pressure (JNC-VI). Am J Med Sci 1999; 318: 357–364.
9. Cooper RS, Liao Y. Is hypertension among blacks more severe or simply more common? Circulation 1992; 85 (abstract):12.
10. Diex-Roux A, Merkin SS, Arnett D, Chambless L, Massing M, Nieto FJ, Sorlie P, Szklo M, Tyroler HA, Watson RL. Neighborhood of residence and incidence of coronary heart disease. N Engl J Med 2001; 345: 99–106.
11. Sorlie P, Rogot E, Anderson R, et al. Black–white mortality differences by family income. Lancet 1992; 340:346–350.
12. Gillum RF. The epidemiology of cardiovascular disease in black Americans. N Engl J Med 1996; 335: 1597–1599.
13. Hypertension Detection and Follow-up Program Cooperative Group. Five year

findings of Hypertension Detection and Follow-up Program. II. Mortality by race, sex, and age. JAMA 1979; 242:2572–2576.
14. Hall WD, Ferrario CM, Moore MA, et al. Hypertension-related morbidity and mortality in the southeastern United States. Am J Med Sci 1997; 31: 195–209.
15. Poulter NR, Khaw KT, Hopwood BEC, et al. The Kenyan Luo migration study: observations on the initiation of a rise in BP. Br Med J 1990; 300; 967–972.
16. Cooper RS, Rotimi CN, Ward R. The puzzle of hypertension in African-Americans. Sci Am 1999; 280: 56–63.
17. Karanja NM, McCullough ML, Kumanyika SK, Pedula KL, Windhauser MM, Obarzanek E, Lin PH, Champagne CM, Swain JF. Pre-enrollment diets of Dietary Approaches to Stop Hypertension trial participants. DASH Collaborative Research Group. J Am Diet Assoc 1999; 99: S28–S34.
18. Ford ES. Race, education, and dietary cations: findings from the Third National Health and Nutrition Examination Survey. Ethn Dis 1998; 8: 10–20.
19. Folsom AR, Burke GL, Byers CL, et al. Implications of obesity for cardiovascular disease in blacks: the CARDIA and ARIC studies. Am J Clin Nutr 1991; 53(suppl.): 1604S–1611S.
20. Wofford MR, Andrew ME, Pickett RA, Brown CA, Wyatt SW, King DS, Jones DW. Obesity hypertension in the atherosclerosis risk in communities cohort: implications of obesity guidelines. J Clin Hypertens 1999;1:27–32.
21. Strauss RS, Pollack HA. Epidimic increase in childhood overweight. JAMA 2001; 286:1986–1998
22. Jones DW, Kim JS, Andrew ME, Kim SJ, Hong YP. Body mass index and blood pressure in Korean men and women: the Korean National Blood Pressure Survey. J Hypertens, 1994; 12: 1433–1437.
23. Hall JE, Brands MW, Henegar JR, et al. Abnormal kidney function as a cause and a consequence of obesity hypertension. Clin Exp Pharmacol Physiol 1998; 25: 58–64.
24. Gottdiener JS, Reda DJ, Materson BJ, et al. Importance of obesity, race and age to the cardiac structural and functional effects of hypertension: the Department of Veterans Affairs Cooperative Study Group on Antihypertensive Agents. J Am Coll Cardiol 1994; 24:1492–1498.
25. Anderson PJ, Chan JC, Chan YL, et al. Visceral fat and cardiovascular risk factors in Chinese NIDDM patients. Diabetes Care 1997; 20: 1854–1858.
26. Metcalf PA, Scragg RK, Dryson E. Associations between body morphology and microalbuminuria in healthy middle-aged European, Maori and Pacific Island New Zealanders. Int J Obes Relat Metab Disord 1997; 21: 203–210.
27. Conlin PR, Chow D, Miller ER 3rd, Scetkey LP, Lin PH, Harsha DW, Moore TJ, Sacks FM, Appel LJ. The effect of dietary patterns on blood pressure control in hypertensive patients: results from the Dietary Approaches to Stop Hypertension (DASH) trial. Am J Hypertens 2000; 13: 949–955.
28. Greenland P. Beating high blood pressure with low-sodium DASH. N Engl J Med 2001; 344: 3–10.

29. Svetkey LP, Simons-Morton D, Vollmer WM, Appel LJ, Conlin PR, Ryan DH, Ard J, Kennedy BM. Effects of dietary patterns on blood pressure: subgroup analysis of the Dietary Approaches to Stop Hypertension (DASH) randomized clinical trial. Arch Int Med 1999;159: 285–293.
30. Sacks FM, Svetkey LP, Vollmer WM, Appel LJ, Bray GA, Harsha D, Obarzanek E, Conlin PR, Miller ER 3rd, Simons-Morton DG, Karanja N, Lin PH; DASH-Sodium Collaborative Research Group. Effects on blood pressure of reduced dietary sodium and the Dietary Approaches to Stop Hypertension (DASH) diet. DASH-Sodium Collaberative Research Group. N Engl J Med 2001; 344: 3–10.
31. Fleet JC. DASH without the dash (of salt) can lower blood pressure. Nutr Rev 2001;59: 291–293.
32. Veterans Administration Cooperative Study Group on Antihypertensive Agents. Urinary and serum electrolytes in untreated and white hypertensives. J Chron Dis 1987; 9: 839–847.
33. Luft FC, Miller JZ, Grim CE, et al. Salt sensitivity and resistance of BP. Hypertension 1991; 17(suppl. 1): 102–108.
34. Falkner B, Hulman S, Kushner H. Hyperinsulinemia and BP sensitivity to sodium in young blacks, J Am Soc Nephrol 1992; 3: 940–946.
35. Weinberger MH. Salt sensitivity of blood pressure in humans. Hypertension 1996; 27: 481–490.
36. Weinberger MH, Fineberg NS. Sodium and volume sensitivity of blood pressure: age and pressure change over time. Hypertension 1991; 18:67–71.
37. Langford HG, Watson RL, Potassium and calcium intake, excretion, and homeostasis in blacks, and their relation to blood pressure. Cardiovasc Drug Ther 1990; 4: 403–406.
38. Rocchini AP, Key J, Bondie D, et al. The effect of weight loss on the sensitivity of blood pressure to sodium in obese adolescents. N Engl J Med 1989; 321: 580–585.
39. Alderman MH, Madhavan S, Cohen J, et al. Low urinary sodium is associated with greater risk of myocardial infarction among treated hypertensive men. Hypertension 1995; 25: 1144–1152.
40. Alderman MH. The great salt war. Am J Hypertens 1997; 10: 584–585.
41. Cutler JA, Follmann D, Allender PS, Randomized trials of sodium reduction: an overview. Am J Clin Nutr 1997; 65(suppl.): 643S–651S.
42. Dyer AR, Elliot P, Shipley M, et al. Body mass index and associations of sodium and potassium with blood pressure in INTERSALT. Hypertension 1994; 23: 729–736.
43. Geleijnse JM, Hofman A, Witteman JCM, et al. Long-term effects of neonatal sodium restriction on blood pressure. Hypertension 1996; 29: 913–917.
44. Veterans Administration Cooperative Study Group on Antihypertensive Agents. Urinary and serum electrolytes in untreated black and white hypertensives. J Chron Dis 1987; 40: 839–847.
45. Whelton PK, He J, Cutler JA, et al. Effects of oral potassium on blood pressure. JAMA 1997; 277: 1624–1632.

46. Tobian L, Sugimoto T, Everson T. High K diets protect arteries, possibly by lowering renal papillary Na and thereby increasing interstitial cell secretion (abstract). Hypertension 1992; 20: 403.
47. Khaw K-T, Barrett-Connor E. Dietary potassium and stroke-associated mortality. A 12-year prospective population study. N Engl J Med 1987; 316: 235–240.
48. Jones DW, Miller ME, Wofford MR, Anderson DC, Cameron ME, Willoughby DL, Adair CT, King NS. The effect of weight loss intervention on antihypertensive medication requirements in the HOT Study. Am J Hypertens 1999; 12: 1175–1180.
49. Stevens J, Kumanyika SK, Keil JE. Attitudes toward body size and dieting: differences between elderly black and white women. Am J Pub Health 1994; 84: 1322–1325.
50. Kumanyika SK. Special issues regarding obesity in minority populations. Ann Int Med 1993; 119: 650–654.
51. Kumanyika SK, Charleston JB. Lose weight and win: a church-based weight loss program for blood pressure control among black women. Patient Educ Couns 1992; 19: 19–32.
52. Kumanyika SK. The impact of obesity on hypertension management in African Americans. J Health Care Poor Underserved 1997; 8: 352–364.
53. Kumanyika SK. Minisymposium on obesity: overview and some strategic considerations. Ann Rev Pub Health 2001; 22: 293–308.
54. Johnson EH, Brandsond D, Everett J, Lollis CM. Obesity and hypertension among African Americans: do African American primary care providers address these conditions when secondary to primary illness? J Natl Med Assoc 1996; 88: 225–229.
55. Tucker K. Dietary patterns and blood pressure in African Americans. Nutr Rev 1999; 57: 356–358.
56. Conlin PR. Dietary modification and changes in blood pressure. Curr Opin Nephrol Hypertens 2001; 10: 359–363.
57. Kokkinos PF, Narayan P, Colleran JA, et al. Effects of regular exercise on blood pressure and left ventricular hypertrophy in African-American men with severe hypertension. N Engl J Med 1995; 333: 1462–1467.
58. Schneider RH, Staggers F, Alxander CN, Sheppard W, Rainforth M, Kondwani K, Smith S, King CG. A randomised controlled trial of stress reduction for hypertension in older African Americans. Hypertension 1995; 26: 820–827.
59. James SA, Kaufman JS, Raghunathan TE, et al. Five year hypertension incidence in African Americans: the contribution of socioeconomic status, perceived stress, and John Henryism (abstract). Am J Hypertens 1996; 9: 19A.
60. Bond V, Mills RM, Caprarola M, Vaccaro P, Adams RG, Blakely R, Roltsch M, Hatfield B, Davis GC, Franks BD, Fairfax J, Banks M. Aerobic exercise attenuates blood pressure reactivity to cold pressor test in normotensive, young adult African-American women. Ethn Dis 1999; 9: 104–110.
61. Murphy JK, Alpert BS, Walker SS. Consistency of ethnic differences in

children's pressor reactivity: 1987 to 1992. Hypertension 1994; 23(suppl. I): I152–I155.
62. Calhoun DA, Mujtinga ML, Collins AS, et al. Normatensive blacks have heightened sympathetic response to cold pressor test. Hypertension 1993; 22: 801–805.
63. Park MK, Menard SW, Schoolfield J. Prevalence of overweight in a triethnic pediatric population of San Antonio, Texas. Int J Obes Relat Metab Disord 2001; 25: 409–416.
64. Crespo CJ, Loria CM, Burt VL. Hypertension and other cardiovascular disease risk factors among Mexican Americans, Cuban Americans, and Puerto Ricans from the Hispanic Health and Nutrition Examination Survey. Public Health Rep 1996; 111 (suppl. 2): 7–10.
65. Appel LJ. The role of diet in the prevention and treatment of hypertension. Curr Atheroscler Rep 2000; 2: 521–528.

17

Policies for Prevention and Treatment of Hypertension

Edward D. Frohlich
Alton Ochsner Medical Foundation, New Orleans, Louisiana, U.S.A.

Edward J. Roccella and Claude Lenfant
National Heart, Lung, and Blood Institute, Bethesda, Maryland, U.S.A.

> *Any plan or course of action adopted by Government, business organizations or the like designed to influence and determine decisions, actions, or other matters* [1].

INTRODUCTION

A discussion of the health policies is appropriate for any text concerned about the issues of prevention and treatment of diseases in the United States, or for that matter, for any national population or health care organization. Broad sociological, economic, political, fundamental, and clinical research issues that ultimately effect patient care are brought to focus by clear health policies for disease prevention and management. Since the American population is increasingly one of advancing age, prevention and treatment of disease have become of primary importance. Health policy transcends the myriad of issues considered by local and federal legislative bodies, governmental executive departments, and insurance and third-party reimbursors for health care, and of course, health care professional organizations. Development of health care policies is thus necessary to bring together the many societal issues that impinge upon diagnosis, treatment, and follow-up care. Furthermore, there is no more important group of diseases demanding well-conceived approaches than cardiovascular diseases. Diseases of the cardiovascular system account for one out of every two deaths in the United States and are responsible for the greatest number of hospitalizations for Medicare recipients in this country [2]. Of particular value for this discussion is the overall problem of the hypertensive diseases.

The National High Blood Pressure Education Program (NHBPEP) will soon celebrate its thirtieth anniversary. Administered by the National Heart, Lung, and Blood Institute (NHLBI), the NHBPEP is a coalition of professional and voluntary organizations, state health departments, community cardiovascular disease programs, local health agencies, and civic groups. Guided by the advice and consensus of a coordinating committee comprising representatives from 45 professional, voluntary, and federal agencies, the program has succeeded in reducing the prevalence of—and gaining control of—hypertension in the United States [3].

In the first two decades of the NHBPEP, policy concentrated on the detection and treatment of hypertension, with special emphasis on those individuals who had the highest levels of blood pressure. This policy of clinical guidelines is exemplified by the Sixth Report of the Joint National Committee on Prevention, Detection, Evaluation, and Treatment of High Blood Pressure (JNC6)[4]. The NHLBI and its partners remain involved in developing clinical guidelines as a natural extension of the federal mandate to improve the health of the people of the United States by conducting research, investigations, experiments, and demonstrations relating to the cause, prevention, and methods of diagnosis and treatment of diseases of the heart and circulation, including high blood pressure. Congress has indicated that the NHLBI's obligation to the public is unfulfilled even though a research project was successfully completed, thus the NHLBI was directed to develop and implement methods for public and professional education on disease awareness, prevention, and control to reduce cardiovascular morbidity, mortality, and health care costs, and to provide updated, peer-reviewed educational programs and publications. In the area of hypertension, these efforts have provided a model for the development of World Health Organization [5] and other national educational publications [6,7], each with its own guidelines, recommendations, and justification.

THE NEED FOR POLICIES

Guidelines and the development of clinical policies are the logical first steps in translating basic research advances into public health benefits. The full value of the many cardiovascular disease clinical trials and other studies could never be achieved without the final step of transferring the results to medical practice, primarily through clinical guidelines and education programs, hence guidelines and education programs are viewed as natural opportunities to translate research findings to practicing health care professionals. This process of translating research for clinical care purposes is all the more critical today because of the remarkable proliferation of information from clinical trials and studies.

The world was stunned by the death of President Franklin Delano Roosevelt at the age of 63 from hypertension, a disease that could not then be treated because of the lack of effective therapy. In the years following his death, medical science generated information at a seemingly exponential rate resulting in more than 50 antihypertensive agents available to treat patients with all forms of severity of hypertension [4]. Virtually every large-scale clinical trial demonstrating the efficacy of lowering blood pressure was conducted in the last 35 years. In addition, lifestyle modification methods have been tested, developed, and shown to lower blood pressure in the less severe forms of hypertension dramatically. They are facilitated by the effectiveness of antihypertensive agents [8–10].

Never before has the production of scientific information been as great as it has been in the past three decades. This is evidenced by the vast number of hypertension clinical trials, the numbers of societies and scientific programs exclusively or largely dedicated to conducting scientific conferences and education programs dealing with hypertension prevention and management, and the number of scientific journals devoted to reporting hypertension research results, as well as the proliferation of scientific papers regarding some aspect of hypertension. Evidence of the effectiveness of blood pressure-lowering therapy has been increasingly documented and extended to older people, including those with isolated systolic pressure elevation, those with so-called mild forms of hypertension, and even those individuals with lower levels of blood pressure who have coexisting cardiovascular conditions, such as diabetes mellitus, hyperlipidemia, and obesity [11,12]. This has increased the number and type of people being treated for hypertension and related disorders. This proliferation of information, and the need to extend treatment to different portions of the population who present with a variety of cardiovascular risk factors and comorbidities, has placed increased demands on and required decisions from the medical community. Changes in the health care delivery system have created a natural demand for the treatment to be more evidence-based and more efficient. Developing clinical guidelines presents a cost-effective way to synthesize the large and ever-growing body of scientific information to improve the effectiveness, efficiency, and facility for treatment. These guidelines have been designed to reduce inappropriate practice treatment variation patterns so that all patients can benefit from the existing scientific findings.

CONSIDERATIONS FOR POLICY DEVELOPMENT

Clinical guidelines and policies employ a range of methods, from highly quantitative analyses to group consensus, in order to develop recommendations. Each method has its place in guidelines development. Regardless of the method used, the promulgated guidelines should describe the method to arrive at its conclusions, serving to appreciate the context of the guidelines and their development to better judge the credibility of the published policy. The guideline method description should be clear enough to permit other groups to use the same methods with a reasonable expectation of reaching similar conclusions. Most policy makers and health care practitioners agree that clinical guidelines should be based on the available scientific evidence following a careful review of the existing scientific literature. Meaningful decisions about health care should rely on valid reviews of the existing literature. On the other hand, good literature reviews may provide a conclusion that is statistically significant, but may of itself be clinically irrelevant. Careful assessment of the needs of people using existing health services must remain important in developing guidelines. Additionally, once formulated, guidelines should try to employ the views of patient preferences.

In developing clinical guidelines, randomized controlled trials (RCTs) remain the best source of evidence for clinical practice, and they should be used when available. They have limitations, however, including short to moderate duration, whereas the benefits of therapy will accrue over a lifetime. Most RCTs lack a true placebo group, and so underestimate the beneficial effect of the therapy. It must be acknowledged that RCTs do not represent true clinical practice because some patients, typically those at higher risks, are excluded from the trials, including patients with a recent stroke, myocardial infarction, or with a specific need for the study drug. The study cohort may thus be at a lower risk than the general practice population.

Randomized control trials focus primarily on a priori end points and not necessarily on the other benefits of therapy. JNC-6 suggests that in considering the evidence to formulate clinical policy, absolute rather than relative changes should be used, because benefits derived from treating hypertension (or any chronic disease) depend on absolute risk [6]. Those patients who are at greater risk will therefore achieve greater benefit. Randomized control trials also provide information regarding the reduction in the numbers of cardiovascular events over a specific time. The inverse of absolute risk reduction is the number of patients needed to be treated (NNT) during a specific time interval, usually 5 years, to prevent one event. This may seem clinically attractive, but it does not present a challenge. Because age and previous cardiovascular disease and risk factors are the most powerful predictors of outcomes, there is a strong possibility that measurement and reduction of modifiable risk factors would be recommended only in the elderly or in those who have already experienced a cardiovascular event. Other considerations relate to 5-year survival, what really concerns the middle-aged hypertensive patient, and whether or not the clinician should consider a longer-term perspective and longer-term benefit of disease-free life when dealing with younger hypertensive patients.

Consider the data on the incidence of congestive heart failure from the Framingham Heart Study (Fig. 1). If decisions to treat are based on 5-year follow-up data—that is, the difference in the number of events between those with normal blood pressure and stage 1 hypertension at the 5-year mark—one could argue that the benefit of treatment would be relatively small, and the recommendation might be to not treat the hypertension. At 10 years, however, the difference is actually quite large, and the recommendation would be to favor treatment. Some individuals therefore may take the position to wait until the tenth year before treating, thereby preventing unnecessary drug medication for a decade or so. If treatment were not started until year 10, however, one must consider whether there would be any organ left to preserve. Will treating the patient beginning at year 10 reverse the risk of an event back to zero? Will the quality of life in the succeeding 10 years be as fruitful? Guidelines should help busy practicing clinicians consider these

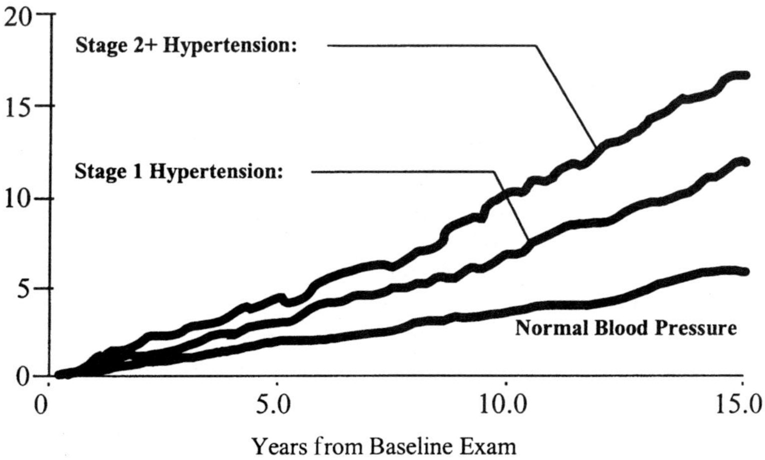

FIGURE 1 Cumulative incidence of congestive heart failure. *Source*: Framingham Heart Study.

issues, but they should not make the specific management decision for the physician or his patient.

In the final analysis, specific therapeutic decisions must be based on the specific patient and the judgment of his or her physician. The responsible physician's judgment must remain paramount.

THE NEED FOR PRIMARY PREVENTION POLICIES

Until recently, blood pressure-related risk reduction efforts have almost uniformly revolved around the paradigm of hypertension detection and treatment. This is because high blood pressure was among the most common and important of the risk factors underlying the major cardiovascular–renal diseases. In Western societies, however, hypertension and the prevalence of high blood pressure as well as the complications have been related to the fact that blood pressure rises progressively with age [13]. In addition, despite the benefits of treating hypertension, this approach has never prevented all blood pressure-related cardiovascular diseases in society. This is because vascular complications occur prior to the establishment of clinical hypertension, and there is a continuous blood pressure–cardiovascular disease risk relationship that is present even though a patient's blood pressure may fall within a normotensive range.

In the Multiple Risk Factor Intervention Trial, the adjusted relative risk of cardiovascular mortality for those in the systolic range of 140 to 160 mmHg is about twice the risk of those in the systolic pressure range of 120 to 129 mmHg [13]. It has been concluded that the higher the blood pressure, the greater the inherent risk for cardiovascular disease, strokes, renal disease, and all-cause mortality. In addition, there is no way to guarantee that all patients with high blood pressure can be detected and adequately treated. Regardless, damage to the heart, brain, fundi, and kidney also occurs at these lower ranges, and may often be present before antihypertensive therapy is initiated. Furthermore, even though the cardiovascular mortality rate at the lower levels of the systolic range of 120 to 129 mmHg is relatively small, there is a significant portion of the population whose blood pressures fall within this range [3], thus the overall number of people with the potential for increased cardiovascular and renal events is large.

Many of the treatment regimens for high blood pressure may be expensive and may be priced beyond the reach of some patients. Almost all treatments carry the potential for some adverse effects, thus treating hypertension represents an important but less than ideal response to the population at large with potential hypertensive and other cardiovascular disease.

Over the years, hypertensive and atherosclerotic cardiovascular diseases have entered into an exciting new phase, moving from those efforts that promoted secondary prevention of the disease outcomes to the promising era of primary prevention, moving from medical and, when necessary, surgical treatments, to specific areas of lifestyle modifications and the employment of those pharmacological agents that show great promise and excitement for primary prevention.

To be fully successful with primary prevention, a major effort in education of health care professionals is essential, but to be truly effective, educational programs for the public must be instituted so that all groups, those less educated as well as those with higher levels of education, can be made aware of the impact of disease and of the lifestyle modifications that can prevent hypertension. Such educational programs must communicate (1) the need for cessation of use of all tobacco products (to reduce overall cardiovascular risk); (2) the importance of achieving an ideal body weight; (3) the need to restrict alcohol intake to no more than one ounce of ethanol (or its equivalent) daily; (4) to have periodic medical screenings for hypertension, hyperlipidemias, diabetes mellitus, and cardiac enlargement and other cardiovascular risk factors; (5) to follow a regular and active exercise program; and (6) to be aware that an excessive daily dietary sodium intake (the current recommendations no more than 100 mEq or 2.4 g of sodium [14]) may exacerbate the tendency to elevate arterial pressure or serve to add to volume overload of the heart if the patient is predisposed to develop cardiac failure.

Clearly, the lifestyle modifications are valuable for any good disease prevention program for the general public, but particularly if there is a family history of hypertension or premature death from cardiovascular diseases. Encouraging patients to follow the lifestyle modifications should be part of the daily practice of medicine by all health care providers, whether generalists or physicians in specialty practices. It is particularly fortunate that these primary prevention measures are pertinent to both hypertensive disease and atherosclerotic cardiovascular disease. These lifestyle modifications are of major importance today, as (1) overweight and obesity are among the more common risks in the general public today; (2) the detection of hypertension, hyperlipidemias, and diabetes mellitus is a relatively simple measure, and they are the major modifiable risk factors for coronary heart disease; (3) tobacco consumption remains ubiquitous and is increasing in certain populations (e.g., the young, women); and (4) the employment of these risk-reducing lifestyle modifications is relatively simple and straightforward.

PRIMARY PREVENTION STRATEGIES

Preventing hypertension thus provides a meaningful way to stop the continuing costly cycle of managing hypertensive patients and their complications, and the associated lost productivity to society. Two strategies can be

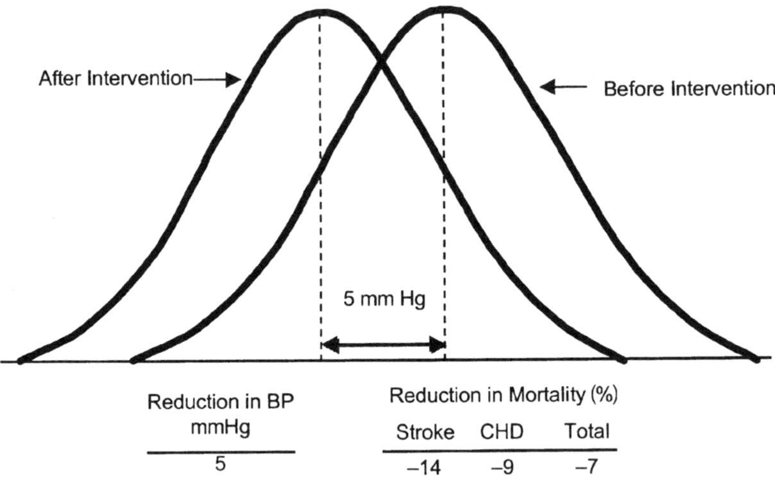

FIGURE 2 Systolic blood pressure distributions. *Source*: NHBPEP working group report in primary prevention in hypertension (1993).

employed: (1) a population-based strategy that aims to achieve a reduction in the average of blood pressure, and (2) a targeted strategy focusing special effort to lower blood pressure of at-risk populations with greater potential to develop significant disease. The targeted strategy would focus on people with high normal blood pressure, people with a family history of hypertension, African Americans, and individuals with one or more risk factors that contribute to an increased blood pressure.

The distribution of blood pressure within a population fits a bell-shaped curve (Fig. 2). Small reductions in the population's average blood pressure levels has the very real potential to produce not only a substantial reduction in hypertension prevalence, but also a remarkable large decrease in cardiovascular risk. Reducing the average arterial pressure among the entire at-risk population will have significant benefits. It has been calculated that on average, a 5 mmHg reduction in blood pressure could reduce stroke, coronary heart disease, and total mortality by 14%, 9%, and 7%, respectively [15]. Lifestyle modifications that can be used for both the entire population and the targeted populations include the measures identified previously.

Dietary Sodium and Caloric Restriction

It has been estimated that 50% of dietary sodium intake comes from processed, canned, or frozen foods [16]. In most acculturated societies, people consume between 6 to 12 g (or more) of salt per day. This amount exceeds the physiological need for salt, and is far greater than the typical salt consumption of primitive societies. The preponderance of evidence from observational studies documents the relationship between various measures of salt intake and blood pressure; the higher the dietary sodium intake the greater the chance of having a clinically significant elevated arterial pressure. A number of clinical trials and feeding studies have demonstrated that reducing dietary sodium intake will decrease blood pressure rather dramatically [9,17]. Some portions of the population, such as African Americans and the elderly, may experience even greater blood pressure reductions by reducing salt intake [10]. The obvious challenge is that because of the ubiquitous nature of sodium and abundance of calories in processed and fast foods, the potential for reduction of sodium and caloric intake exceeds the capability of intervention studies and what can be accomplished in contemporary society. In addition, recent studies have shown that increased dietary sodium intake will promote fibrosis of the heart and kidneys, thereby adding to the risk of target organ functional impairment over and above the elevation of blood pressure [18].

Public policies promoting public education and increasing demand for lower sodium and lower calorie foods could have a very meaningful benefit toward reducing the morbidity and mortality associated with hypertensive disease. In public education programs, messages should be targeted to reach certain segments of the population. For example, school curricula and extracurricular activities provide splendid opportunities to promote the adoption of healthy eating habits. The benefits of such efforts would be enormous, since there are approximately 50 million Americans with hypertension and vastly more who are at risk [19]. Moreover, the problem of overweight and obesity in our society has achieved "epidemic" proportions [7].

Manufacturers of processed foods have an outstanding opportunity to improve the health of our population by lowering the population's average good pressures and risk of target organ damage by reducing the calories and sodium content of processed foods. This can be achieved, especially with convenience foods such as frozen dinners and soups, as well as in cereals, breads, and dairy products. The labeling of calories and the sodium content of foods has benefited another public policy activity, which has helped consumers make wise food choices. Supermarkets can also assist in public policy activities by providing shelf labels indicating the sodium and calorie content of foods, and they can distribute educational materials to their customers. Restaurants, cafeterias, and fast food outlets can help influence the amount of sodium consumed by customers by reducing the amount of sodium added to their products. Food service operators should be encouraged to label, serve, and promote selections lower in sodium and calorie content, as well as provide salt substitutes when appropriate.

Promoting Physical Activity

Another key element in the primary prevention of hypertension is promoting physical activity, especially in schools, work sites, and community facilities. Regular programs of moderate physical activity; that is, 30 min most days a week, can contribute to the reduction of excess body weight and cardiovascular risk [4,7]. The public should be made aware of how increasing physical activity is an important part of overall lifestyle change. Policies to promote increased physical activity would include increased lighting in parks, stairwells, and parking lots so that the public feels secure about walking and exercising in these environments.

CONCLUSION

Over the past 30 years, there has been both the initial publication and six subsequent (JNC) reports issued on the prevention, detection, evaluation, and treatment of the hypertensive patient that have been formulated and published through the NHBPEP. These periodic reports and other state-of-the-art working group publications dealing with specific hypertension-related issues represent a consensus of thinking concerning a variety of hypertension-related subjects. Indeed, consensus documentation may explain the subtle variances from similar reports by other nationally and internationally constituted bodies. The reported scientific literature (be it from randomized control trials, meta-analyses, retrospective analyses, prospective follow-up studies, cross-sectional population studies, case studies, or other clinical intervention reports) presents evidence supporting the need for evaluation and treatment. Of paramount importance, these developed policy statements have provided the message that all patients with hypertension must be detected, carefully evaluated, and continually treated with periodic follow-up so that hypertensive disease and its sequelae can be controlled. The result will be reduced complications, hospitalizations, and overall costs to society.

Finally, it is important to stress that the health care policies and guidelines referred to in this discussion should not be considered as having the "weight of law." They should serve primarily as focal points and guides for health care professionals to consider in their overall patient care and management. Patients present with multiple risk factors, different family histories and different demographic situations, and of course, their underlying disease mechanisms are varied. Guidelines and policies cannot anticipate all these variables in one patient; therefore the responsible physician's judgment must remain paramount.

REFERENCES

1. Merriam Webster's New Collegiate Dictionary. Springfield, MA: Merriam-Webster, 1977.
2. National Heart, Lung, and Blood Institute. Morbidity & Mortality: 2000 Chart Book on Cardiovascular, Lung and Blood Diseases. Bethesda, MD: National Institutes of Health, 2000: chart 3–4.
3. Burt VL, Cutler JA, Higgins M, Horan MJ, Labarthe D, Whelton P, et al. Trends in the prevalence, awareness, treatment, and control of hypertension in the adult U.S. population: data from the health examination surveys, 1960 to 1991. *Hypertension* 995;26(1):60–69.
4. The Sixth Report of the Joint National Committee on Prevention, Detection, Evaluation, and Treatment of High Blood Pressure. *Arch Int Med* 1997; 157: 2413–2446.
5. 1999 World Health Organization–International Society of Hypertension Guidelines for the Management of Hypertension. Guidelines Subcommittee. *J Hypertens* 1999; 17:151–183.
6. Executive Summary of the Third Report of the National Cholesterol Education Program (NCEP) Expert Panel on Detection, Evaluation, and Treatment of High Blood Cholesterol in Adults (Adult Treatment Panel III) *JAMA* 2001; 285(19):2486–2497.
7. Clinical guidelines on the identification, evaluation, and treatment of overweight and obesity in adults—the Evidence Report. National Institutes of Health. *Obes Res* 1998, 6(suppl. 2): 51S–209S.
8. Appel LJ, Moore TJ, Obarzanek E, Vollmer WM, Svetkey LP, Sacks FM, et al. A clinical trial of the effects of dietary patterns on blood pressure. DASH Collaborative Research Group. *N Engl J Med* 1997, 336:1117–1124.
9. Sacks FM, Svetkey LP, Vollmer WM, Appel LJ, Bray GA, Harsha D, et al. Effects on blood pressure of reduced dietary sodium and the Dietary Approaches to Stop Hypertension (DASH) diet. DASH-Sodium Collaborative Research Group. *N Engl J Med* 2001; 244:3–10.
10. Whelton PK, Appel LJ, Espeland MA, Applegate WB, Ettinger WH Jr, Kostis JB, Kumanyika S, Lacy CR, Johnson KC, Folmar S, Cutler JA. Sodium reduction and weight loss in the treatment of hypertension in older persons a randomized controlled trial of nonpharmacologic interventions in the elderly (TONE). TONE Collaborative Research Group. *JAMA* 1998; 279:839–846.
11. Prevention of stroke by antihypertensive drug treatment in older persons with isolated systolic hypertension. Final results of the Systolic Hypertension in the Elderly Program (SHEP). SHEP Cooperative Research Group. *JAMA* 1991;265:3255–3264.
12. Hansson L, Zanchetti A, Carruthers SG, Dahlof B, Elmfeldt D, Julius S, et al. Effects of intensive blood-pressure lowering and low-dose aspirin in patients

with hypertension: principal results of the Hypertension Optimal Treatment (HOT) randomized trial. HOT Study Group. *Lancet* 1998;351:1755–1762.
13. Neaton JD, Wentworth D. Serum cholesterol, blood pressure, cigarette smoking, and death from coronary heart disease. Overall findings and differences by age for 316,099 white men. Multiple Risk Factor Intervention Trial Research (MRFIT) Group. *Arch Int Med* 1992; 152:56–64.
14. Statement from the National High Blood Pressure Education Program Coordinating Committee Regarding the Consumption of Dietary Salt. Bethesda, MD: National Heart, Lung, and Blood Institute, 1999.
15. Stamler R. Implications of the INTERSALT Study. Hypertension 1991; 17 (suppl. I):16–20.
16. James WP, Ralph A, Sanchez-Castillo CP. The dominance of salt in manufactured food in the sodium intake of affluent societies. *Lancet* 1987; 1: 426–429.
17. Cutler JA, Follmann D, Allender PS. Randomized trials of sodium reduction: an overview. *Am J Clin Nutr* 1997; 65(suppl.):643S–651S.
18. Ye HCM, Burrell LM, Black MJ, Wu LL, Dilley RJ, Cooper ME, Johnston CI. Salt induces myocardial and renal fibrosis in normotensive and renal hypertensive rats. *Circulation* 1998; 98:2621–2628.
19. Wotz M, Cutler J, Roccella EJ, Rohde F, Thom T, Burt V. Statement from the National High Blood Pressure Education Program prevalence of hypertension. *Am J Hypertens* 2000; 13(1 Pt. 1):103–104.

Index